AF823663

Contemporary Rheumatology

Series Editor
Yasser El Miedany, Gravesend, UK

Everyday rheumatologists are faced with new challenges pertaining to the management of both common as well as uncommon rheumatic disorders. The series, Contemporary Rheumatology, will explore new frontiers in rheumatology. It will cover both basic and clinical sciences and provide a state-of-the art approach to the diagnosis and management of different inflammatory as well as non-inflammatory conditions. This series will highlight emerging fields, treatments, and research in rheumatology from precision medicine to the use of cannabinoids in treatment of rheumatic diseases. By gathering key information on state-of-the-art care for practitioners of rheumatology, this series aims to support clinicians in developing new treatment plans for patients diagnosed with rheumatic diseases typically treated with more traditional approaches. In addition to demystifying newer technology and research in rheumatology, this series will also explore connections between rheumatic diseases and other disorders and medical specialties, such as osteoporosis in renal failure, the genetic factors to rheumatic diseases, and the bridge between rheumatic disease and sexual health. Patients with rheumatic conditions may be at increased risk for other chronic diseases, and it is crucial to those patients to have informed clinicians across specialties. These volumes will enable physicians outside the realm of rheumatology to better treat patients in their care who also suffer from rheumatic diseases. Research in rheumatology moves quickly, and there is continued focus on advancements in research and treatment. This series provides space in the rheumatology book program at Springer to track progress made in the field with series editor Dr. Yasser El Miedany, a leader in rheumatology, and continually provide state-of-the-art titles in the area.

Jeimylo de Castro • Yasser El Miedany
Editors

Advances in Chronic and Neuropathic Pain

Springer

Editors
Jeimylo de Castro
SMARTMD Philippines
Centuria Medical Makati
Makati City, Philippines

Yasser El Miedany
Institute Medical Sciences
Canterbury Christ Church University
Canterbury, Kent, UK

ISSN 2662-7531 ISSN 2662-754X (electronic)
Contemporary Rheumatology
ISBN 978-3-031-10686-6 ISBN 978-3-031-10687-3 (eBook)
https://doi.org/10.1007/978-3-031-10687-3

© The Editor(s) (if applicable) and The Author(s), under exclusive license to Springer Nature Switzerland AG 2022
This work is subject to copyright. All rights are solely and exclusively licensed by the Publisher, whether the whole or part of the material is concerned, specifically the rights of translation, reprinting, reuse of illustrations, recitation, broadcasting, reproduction on microfilms or in any other physical way, and transmission or information storage and retrieval, electronic adaptation, computer software, or by similar or dissimilar methodology now known or hereafter developed.
The use of general descriptive names, registered names, trademarks, service marks, etc. in this publication does not imply, even in the absence of a specific statement, that such names are exempt from the relevant protective laws and regulations and therefore free for general use.
The publisher, the authors, and the editors are safe to assume that the advice and information in this book are believed to be true and accurate at the date of publication. Neither the publisher nor the authors or the editors give a warranty, expressed or implied, with respect to the material contained herein or for any errors or omissions that may have been made. The publisher remains neutral with regard to jurisdictional claims in published maps and institutional affiliations.

This Springer imprint is published by the registered company Springer Nature Switzerland AG
The registered company address is: Gewerbestrasse 11, 6330 Cham, Switzerland

Foreword

Pain is a condition that has confounded doctors and patients for millennia. Neuropathic pain, which reflects damage to the nerves themselves, has been particularly difficult to treat. As a practicing interventional pain, physician as well as a former pain fellowship director, I deal with the diagnosis and treatment of chronic and neuropathic pain every day. Dr. Jeimylo (Jim) de Castro and I have worked together for many years, through the World Institute of Pain (WIP), the Certified Interventional Pain Sonographer (CIPS) certification program, and the Philippine Academy of Rehabilitation conferences. He is a CIPS, a diplomate of the American Academy of Regenerative Medicine (DABRM, a diplomate of the Philippine Board of Rehabilitation Medicine, and chair of his rehabilitation department in Santa Rosa City, Philippines. Yasser El Miedany is a professor of rheumatology at Canterbury Christ Church University in the UK, and he is a fellow of both the American and British rheumatologic societies.

Over the last few years, our understanding of the causes and treatments of various pain conditions, including neuropathic pain, has grown exponentially. Unfortunately, such information is scattered across multiple journals and textbooks. In this new book *Advances in Chronic and Neuropathic Pain*, Drs. de Castro and Miedany have gathered an international group of pain physicians to describe our current understandings regarding the pathophysiology, diagnosis, and treatment of chronic and neuropathic pain.

In this book, you will find sections on the influence of age on pain ("Pain in children and young adults"; "Pain in older adults") as well as current information on a variety of pain conditions such as cancer, degenerative disease, peripheral neuropathy, and phantom limb pain. There are sections on the pharmacologic, non-pharmacologic, and interventional treatment on pain. The editors have also included sections on diagnosis and outcome assessment.

As the body of knowledge regarding pain grows, it is important for clinicians to have an available comprehensive reference, where the improvements in understanding are gathered in one location. This book is well designed for the young physicians studying for certification examinations, as well as for the established physicians ready to update their understanding of the current state of chronic and neuropathic assessment and treatment. I congratulate the editors on this impressive book and I am honored to have been asked to write this foreword.

Pain and Headache Center
Eagle River, AK, USA

Andrea Trescot, MD, DABIPP, FIPP, CIPS

Preface

Chronic and neuropathic pain is a complex spectrum of symptoms affecting the nerves of both children and adults. The International Association for the Study of Pain (IASP) defines it as pain caused by a lesion or disease of the somatosensory system. It may have a central or peripheral origin. Furthermore, pain that is longer than 3 months is considered chronic pain. Due to the ubiquitous and subjective nature of pain as a clinical manifestation, it is often difficult to identify the presence of neuropathic pain during the nascent phase of the disease. Therefore, clinical-based validated screening tools with an anatomical distribution of the extent of pain are used to determine the certainty of the disease. This is designed to help practitioners establish the existence of neuropathic pain and thus aid in the formulation of the treatment. Diagnostic testing protocols in the form of pain questionnaires, validated screening tools, confirmatory tests for nerve damage, sensory testing, and neurophysiological techniques are available to help in the diagnosis and can complement the findings seen during clinical history taking and physical examination. Recently, composite pain biomarkers were identified to help us understand specific pain mechanisms which can guide clinicians in the diagnosis and management of this condition.

The normal course of this condition varies from patient to patient. A French study, however, documented and followed the course of neuropathic pain and on average may take about 23 months from its onset to its diagnosis. However, an additional 20 months are needed before a patient can be referred to a pain center. These centers may not be readily available in some countries such that primary physicians may refer these patients initially to pain specialists, neurologists, rheumatologists, oncologists, and even physiatrists with the hope that eventually appropriate management may be provided to abate the symptoms of the patients. A single or a combination of drugs like calcium channel antagonists (Pregabalin and Gabapentin), tricyclic antidepressants, opiates, SNRIs, steroids, and NSAIDs medications are commonly used to address pain. More specific medications are given once the diagnosis of neuropathic pain is established. While these medications provide immediate relief, they have not been proven to deliver the needed lasting effects. Hence, considerations of more effective and advanced guided interventions by means of fluoroscopy and ultrasound come into play. These modalities facilitate the delivery of medications to their target site more effectively. With these challenges in mind, we have worked along with world experts to tackle the problems of chronic and neuropathic pain, its diagnosis, clinical manifestations, and treatments. The role of both pharmacologic and non-pharmacologic therapies is initially given emphasis. More advanced approaches are introduced in this book for challenging patients with intractable pain using modalities to assess the sources and sites of pain. Ultrasound and fluoroscopy are effective modalities to guide interventional procedures among practitioners. We have also included regenerative therapies with their promising effects as a new intervention for chronic neuropathic pains.

The book is structured by introducing a classification of chronic pain together with the challenges that every practitioner is dealing with. An in-depth discussion of the pathophysiology of chronic and neuropathic pains is included to provide readers with an appreciation of the disease process. The unique and peculiar clinical manifestation of this disease among children and adults provides a distinct understanding of how this disease affects different age groups and thus, enables practitioners to achieve a different perspective in terms of assessment and treatment.

Although neuropathic pain is a disease with a lesion in the somatosensory system, other diseases can mimic its presentation. Our authors, therefore, have included those diseases which have distinct peripheral nerve lesions as opposed to those with chronic clinical presentation of pain that may not have injuries involving the peripheral nerves. These include cancer pain, degenerative diseases, complex regional pain syndromes, neuropathic pain syndromes, and fibromyalgias. With the constantly evolving understanding of this disease, modifications may inevitably change the approach to assessing the symptoms of this disease while trying to differentiate what is purely neuropathic versus those which are simply nociceptive in nature due to the absence of nerve injuries.

The clinical assessment and diagnostic testing form a critical part of neuropathic pain management. In fact, the success of the treatment wholly or partially depends on the diligence one puts into this part of clinical evaluation. Outcome measures evaluate the patient prior to an intervention, the degree by which the patient responds to the treatment, and the risk categorization of the patient, thus providing us information on how effectively the treatment has impacted the course of the pain experienced by the patient.

With all the research being done to understand chronic and neuropathic pain, treatment options are still evolving. For the last five years, we have seen new therapies coming into the scene and providing us with a helpful guide on how to control pain if unable to treat it effectively. However, we cannot entirely dismiss the contribution of existing medications and other non-pharmacologic treatments in regulating neuropathic pain. Thus, our authors have meaningfully presented treatment options and protocols for the different stages of the disease and the level of severity of the disease with added precautionary measures when deleterious effects are observed during its prolonged administration. The use of image-guided interventional procedures such as fluoroscopy or ultrasound improves the outcome of pain relief as it targets specific lesions causing the pain. The portability and dynamic feature of ultrasound makes it a preferred modality for most interventional procedures.

Recently, regenerative therapies have positively been shown to be beneficial for pain attenuation by reducing the inflammatory state of the injured nerve and ultimately inducing tissue repair. However, more studies are needed to fully understand the therapeutic mechanisms for effective treatment. These advances have added value to the existing regimen of pain control mechanisms in addressing neuropathic pain.

I hope that the advances written in this book take us closer to the hope stated in the "Good Book." To wit, "neither shall there be any more pain; for the former things are passed away." Revelation 21:4.

I would like to thank my mentor and colleague, Dr. Yasser El Miedany for the opportunity to write this book with him and to all the chapter authors who have diligently contributed their time and skill to make this project possible. I also would like to thank my wife, Kyna de Castro, and my two kids, Rafael Bennett and Zarah Francine for the inspiration they have given me while preparing this book. And most of all, I thank our Almighty God for the discernment and wisdom for a project I could not possibly do without.

Silang, Cavite, Philippines Jeimylo de Castro

Contents

Part I
Understanding Chronic and Neuropathic Pain

Chapter 1
Classification of Chronic Pain

Troy Henning, Steven Stanos, and Wilson Chang

Types of Pain

Pain is a common reason for which the worldwide population seeks medical care. In 2001, a Study of the Finish health system found that 40% of the visits to a primary care provider were related to the management of pain [1]. In 2017, Murphy et al. performed a multivariate analysis of diagnostic codes (ICD-9) in the United States from 2000 to 2012 and found the prevalence of chronic pain to be 10.4% [2]. Chronic pain and pain related suffering has long been recognized as a national health problem with significant impact on physical health, emotional functioning, and costs to society. Chronic pain, besides being a common reason for people to seek medical care [3], has been linked to restrictions in mobility, daily function, affective distress (anxiety, depression), and poor perceived health or lower quality of life [4, 5]. Data from the National Health Interview Survey (NHIS) reported that "chronic pain", described as pain experienced on most days or every day in the past 6 months, impacted 50 million Americans [5, 6]. The survey also defined

T. Henning (✉)
Medical Director Sports and Performance Medicine, Swedish Medical Center, Seattle, WA, USA
e-mail: Troy.henning@swedish.org

S. Stanos
Medical Director Rehabilitation and Performance Medicine, Swedish Medical Center, Seattle, WA, USA
e-mail: Steven.stanos@swedish.org

W. Chang
Pain Medicine, Swedish Medical Center, Seattle, WA, USA
e-mail: Wilson.chang@swedish.org

© The Author(s), under exclusive license to Springer Nature Switzerland AG 2022

J. de Castro, Y. El Miedany (eds.), *Advances in Chronic and Neuropathic Pain*, Contemporary Rheumatology, https://doi.org/10.1007/978-3-031-10687-3_1

"high-impact chronic pain", chronic pain limiting life or work activities on most days or every day during the past 6 months, impacting 20 million US adults [6, 7].

The International Association for the study of Pain defines pain as an "unpleasant sensory or emotional experience associated with actual or potential tissue damage or described in terms of such damage" [8, 9]. The categorization or classification system used in the diagnosis of pain is an ever evolving process as the interrelatedness of diseases, pain, and biopsychosocial influences have been realized all while keeping pace with the latest iteration of the International Classification of Diseases, ICD-11 [10–12]. This chapter will provide some historical reference to the evolution of how pain is classified and review some of the basic definitions.

In 1980, Dr. Loeser described four broad categories of pain: nociception, perception of pain, suffering and pain behaviors (Table 1.1) [13]. Behind each of these categories are anatomic, physiologic and psychologic substrates that transform pain from a neurochemical signal to an adverse experience incorporating behavioral changes [8]. Additionally, pain can be further stratified based upon its timetable of manifestation: transient, acute and chronic (Table 1.2) [8]. Lastly, an individual's pain perception is intricately related to the chronicity of the painful experience as outlined in Table 1.2.

Since the early 1990s, a mechanistic-based pain classification system characterized by a relatively dichotomous approach distinguishing primarily nociceptive pain (pain arising from actual or threatened damage to non-neural tissues and primarily related to activation of nociceptors) from neuropathic pain (pain arising from a lesion or disease affecting the somatosensory system). A third group, "mixed pain", was less well defined and could include pain conditions that shared both nociceptive

Table 1.1 Categories of pain

Nociception	Detection of tissue damage by A delta and C fibers. Can be influenced by inflammatory and neural changes in their immediate environment.
Perception of pain	Triggered by a noxious stimulus such as injury or disease. Acutely associated with specific autonomic and somatic reflexes which are not involved in chronic pain. Intensity of pain is not directly tied to amount/extent of tissue damage.
Suffering	Negative response induced by pain, fear, anxiety or stress.
Pain behaviors	Things that a person can or cannot do because of pain and suffering.

Table 1.2 Chronicity of pain

Transient	Activation of nociceptive transducers in absence of tissue damage. A brief experience that does not drive one to seek medical care.
Acute	Substantial injury to tissue with activation of nociceptive transducers at site of injury. The body is capable of healing allowing the pain to stop prior to complete healing. Seen after trauma, procedures/surgery and some diseases. The patient may seek medical care depending on the extent of tissue injury or degree of pain.
Chronic	It is not time defined but more related to inability of the body to restore physiologic functions to normal homeostatic level. Maybe perpetuated by factors other than tissue injury and last beyond healing phase. The patients' perception of pain may persist beyond treatment.

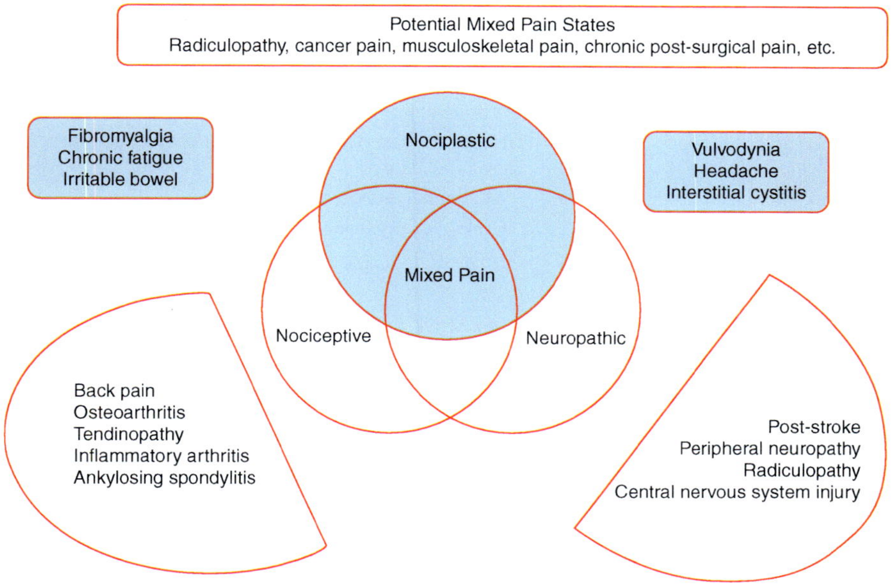

Fig. 1.1 Potential Mixed Pain States. (Adapted from Freynhagen et al. [14])

and neuropathic pain characteristics and/or conditions that did not exhibit signs or symptoms of any actual or threatened tissue damage, nor evidence of the somatosensory system, including fibromyalgia and visceral pain conditions like irritable bowel syndrome (Fig. 1.1) [14]. With the evolution of the understanding of peripheral and central sensitization, a need to clarify and better define mixed pain syndromes evolved. In 2017, the IASP approved this third descriptor to be defined as "nociplastic" pain [15]. It represents activation of nociception in the absence of identifiable actual or threatened tissue damage that would stimulate peripheral nociceptors or, no evidence for disease/injury of the somatosensory system that may would explain the pain [15].

An additional effort initiated in 2013 by the American Pain Society and federal research groups worked to develop a consensus on nomenclature to improve assessment and the study of pain conditions, the Analgesic, Anesthetic, and Addiction Clinical Trial Translations Innovations Opportunities and Networks (ACTTION) , described as the ACTTION-APS Pain Taxonomy (AAPT) . The inspiration and framework for organizing the taxonomy were derived from the formation of the Diagnostic and Statistical Manual of Mental Disorders (DSM) and the International Classifications of Headache Disorders (ICHD) [10]. The AAPT recognized that a taxonomy should be based on best currently available evidence and incorporate the biopsychosocial—assessment of interaction of physical, psychological/behavioral, social, and cognitive measures—model. Their aims where to provide a living framework to develop common terminology that could help direct clinical care, research, and education while aligning with international classifications of diseases (ICD)

Table 1.3 Categories of pain, adopted from AAPT Table 1.2

Peripheral and central nervous system	Neuropathic pain
Musculoskeletal	Arthritis, axial pain, myofascial, chronic wide-spread, fibromyalgia
Orofacial and head pain	Headache disorders, temporomandibular and other orofacial pain
Visceral, pelvic and urogenital	Abdominal, pelvic, urogenital pain
Disease associated pain not otherwise classified	Examples: malignancy, infectious disease

Table 1.4 Dimensions of pain, adopted from AAPT Table 1.3

Dimension	Description
1. Core diagnostic criteria	Symptoms and signs along with diagnostic tests and differential diagnosis
2. Common features	Pain characteristics, nonpainful features, epidemiology
3. Common medical comorbidities	Associated diseases
4. Neurobiological, psychosocial and functional consequences	Consequences related to chronic pain
5. Putative neurobiological and psychosocial mechanisms, risk factors and protective factors	How these impact pain

codes [10]. The AAPT recommended organizing chronic pain disorders into the following categories: (1) peripheral and central nervous system, (2) musculoskeletal system, (3) orofacial and head pain system, (4) visceral, pelvic, and urogenital pain, (5) disease associated pains not classified elsewhere (Table 1.3) [10]. This organization shed light on organ-based classification system of pain that were not previously present. Each category is further defined by five dimensions: (1) core diagnostic criteria, (2) common features, (3) common medical comorbidities, (4) neurobiological, psychosocial and functional consequences, (5) putative neurobiological and psychosocial mechanisms, risk and protective factors (Table 1.4) [10]. These dimensions consolidate the spectrum of pain involving its epidemiology, signs and symptoms, associated medical co-morbidities, as well as the consequences of pain and how it affects the individual.

In 2015, the International Association for the Study of Pain (IASP) established a taskforce to develop a classification system for chronic pain aligning it with the International Classification of Diseases (ICD) version 11 (ICD-11). Chronic pain disorders were divided into seven categories: (1) chronic primary pain, (2) chronic cancer pain, (3) chronic posttraumatic and postsurgical pain, (4) chronic neuropathic pain, (5) chronic headache and orofacial pain, (6) chronic visceral pain, (7) chronic musculoskeletal pain (Table 1.5) [11]. The World Health Organization (WHO) also allows for optional specifiers or extension codes to be used with any of the seven categories of chronic pain. These extensions help demonstrate how pain severity and the temporal course of chronic pain negatively impact the social and psychological welling being of the patient [12].

Table 1.5 IASP classification systemfor chronic pain related to ICD-11

Chronic primary pain: pain in one or more regions	>3 months of persistent or recurrent pain. Associated with functional or emotional distress/disability
Chronic cancer pain: caused by the cancer or associated treatments	Subdivided by location (visceral or musculoskeletal), intermittent or continuous presentation
Chronic postsurgical and posttraumatic pain	Pain lasting more than 3 months after the procedure or trauma and not explained by another cause
Chronic neuropathic pain	History of injury or disease of the central or peripheral somatosensory system supported by diagnostic exam (imaging, biopsy, neurophysiologic or laboratory test). Positive (hyperalgesia/allodynia/paresthesia) and negative (anesthesia/weakness) features must be present
Chronic headache/orofacial pain	Pain present ε 50% of days in past 3 months
Chronic visceral pain	Subdivided by etiology: persistent inflammation, vascular (ischemia/thrombotic), obstruction/distension, traction/compression, combinations if injury and referral from other locations. Typically presents as referred pain along a somatic reference zone
Chronic musculoskeletal pain	Nociceptive pain caused by injury to the musculoskeletal tissue through inflammation, infection, metabolic, autoimmune or mechanical insult

In 2018, the aforementioned taskforce formed by IASP refined the classification system for chronic pain disorders by dividing the 2015 scheme into chronic primary pain and secondary pain syndromes [12]. The definition of chronic primary pain remained the same but now included subdivisions of widespread, complex regional, primary headache or orofacial, visceral and musculoskeletal pain. They define secondary pain syndromes as those related to a primary disease entity where pain can be a presenting feature (Fig. 1.2). This secondary syndrome/diagnosis allows the pain to be considered as a separate diagnosis entity even after the primary disease has been successfully treated. Additionally, given that a type of pain may fit with multiple causes/categories the ICD-11 model of multiple parenting framework allows for flexibility in relating diagnoses. For example, a subordinate diagnosis (chemotherapy induced peripheral polyneuropathy) may match with multiple primary diagnoses (chronic cancer pain and chronic neuropathic pain) [12]. While upgrading the classification system the taskforce continued their aim of helping scientists and clinicians have a diagnostic framework from which research and treatment approaches can be developed while aligning with the ICD-11 model [11, 12].

Since adoption of the ICD-11 in 2019 by the World Health Authority, Barke et al. have field tested the properties of the ICD-11 compared to the ICD-10 version using vignette cases on trained providers [16]. The ICD-11 version was found to be more accurate, less ambiguous and easier to apply [16]. When used in a tertiary care pain clinic, the ICD-11 version was found to provide more detailed diagnoses and be more applicable to clinical care, research and aid in the allocation of resources [17].

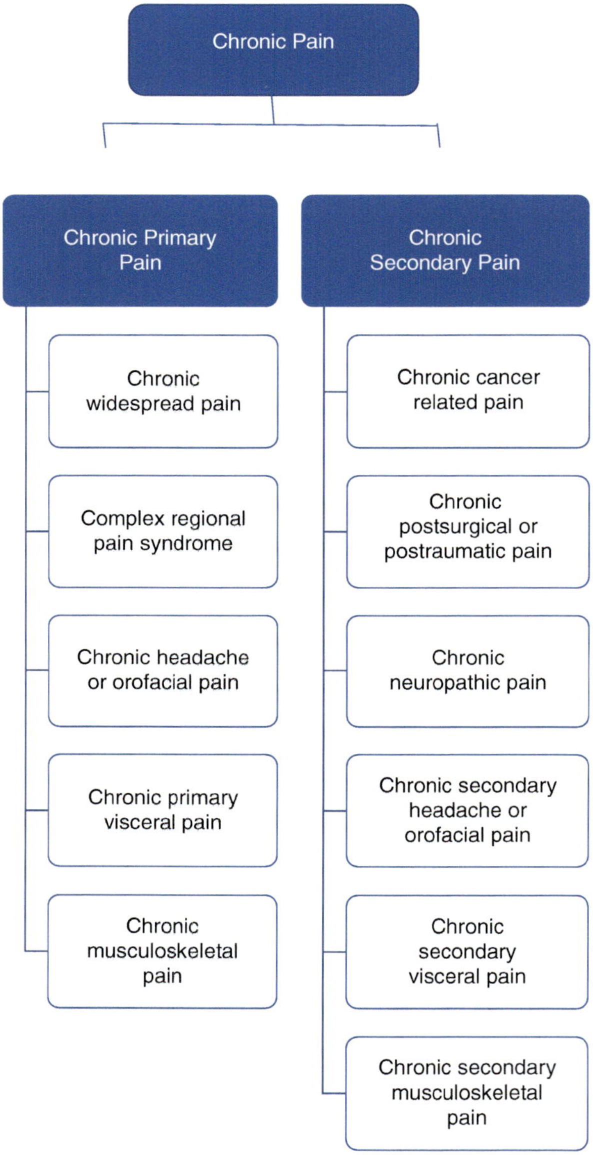

Fig. 1.2 2019 IASP classification of chronic pain

For simplicity and rapid review of material, commonly used clinical terms related to pain are presented in Table 1.6.

In conclusion the 2019 IASP taskforces pain classification scheme provides the most recent working model for categorizing pain types. This living framework strives to provide clinicians and researchers an effective communication platform from which research and clinical care for painful disorders can continue to evolve

Table 1.6 Commonly used clinical definitions related to pain [18]

Noxious stimulus	Tissue damaging stimulus
Pain threshold	Lowest degree of stimulus that is perceived as pain
Pain tolerance	Highest degree of pain an individual can tolerate
Paresthesia	Abnormal sensation that is either elicited or occurs spontaneously
Hypoalgesia	Blunted response to a stimulus which is normally painful
Hypoesthesia	Lowered sensitivity to a given stimulus excluding special senses
Hyperpathia	Painful, heightened reaction to a stimulus
Hyperalgesia	Elevated response to a painful stimulus
Hyperaesthesia	Lower threshold and heightened response to a stimulus excluding special senses
Dysesthesia	Spontaneous or elicited unpleasant abnormal sensation
Causalgia	A painful syndrome related to nerve injury characterized by allodynia, burning pain and hyperpathia
Anaesthesia dolorosa	Pain perceived in a region that was anesthetized
Analgesia	Absence of pain to a normally painful stimulus
Allodynia	Painful response to a normally nonpainful stimulus

as new discoveries in the field are achieved. A related and updated mechanistic classification of pain has included "nociceptive", "neuropathic", and "nociplastic" pain to better describe and represent an improved understanding of the complex pathophysiologic and psychologic mechanisms underlying acute and chronic pain and pain related suffering [19].

References

1. Mäntyselkä P, Kumpusalo E, Ahonen R, et al. Pain as a reason to visit the doctor: a study in Finnish primary health care. Pain. 2001;89(2–3):175–80.
2. Murphy KR, Han JL, Yang S, et al. Prevalence of specific types of pain diagnoses in a sample of United States adults. Pain Physician. 2017;20(2):E257–68.
3. Schappert SM, Burt CW. Ambulatory care visits to physician offices, hospital outpatient departments, and emergency departments: United States, 2001-02. Vital Health Stat. 2006;(159):1–66.
4. Gureje O, Von Korff M, Simon GE, Gater R. Persistent pain and well-being: a World Health Organization study in primary care. JAMA. 1998;280(2):147–51.
5. Smith BH, Elliott AM, Chambers WA, Smith WC, Hannaford PC, Penny K. The impact of chronic pain in the community. Fam Pract. 2001;18(3):292–9.
6. Dahlhamer J, Lucas J, Zelaya C, et al. Prevalence of chronic pain and high-impact chronic pain among adults—United States, 2016. Morb Mortal Wkly Rep. 2018;67(36):1001.
7. Nahin RL. Estimates of pain prevalence and severity in adults: United States, 2012. J Pain. 2015;16(8):769–80.
8. Loeser JD, Melzack R. Pain: an overview. Lancet. 1999;353(9164):1607–9.
9. Merskey H, Bogduk N. Classification of chronic pain. Seattle: International Association for the Study of Pain Press; 1994.

10. Fillingim RB, Bruehl S, Dworkin RH, et al. The ACTTION-American Pain Society Pain Taxonomy (AAPT): an evidence-based and multidimensional approach to classifying chronic pain conditions. J Pain. 2014;15(3):241–9.
11. Treede R-D, Rief W, Barke A, et al. A classification of chronic pain for ICD-11. Pain. 2015;156(6):1003–7.
12. Treede RD, Rief W, Barke A, et al. Chronic pain as a symptom or a disease: the IASP classification of chronic pain for the international classification of diseases (ICD-11). Pain. 2019;160(1):19–27.
13. Loeser J. Perspectives on pain. In: Clinical pharmacology & therapeutics. Berlin: Springer; 1980. p. 313–6.
14. Freynhagen R, Parada HA, Calderon-Ospina CA, et al. Current understanding of the mixed pain concept: a brief narrative review. Curr Med Res Opin. 2019;35(6):1011–8.
15. Pain IAftSo. IASP terminology. 2018. https://www.iasp-pain.org/Education/Content.aspx?ItemNumber=1698.
16. Barke A, Korwisi B, Jakob R, Konstanjsek N, Rief W, Treede R-D. Classification of chronic pain for the international classification of diseases (ICD-11): results of the 2017 international WHO field testing. Pain. 2021;163(2):e310–8.
17. Zinboonyahgoon N, Luansritisakul C, Eiamtanasate S, et al. Comparing the ICD-11 chronic pain classification with ICD-10: how can the new coding system make chronic pain visible? A study in a tertiary care pain clinic setting. Pain. 2021;162(7):1995–2001.
18. Lindblom U. Pain terms: a current list with definitions and notes on usage. Pain Suppl. 1986;3:S215–21.
19. Stanos S, Brodsky M, Argoff C, et al. Rethinking chronic pain in a primary care setting. Postgrad Med. 2016;128(5):502–15.

Chapter 2
The Challenge in Dealing with Chronic and Neuropathic Pain

Tolga Ergönenç, Rehab Mahmoud Salem, Rania Elsaied Elkholy, and Abdallah El-Sayed Allam

Introduction

Pain is as old as life itself, and it is a sensation that is universally experienced regardless of race, gender, or age. Acute pain serves as a protective mechanism, alerting the body to the possibility of actual tissue damage. A complex physiological system ensures that such warnings are taken seriously and those appropriate responses are initiated. When the patient is treated, the acute pain subsides. The situation becomes more complicated when the pain becomes a part of the disease process, as in chronic pain conditions. The pathophysiology, diagnosis, and definition of chronic pain are different. For some chronic pain conditions, the diagnosis is based solely on the patient's subjective symptoms, for which there is no known organic cause. Acute pain relief medications like opioids and non-steroidal anti-inflammatory drugs (NSAIDs) may be ineffective at relieving chronic pain in this situation. The use of additional painkillers, typically used for depression, seizures,

T. Ergönenç (✉)
Department of Anesthesiology and Reanimation, Palliative Care, Republic of Turkey Ministry of Health Akyazi Hospital, Sakarya, Turkey

Morphological Madrid Research Center (MoMaRC), Madrid, Spain
e-mail: tolga.ergonenc@saglik.gov.tr

R. M. Salem · R. E. Elkholy
Department of Physical Medicine, Rheumatology and Rehabilitation, Tanta University Hospitals and Faculty of Medicine, Tanta University, Tanta, Egypt
e-mail: rehab.salem@med.tanta.edu.eg

A. E.-S. Allam
Morphological Madrid Research Center (MoMaRC), Madrid, Spain

Department of Physical Medicine, Rheumatology and Rehabilitation, Tanta University Hospitals and Faculty of Medicine, Tanta University, Tanta, Egypt

© The Author(s), under exclusive license to Springer Nature Switzerland AG 2022

J. de Castro, Y. El Miedany (eds.), *Advances in Chronic and Neuropathic Pain*, Contemporary Rheumatology, https://doi.org/10.1007/978-3-031-10687-3_2

or local anesthesia, are increasingly being used to treat many types of chronic pain, especially neuropathies. Nevertheless, side effects can be severe, and their use may not completely alleviate pain. Chronic pain presents a unique set of challenges for healthcare professionals because it necessitates a rational and pragmatic approach to management. One thing is for sure, despite all the confusion. A surprising number of people suffer from chronic pain. Chronic pain should be addressed as an essential public health problem [1].

Establishing Reasonable Anticipation

Chronic pain management is a long-term process. Starting with realistic expectations and developing a long-term strategy that recognizes the complexity of the problem are essential steps for both doctors and patients. Patients with hypertension do not expect to achieve control after a single course of treatment; instead, they expect a long-term strategy that includes diet, exercise, medication, education, and preventative measures, among others. Similarly, patients with chronic pain (and their physicians) should anticipate a long-term, versatile approach. Iatrogenic situations can arise when a patient has unrealistic expectations of "quick pain relief." This can result in unnecessary drug therapy, dose-escalation, and over-enthusiastic interventions by clinicians seeking short-term gains.

Accepting That Pain Medications Have Their Limitations

When it comes to treating chronic pain, all of the commonly prescribed analgesics have significant drawbacks. Examples include long-term use of paracetamol, which has been shown to cause liver function changes, and non-steroidal anti-inflammatory drugs, which have been linked to potentially serious renal, gastrointestinal, and cardiovascular side effects [2].

Prescription rates for opioid analgesics have increased dramatically over the past 15 years in many countries. Although well-known side effects such as constipation and sedation (particularly in older people) may occur, when opioids are used for a prolonged period in combination with other medications, tolerance, hyperalgesia, dependence, and misuse may occur as a result. When opioids are indicated, they can and should be used; however, a treatment that does not include opioids should not be considered incomplete.

More than ever, the concept of a comprehensive pain management strategy is becoming increasingly valuable. Patients with chronic pain are often referred to primary care clinicians, surgeons, and emergency department doctors. These clinicians play a critical role in initiating and developing a long-term strategy for pain management, which may include prompt referral to pain specialists. Some other vital components of a comprehensive management plan include treating underlying conditions; using a variety of medications to maximize effectiveness while minimizing side effects, such as muscle relaxants, antidepressants, and topical agents, in addition to conventional analgesics; incorporating psychological interventions and physical therapy; and considering integrative approaches, such as acupuncture, medical ozone therapy, and mind-body therapy [3, 4].

The goal of chronic pain management is not to eliminate the defensive signal entirely, but to adjust the threshold so that it does not become excessive. This is probably the most difficult goal in chronic pain management, and it has been and will continue to be the focus of decades of effort in the field of pain research.[5, 6].

Epidemiology of the Chronic Pain

Multiple studies show that chronic pain is a common condition among the general population, and that it can have a negative impact on the individual's health, employment, and quality of life [7].

Chronic pain, which is typically defined as pain that lasts longer than 3 months, is prevalent throughout the world, affecting roughly 20% of the global population on average.

Estimates of chronic pain prevalence vary significantly across developed and developing countries, owing to differences in study methodology, definitions of chronic pain, and cultural differences in willingness to report pain. In the majority of studies, the female gender and older age group have been found to be associated [8].

It is difficult to determine whether the global prevalence of chronic pain is increasing based on the data currently available. Chronic pain is rarely experienced in isolation; rather, it is frequently accompanied by coexisting mental and physical health problems [9].

Numerous countries are experiencing an increase in the prevalence of comorbid chronic conditions such as obesity and diabetes. Chronic pain is likely to increase in prevalence in societies that promote unhealthy lifestyles [10].

Classification of the Chronic Pain

Pain classifications based on mechanisms have evolved over time. Traditionally, pain mechanisms were classified as nociceptive or neuropathic. This classification system worked admirably well for acute and cancer-related pain. Many patients with chronic non-cancer pain (CNCP) had no clear source for ongoing tissue damage or disease, and a nerve injury or pathology could not be demonstrated. It was discovered that chronic pain was frequently caused by nervous system sensitization or a loss of descending inhibition.

The 2019 classification, an updated version of the International Classification of Diseases 11, distinguishes between primary pain, which is caused by nervous system dysfunction, and secondary pain, which is caused by an underlying injury or disease process [11].

The new classification of chronic pain as a "somatic symptom disorder" and a mental health problem, when it is not associated with a physical disease process, is a positive step in the right direction.

Neuroscience of the Chronic Pain

We can think of the nervous system as serving as a link between our conscious minds and our physical bodies. Our physical well-being is connected to our mental and emotional well-being via the nervous system, and vice versa [12].

Since gate control theory first proposed that nociceptive impulses to the brain are modulated rather than transmitted directly to the brain, our understanding of the nervous system's role in pain has continued to evolve [13].

The neural system which underlying pain is intricate and multilayered. There are nociceptive, cognitive, and affective networks involved, all of which can undergo structural and functional changes in the presence of chronic pain. Nociceptive information is processed by the primary and secondary somatosensory cortexes, the anterior cingulate cortex, the anterior and posterior insula, the medial and ventrolateral thalamus, and the hypothalamus. The limbic system, which includes the amygdala, nucleus accumbens, and hippocampus, is involved in emotions and motivation and communicates with cortical systems, including prefrontal cortical circuitry, during the evaluation of pain experience [14].

Cervero and Laird proposed a three-stage pain model. The processing of brief, acute noxious stimuli are included in stage 1. When the noxious stimulus is intense or prolonged, inflammation and tissue injury occur in stage 2. Stage 3 pain refers to abnormal pain states that are typically characterized by damage to either peripheral or central nervous system components, also known as neuropathic pain. Although each of these three stages of pain has its own physiology, there is evidence that they are all related [15].

Tissue damage and nociceptive responses have a strong correlation in normal circumstances.

However, some changes may occur that shift the system's functioning toward the neuropathic end, where the correlation between observable injury and nociceptive responses is low. Variations in the quantity and quality of noxious input cause these changes, which distort the functioning of the sensory pain system. As a result, pain loses its protective function and becomes the problem itself [15].

Assessment of Chronic Non-malignant and Malignant Pain

Chronic pain is often a sign of an underlying disease process when it comes to diseases like cancer, which has a high mortality rate [16].

It is possible for chronic pain to be linked to both disease and treatment. According to various epidemiological surveys, 20–25% of cancer patients have chronic pain related to chemotherapy, radiation therapy, or surgery [17].

As a result of their treatment, some of these patients have been cured of cancer, but they are still in excruciating pain. Chronic pain can be caused by AIDS, arthritis, sickle cell anemia, and many other medical conditions. Low back pain, failed back surgery, and chronic headache that does not exhibit classic migraine symptoms are examples of chronic pain disorders as well. Chronic pain without a specific diagnosis falls into this category. To alleviate symptoms, the psychological complications of the disease and rehabilitation approaches should all be addressed in treatment [16].

Diagnosing chronic nonmalignant pain necessitates ruling out other possible causes. A clinical evaluation is required in most cases to make a diagnosis. Various clinical parameters should be used throughout the intervention to assess the effectiveness of any treatment and to maintain the patient's health status [18].

Challenges in Chronic Pain Management

Patient-Related Challenges

Eduardo Bruera et al. observed patient-related barriers in Canada many years ago. They investigated refractory pain using "prognostic factors" to identify patients for whom managing cancer pain with opioids was difficult. The following factors were associated with poor prognosis: incident or movement-related pain, neuropathic pain, severe psychological distress, a history of alcohol or drug abuse, or a recent history of opioid tolerance [19].

Health System-Related Challenges

A global health system challenge is the medical system's general failure to integrate palliative care and pain management goals into primary disease treatment. The underlying medical condition must be treated in order for pain management to be successful [18].

Multidisciplinary Approach Challenges

Because chronic pain is so complex, medical treatment alone or single-professional approaches may be ineffective, and multidisciplinary treatment may be required [20].

Pain management programs for chronic pain conditions are being developed all over the world, and there is a great demand for multidimensional management strategies, particularly in the case of chronic pain of neuropathic origin [21, 22].

The treatment options available to patients suffering from chronic pain, in contrast to the treatment options available to patients suffering from most forms of acute, peripheral, or nociceptive pain, frequently provide only short-term or partial relief from symptoms [23].

Interdisciplinary pain management is frequently offered as a last resort at a very late stage of treatment, after all other options have been exhausted and no longer work [24].

Most of these interdisciplinary interventions are aimed at getting people back to work, but they also teach cognitive-behavioral skills to help people better deal with pain from their own point of view. There is strong evidence that intensive bio-psychosocial rehabilitation with a functional restoration approach can improve both pain and function in chronic back pain patients [25].

References

1. Holden JE, Pizzi JA. The challenge of chronic pain. Adv Drug Deliv Rev. 2003;55(8):935–48. https://doi.org/10.1016/S0169-409X(03)00097-8.
2. Gupta A, Bah M. NSAIDs in the treatment of postoperative pain. Curr Pain Headache Rep. 2016;20(11):62. https://doi.org/10.1007/S11916-016-0591-7.
3. Qaseem A, Wilt TJ, McLean RM, Forciea MA, Clinical Guidelines Committee of the American College of Physicians, Denberg TD, Barry MJ, Boyd C, Chow RD, Fitterman N, Harris RP, Humphrey LL, Vijan S. Noninvasive treatments for acute, subacute, and chronic low back pain: a clinical practice guideline from the American College of Physicians. Ann Intern Med. 2017;166(7):514–30. https://doi.org/10.7326/M16-2367.
4. Mao J, Gold MS, Backonja M. Combination drug therapy for chronic pain: a call for more clinical studies. J Pain. 2011;12(2):157–66. https://doi.org/10.1016/J.JPAIN.2010.07.006.
5. Mao J. Current challenges in translational pain research. Trends Pharmacol Sci. 2012;33(11):568–73. https://doi.org/10.1016/J.TIPS.2012.08.001.
6. Mao J, Kitz RJ. Challenges of managing chronic pain. BMJ. 2017;356:j741. https://doi.org/10.1136/BMJ.J741.
7. Smith BH, Elliott AM, Alastair Chambers W, Smith WC, Hannaford PC, Penny K. The impact of chronic pain in the community. Fam Pract. 2001;18(3):292–9. https://doi.org/10.1093/fampra/18.3.292.
8. Tsang A, von Korff M, Lee S, Alonso J, Karam E, Angermeyer MC, Borges GLG, Bromet EJ, de Girolamo G, de Graaf R, Gureje O, Lepine JP, Haro JM, Levinson D, Oakley Browne MA, Posada-Villa J, Seedat S, Watanabe M. Common chronic pain conditions in developed and developing countries: gender and age differences and comorbidity with depression-anxiety disorders. J Pain. 2008;9(10):883–91. https://doi.org/10.1016/J.JPAIN.2008.05.005.

9. Bruggink L, Hayes C, Lawrence G, Brain K, Holliday S. Chronic pain: overlap and specificity in multimorbidity management. Aust J Gen Pract. 2019;48(10):689–92. https://doi.org/10.31128/AJGP-06-19-4966.
10. Rajappa H, Hayes C. People, medicine, and society: an overview of chronic pain management. Arch Med Health Sci. 2020;8(1):68. https://doi.org/10.4103/AMHS.AMHS_108_20.
11. Treede RD, Rief W, Barke A, Aziz Q, Bennett MI, Benoliel R, Cohen M, Evers S, Finnerup NB, First MB, Giamberardino MA, Kaasa S, Korwisi B, Kosek E, Lavand'Homme P, Nicholas M, Perrot S, Scholz J, Schug S, et al. Chronic pain as a symptom or a disease: the IASP classification of chronic pain for the international classification of diseases (ICD-11). Pain. 2019;160(1):19–27. https://doi.org/10.1097/J.PAIN.0000000000001384.
12. Siddall PJ. Neuroplasticity and pain: what does it all mean? Med J Aust. 2013;198(4):177–8. https://doi.org/10.5694/MJA13.10100.
13. Melzack R, Wall PD. Pain mechanisms: a new theory. Science. 1965;150(3699):971–9. https://doi.org/10.1126/SCIENCE.150.3699.971.
14. Tajerian M, David Clark J. Nonpharmacological interventions in targeting pain-related brain plasticity. Neural Plast. 2017;2017:2038573. https://doi.org/10.1155/2017/2038573.
15. Cervero F, Laird JMA. From acute to chronic pain: mechanisms and hypotheses. Prog Brain Res. 1996;110:3–15. https://doi.org/10.1016/s0079-6123(08)62561-3.
16. Payne R. Chronic pain: challenges in the assessment and management of cancer pain. J Pain Symptom Manage. 2000;19(1 Suppl):12–5. https://doi.org/10.1016/S0885-3924(99)00123-2.
17. Jacox A, Carr DB, Payne R. New clinical-practice guidelines for the management of pain in patients with cancer. N Engl J Med. 1994;330(9):651–5. https://doi.org/10.1056/NEJM199403033300926.
18. Scascighini L, Sprott H. Chronic nonmalignant pain: a challenge for patients and clinicians. Nat Clin Pract Rheumatol. 2008;4(2):74–81. https://doi.org/10.1038/ncprheum0680.
19. Bruera E, MacMillan K, Hanson J, MacDonald RN. The Edmonton staging system for cancer pain: preliminary report. Pain. 1989;37(2):203–9. https://doi.org/10.1016/0304-3959(89)90131-0.
20. Gatchel RJ, Polatin PB, Mayer TG, Garcy PD. Psychopathology and the rehabilitation of patients with chronic low back pain disability. Arch Phys Med Rehabil. 1994;75(6):666–70. https://doi.org/10.1016/0003-9993(94)90191-0.
21. Gatchel RJ, Okifuji A. Evidence-based scientific data documenting the treatment and cost-effectiveness of comprehensive pain programs for chronic nonmalignant pain. J Pain. 2006;7(11):779–93. https://doi.org/10.1016/J.JPAIN.2006.08.005.
22. Smith BH, Torrance N, Bennett MI, Lee AJ. Health and quality of life associated with chronic pain of predominantly neuropathic origin in the community. Clin J Pain. 2007;23(2):143–9. https://doi.org/10.1097/01.AJP.0000210956.31997.89.
23. Riedel W, Neeck G. Nociception, pain, and antinociception: current concepts. Zeitschrift Fur Rheumatologie. 2001;60(6):404–15. https://doi.org/10.1007/S003930170003.
24. Olason M. Outcome of an interdisciplinary pain management program in a rehabilitation clinic. Work. 2004;22(1):9–15.
25. Guzmán J, Esmail R, Karjalainen K, Malmivaara A, Irvin E, Bombardier C. Multidisciplinary bio-psycho-social rehabilitation for chronic low back pain. Cochrane Database Syst Rev. 2002;(1):CD000963. https://doi.org/10.1002/14651858.CD000963.

Part II
Pathophysiology

Chapter 3
Pathophysiology of Chronic Pain

Kirellos Said Abbas, Abdallah El-Sayed Allam, Felice Galluccio, Ahmed Amine El OUMRI, Abdullah AlKharabsheh, and Ammar Salti

Abbreviations

BDNF	Brain-derived neurotrophic factor
Caspase-6	Cysteine-aspartic acid protease-6
CNS	Central nervous system

K. S. Abbas
Faculty of Medicine, Alexandria University, Alexandria, Egypt

A. E.-S. Allam (✉)
Department of Physical Medicine, Rheumatology and Rehabilitation, Tanta University Hospitals and Faculty of Medicine, Tanta University, Tanta, Egypt

Morphological Madrid Research Center (MoMaRC), Madrid, Spain

F. Galluccio
Morphological Madrid Research Center (MoMaRC), Madrid, Spain

Division of Rheumatology, Medical-Geriatric Department, University Hospital AOU Careggi, Florence, Italy
e-mail: felice.galluccio@momarc.org

A. A. El OUMRI
Departement of Physical Medicine and Rehabilitation, Mohammed VI University hospital Oujda , Immuno Hematology and Cellular Therapy Laboratory, Faculty of Medicine of oujda, Mohammed First University of Oujda, Mohammed VI University hospital Oujda and Faculty of Medicine Mohammed First University of oujda, Oujda, Morocco

A. AlKharabsheh
King Abdullah University Hospital, Jordan University of Science and Technology, Irbid, Jordan

A. Salti
Anesthesia and Interventional Pain Medicine, Cleveland Clinic, Abu Dhabi, UAE

Anesthesiology - Cleveland Clinic Lerner College of Medicine - Case Western Reserve University, Cleveland, OH, USA

© The Author(s), under exclusive license to Springer Nature Switzerland AG 2022

J. de Castro, Y. El Miedany (eds.), *Advances in Chronic and Neuropathic Pain*, Contemporary Rheumatology, https://doi.org/10.1007/978-3-031-10687-3_3

CSF-1	Colony-stimulating factor-1
CX	Connexin
DAMPs	Damage-associated molecular patterns
GABA	Gamma-aminobutyric acid
JAK-STAT	Janus kinase/signal transducer and activator of the transcription
lncRNA	Long non-coding RNAs
MMPs	Matrix metalloproteinases
NMDA	*N*-methyl-D-aspartate
PRR	Pattern-recognition receptors
RAGE	Advanced glycation end products
TNF	Tumor necrosis factors
TRP	Transient receptor potential channels

Introduction

Chronic pain is a clinical status characterized by persistent symptoms of pain e.g., hyperalgesia, allodynia which may persist for longer than 3–6 months. The pathogenesis of chronic pain is not fully understood, and its treatment still represents a significant health problem; 19% of adult European suffer chronic pain and a third of children experienced it in their life [1–3]. The Global Burden of Disease Study estimated pain and its related diseases as the leading cause of disability worldwide [4]. Understanding the underlying pathophysiology of chronic pain is crucial for all healthcare workers involved in pain management. Advancing in age, being female, living in low socioeconomic status, being illiterate, unemployed, obese, drinking too much alcoholic, living a sedentary life, following an unhealthy diet are associated with higher prevalence and intensity of pain according to Mills et al. in their epidemiological review [5].

Normal Physiology

Normal physiology of pain signaling includes transduction (intracellular changes upon ligand activation), transmission (movement of pain signals), modulation (alteration in pain signals), and perception (unpleasant sensory and emotional experience). Any tissue damage or inflammatory reactions affecting the receptors or peripheral fibers will affect the normal physiology, also pain processing in the CNS may be dysregulated. Chronic pain is classified as nociceptor pain and neuropathic according to the type of the noxious agent, they may coexist, and pain sensitization is classified to peripheral or central according to the site of dysregulation [6].

Pathway of the Chronic Pain

Receptors
Nociceptors
Afferent
Small-diameter myelinated A and unmyelinated C nerve fibers.
First-order neurons
Dorsal horn of the spinal cord.
Spinothalamic tract
The major ascending pathway for pain and temperature.
Second-order neurons
Rexed layers I, II, and V.
Third-order neurons
Ventral posterolateral (VPL) nucleus of the thalamus.
Cortex
Signal projected to the primary somatosensory cortex.

Information in the dorsal root ganglion is subjected to modulation by descending signals from the brain stem nuclei [7].

Nociceptors (Pain Receptors)

Nociceptors localize at the somatic body parts (bone, muscle, joints) or visceral body organs. Location of receptors classifies nociceptors pain as somatic; well localized and intense, and visceral pain; poorly localized and diffuse. Nociceptor pain is the body's reaction to a painful stimulus like a muscle sprain or tissue damage [8]. Nociceptors and their related afferent nerves differ according to their function and size in myelination, electrophysiological pattern, surface markers, and gene expression [9].

Neuropathic Pain

Noxious agents to the peripheral nociceptor may be caused by inflammation trauma, cancer, arthritis, and others. Those noxious agents promote an increase in the release of the pain mediators' substances and neurotransmitters such as substance P, prostaglandins, and bradykinins. Depolarization starts at the level of the nociceptors and travels up to the second-order neurons in the spinal cord, and midbrain then to the higher centers and limbic system. Neuropathic pain is chronic pain associated with lesions or dysregulation in the pain pathways. Neuropathic pain may be in the form of dysesthesia, abnormal sensation, allodynia, or pain from non-painful stimuli. Neuropathic pains are more severe and more difficult to treat [6, 10, 11].

Possible Mechanisms and Pathogenesis

Peripheral Sensitization

The presence of peripheral nerve injury increases the sensitivity of the nerve to pain through local release of inflammatory substances, recruiting immune cells, and release of cytokines e.g., TNF and interleukins which potentiate the action of both Na and Ca channels [6, 12, 13]. Activation of receptors on the nociceptor neurons proceeds post-transduction modification on the regulation of ion channels, transient receptor potential channels (TRP), pattern-recognition receptors (PRR), toll-like receptors (TLRs), and receptors for advanced glycation end products (RAGE) [14].

Central Sensitization

Continuous peripheral sensitization leads to changes at the level of CNS named "central sensitization". Central sensitization is associated with reduced pain threshold and modulation in pain pathways at the level of CNS. These modulations in CNS are possible explanations for depression and anxiety attacks associated with chronic pain. It also explains the high prevalence of chronic pain among patients with depression as depression is itself characterized by inflammatory activity [5, 15–17]. Central sensitization is thought to be the reason for neuropathic pain symptoms such as allodynia, hyperalgesia, secondary hyperalgesia, temporal summation, expansion of referred pain region, and defective descending inhibitory control [17–19].

Glial Cells

CNS glial cells play an important role in the pain pathways; reactive changes are seen in astrocytes, microglia, and oligodendrocytes as a sequela of pathological conditions evoking pain [20–22]. Proinflammatory mediators derived from neurons themselves are responsible for microglial cell activation e.g. colony-stimulating factor 1 (CSF1) caspase-6, interleukin-1β, and extracellular proteases damage-associated molecular patterns (DAMPs) [20, 23–26]. Those mediators activate glial cells by binding to pattern-recognition receptors (PRR) [20]. The role of microglial cells in pain can be noticed by the effect of drugs inhibiting their activation [27, 28]. minocycline, propentofylline, and ibudilast [29–31]. Microglia release IL-1β a cytokine seen to be upregulated in chronic pain which enhances NMDA receptors and inhibits GABA transmission [32–35]. Drugs antagonizing its action showed good results in attenuating pain intensity [35–38]. Transmission of ions dramatically increases between glial cells through connexin-43 (CX43) gap junction. This increase is associated with high expression of connexin-43 (CX43) protein [39]. Carbenoxolone as a gap junction inhibitor showed positive results [40]. Matrix metalloproteinases (MMPs) also play a role in the regulation of inflammatory cytokines associated with nerve injury; using tissue inhibitors of MMP showed positive results in attenuating chronic pain [41, 42]. Other mediators like catecholamines and oligodendrocytes precursor cells are seen to be upregulated in chronic pain pathways [22, 43].

Pattern Recognition Receptors (PRP)

Pattern recognition receptors (PRP)) such as TLRs and RAGEs play their role in chronic pain through both peripheral and central sensitization [14]. TLRs are responsible for the induction of proinflammatory mediators and generating biologically active IL-1β. RAGEs are membranous proteins with cytoplasmic domain upon activation they increase transduction and upregulation of cytokines and proinflammatory material [14].

JAK-STAT Pathway

A new therapeutic target is Janus kinase/signal transducer and activator of the transcription (JAK-STAT) pathway. This pathway is very crucial in immune cell activation and cytokine production. Once cytokines bind to JAK receptors they become phosphorylated and translocate to the nucleus where they enhance gene transcription. Those genes are related to numerous cytokines and proinflammatory materials [44, 45].

Cysteinyl-Aspartate-Specific Proteases (CASPs)

They are proteases responsible for initiating cell apoptosis. They are highly expressed in dorsal root ganglions, peripheral nerves, and the brain. In chronic pain, their activation leads to the neuroinflammatory response, cell apoptosis, and microglial cell activation. Injection of CASPs inhibitors showed positive results in alleviating neuropathic pain [46, 47].

Long Non-coding RNAs (lncRNA)

They are transcripts not coding for protein synthesis and found to be highly expressed in the spinal cord and dorsal ganglia in chronic neuropathic pain. Researchers supposed they are involved in cytokine production, activation, and interaction with TLRs to be an important part of neuropathic chronic pain pathways [48, 49].

GABAergic Plasticity

After nerve injuries, changes occur in peripheral nerves and nociceptors leading to pain hypersensitivity. Decrease in GABA inhibition though to be one of the causes and named "neuropathy-induced decrease of GABA synaptic inhibition". Injury through to causes cell apoptosis decreasing GABAergic nerves [50, 51].

Purinergic Signaling in Microglia

Stimulation of P2X4 receptors on the surface of microglia release brain-derived neurotrophic factor (BDNF), this substance dysregulates ion exchanges inverting cell polarity and converting GABA and glycine to the polarizing agent rather than hyperpolarizing agents [52–54].

Mitochondrial Role in the Pathogenesis of Chronic Pain

Recently, mitochondria were found to be involved in the pathogenesis of chronic pain. Increase production of reactive oxygen species (ROS) and superoxide associated with hyperalgesia even without nerve injury. Blocking of ATP-dependent mechanism in mitochondria gave positive results in reducing some types of neuropathic pain [55–57].

Conclusion

Despite the pathogenies of chronic pain is not yet well understood, numerous theories have been proposed and new therapeutic agents have been tried and are anticipated to reach an effective agent in decreasing the burden of chronic pain.

References

1. Fornasari D. Pain mechanisms in patients with chronic pain. Clin Drug Investig. 2012;32(Suppl 1):45–52.
2. Rapo-Pylkkö S, Haanpää M, Liira H. A one-year follow-up study of chronic pain in community-dwelling older adults with and without neuropathic pain. BMC Geriatr. 2017;17(1):152.
3. Huguet A, Miró J. The severity of chronic pediatric pain: an epidemiological study. J Pain. 2008;9(3):226–36.

4. Global, regional, and national incidence, prevalence, and years lived with disability for 328 diseases and injuries for 195 countries, 1990-2016: a systematic analysis for the Global Burden of Disease Study 2016. Lancet (London, England). 2017;390(10100):1211–59.
5. Mills SEE, Nicolson KP, Smith BH. Chronic pain: a review of its epidemiology and associated factors in population-based studies. Br J Anaesth. 2019;123(2):e273–83.
6. Pergolizzi J, Ahlbeck K, Aldington D, Alon E, Coluzzi F, Dahan A, et al. The development of chronic pain: physiological CHANGE necessitates a multidisciplinary approach to treatment. Curr Med Res Opin. 2013;29(9):1127–35.
7. Helme RD, Gibson S, Khalil Z. Neural pathways in chronic pain. Med J Aust. 1990;153(7):400–6.
8. Nicholson B. Differential diagnosis: nociceptive and neuropathic pain. Am J Manag Care. 2006;12(9 Suppl):S256–62.
9. Lallemend F, Ernfors P. Molecular interactions underlying the specification of sensory neurons. Trends Neurosci. 2012;35(6):373–81.
10. Mantyh PW. Cancer pain and its impact on diagnosis, survival and quality of life. Nat Rev Neurosci. 2006;7(10):797–809.
11. Schaible HG, Richter F, Ebersberger A, Boettger MK, Vanegas H, Natura G, et al. Joint pain. Exp Brain Res. 2009;196(1):153–62.
12. Costigan M, Scholz J, Woolf CJ. Neuropathic pain: a maladaptive response of the nervous system to damage. Annu Rev Neurosci. 2009;32:1–32.
13. Zhang N, Oppenheim JJ. Crosstalk between chemokines and neuronal receptors bridges immune and nervous systems. J Leukoc Biol. 2005;78(6):1210–4.
14. Kato J, Agalave NM, Svensson CI. Pattern recognition receptors in chronic pain: mechanisms and therapeutic implications. Eur J Pharmacol. 2016;788:261–73.
15. Edwards RR, Cahalan C, Mensing G, Smith M, Haythornthwaite JA. Pain, catastrophizing, and depression in the rheumatic diseases. Nat Rev Rheumatol. 2011;7(4):216–24.
16. Smart KM, Blake C, Staines A, Doody C. Self-reported pain severity, quality of life, disability, anxiety and depression in patients classified with 'nociceptive', 'peripheral neuropathic' and 'central sensitisation' pain. The discriminant validity of mechanisms-based classifications of low back (±leg) pain. Man Ther. 2012;17(2):119–25.
17. Sandkühler J. Models and mechanisms of hyperalgesia and allodynia. Physiol Rev. 2009;89(2):707–58.
18. Pedersen JL, Andersen OK, Arendt-Nielsen L, Kehlet H. Hyperalgesia and temporal summation of pain after heat injury in man. Pain. 1998;74(2–3):189–97.
19. Pertovaara A, Almeida A. Chapter 13: Descending inhibitory systems. In: Handbook of clinical neurology, vol. 81. Amsterdam: Elsevier; 2006. p. 179–92.
20. Chen G, Zhang Y-Q, Qadri YJ, Serhan CN, Ji R-R. Microglia in pain: detrimental and protective roles in pathogenesis and resolution of pain. Neuron. 2018;100(6):1292–311.
21. Ji R-R, Berta T, Nedergaard M. Glia and pain: is chronic pain a gliopathy? Pain. 2013;154:S10–28.
22. Shi Y, Shu J, Liang Z, Yuan S, Tang SJ. EXPRESS: oligodendrocytes in HIV-associated pain pathogenesis. Mol Pain. 2016;12:1744806916656845.
23. Berta T, Park C-K, Xu Z-Z, Xie R-G, Liu T, Lü N, et al. Extracellular caspase-6 drives murine inflammatory pain via microglial TNF-α secretion. J Clin Invest. 2014;124(3):1173–86.
24. Abbadie C, Bhangoo S, De Koninck Y, Malcangio M, Melik-Parsadaniantz S, White FA. Chemokines and pain mechanisms. Brain Res Rev. 2009;60(1):125–34.
25. Guan Z, Kuhn JA, Wang X, Colquitt B, Solorzano C, Vaman S, et al. Injured sensory neuron-derived CSF1 induces microglial proliferation and DAP12-dependent pain. Nat Neurosci. 2016;19(1):94–101.
26. Ji R-R, Xu Z-Z, Gao Y-J. Emerging targets in neuroinflammation-driven chronic pain. Nat Rev Drug Discov. 2014;13(7):533–48.

27. Raghavendra V, Tanga F, DeLeo JA. Inhibition of microglial activation attenuates the development but not existing hypersensitivity in a rat model of neuropathy. J Pharmacol Exp Ther. 2003;306(2):624–30.
28. Echeverry S, Shi XQ, Yang M, Huang H, Wu Y, Lorenzo LE, et al. Spinal microglia are required for long-term maintenance of neuropathic pain. Pain. 2017;158(9):1792–801.
29. Sweitzer S, Schubert P, DeLeo J. Propentofylline, a glial modulating agent, exhibits antiallodynic properties in a rat model of neuropathic pain. J Pharmacol Exp Ther. 2001;297(3):1210–7.
30. Walters ET. Neuroinflammatory contributions to pain after SCI: roles for central glial mechanisms and nociceptor-mediated host defense. Exp Neurol. 2014;258:48–61.
31. Ellis A, Wieseler J, Favret J, Johnson KW, Rice KC, Maier SF, et al. Systemic administration of propentofylline, ibudilast, and (+)-naltrexone each reverses mechanical allodynia in a novel rat model of central neuropathic pain. J Pain. 2014;15(4):407–21.
32. Binshtok AM, Wang H, Zimmermann K, Amaya F, Vardeh D, Shi L, et al. Nociceptors are interleukin-1β sensors. J Neurosci. 2008;28(52):14062–73.
33. Takeda M, Kitagawa J, Takahashi M, Matsumoto S. Activation of interleukin-1β receptor suppresses the voltage-gated potassium currents in the small-diameter trigeminal ganglion neurons following peripheral inflammation. Pain. 2008;139(3):594–602.
34. Gustafson-Vickers SL, Van Lu B, Lai AY, Todd KG, Ballanyi K, Smith PA. Long-term actions of interleukin-1β on delay and tonic firing neurons in rat superficial dorsal horn and their relevance to central sensitization. Mol Pain. 2008;4:63.
35. Kawasaki Y, Zhang L, Cheng J-K, Ji R-R. Cytokine mechanisms of central sensitization: distinct and overlapping role of interleukin-1β, interleukin-6, and tumor necrosis factor-α in regulating synaptic and neuronal activity in the superficial spinal cord. J Neurosci. 2008;28(20):5189–94.
36. Zhang R-X, Li A, Liu B, Wang L, Ren K, Zhang H, et al. IL-1ra alleviates inflammatory hyperalgesia through preventing phosphorylation of NMDA receptor NR-1 subunit in rats. Pain. 2008;135(3):232–9.
37. Milligan ED, O'Connor KA, Nguyen KT, Armstrong CB, Twining C, Gaykema RP, et al. Intrathecal HIV-1 envelope glycoprotein gp120 induces enhanced pain states mediated by spinal cord proinflammatory cytokines. J Neurosci. 2001;21(8):2808–19.
38. Gabay E, Wolf G, Shavit Y, Yirmiya R, Tal M. Chronic blockade of interleukin-1 (IL-1) prevents and attenuates neuropathic pain behavior and spontaneous ectopic neuronal activity following nerve injury. Eur J Pain. 2011;15(3):242–8.
39. Chen G, Park C-K, Xie R-G, Berta T, Nedergaard M, Ji R-R. Connexin-43 induces chemokine release from spinal cord astrocytes to maintain late-phase neuropathic pain in mice. Brain. 2014;137(8):2193–209.
40. Wang H, Cao Y, Chiang C-Y, Dostrovsky JO, Sessle BJ. The gap junction blocker carbenoxolone attenuates nociceptive behavior and medullary dorsal horn central sensitization induced by partial infraorbital nerve transection in rats. Pain. 2014;155(2):429–35.
41. Ji R-R, Xu Z-Z, Wang X, Lo EH. Matrix metalloprotease regulation of neuropathic pain. Trends Pharmacol Sci. 2009;30(7):336–40.
42. Kawasaki Y, Xu Z-Z, Wang X, Park JY, Zhuang Z-Y, Tan P-H, et al. Distinct roles of matrix metalloproteases in the early- and late-phase development of neuropathic pain. Nat Med. 2008;14(3):331–6.
43. Diatchenko L, Nackley AG, Tchivileva IE, Shabalina SA, Maixner W. Genetic architecture of human pain perception. Trends Genet. 2007;23(12):605–13.
44. Liu H, Yao YM, Yu Y, Dong N, Yin HN, Sheng ZY. Role of Janus kinase/signal transducer and activator of transcription pathway in regulation of expression and inflammation-promoting activity of high mobility group box protein 1 in rat peritoneal macrophages. Shock. 2007;27(1):55–60.
45. Salaffi F, Giacobazzi G, Di Carlo M. Chronic pain in inflammatory arthritis: mechanisms, metrology, and emerging targets—a focus on the JAK-STAT pathway. Pain Res Manag. 2018;2018:8564215.

46. Taylor RC, Cullen SP, Martin SJ. Apoptosis: controlled demolition at the cellular level. Nat Rev Mol Cell Biol. 2008;9(3):231–41.
47. Berta T, Lee JE, Park CK. Unconventional role of caspase-6 in spinal microglia activation and chronic pain. Mediat Inflamm. 2017;2017:9383184.
48. Li Z, Li X, Chen X, Li S, Ho IHT, Liu X, et al. Emerging roles of long non-coding RNAs in neuropathic pain. Cell Prolif. 2019;52(1):e12528.
49. Wu W, Ji X, Zhao Y. Emerging roles of long non-coding RNAs in chronic neuropathic pain. Front Neurosci. 2019;13:1097.
50. Li C, Lei Y, Tian Y, Xu S, Shen X, Wu H, et al. The etiological contribution of GABAergic plasticity to the pathogenesis of neuropathic pain. Mol Pain. 2019;15:1744806919847366.
51. von Hehn CA, Baron R, Woolf CJ. Deconstructing the neuropathic pain phenotype to reveal neural mechanisms. Neuron. 2012;73(4):638–52.
52. Ulmann L, Hatcher JP, Hughes JP, Chaumont S, Green PJ, Conquet F, et al. Up-regulation of P2X4 receptors in spinal microglia after peripheral nerve injury mediates BDNF release and neuropathic pain. J Neurosci. 2008;28(44):11263–8.
53. Coull JA, Beggs S, Boudreau D, Boivin D, Tsuda M, Inoue K, et al. BDNF from microglia causes the shift in neuronal anion gradient underlying neuropathic pain. Nature. 2005;438(7070):1017–21.
54. Inoue K. Purinergic signaling in microglia in the pathogenesis of neuropathic pain. Proc Jpn Acad Ser B Phys Biol Sci. 2017;93(4):174–82.
55. Sui BD, Xu TQ, Liu JW, Wei W, Zheng CX, Guo BL, et al. Understanding the role of mitochondria in the pathogenesis of chronic pain. Postgrad Med J. 2013;89(1058):709–14.
56. Kim HY, Chung JM, Chung K. Increased production of mitochondrial superoxide in the spinal cord induces pain behaviors in mice: the effect of mitochondrial electron transport complex inhibitors. Neurosci Lett. 2008;447(1):87–91.
57. Joseph EK, Levine JD. Mitochondrial electron transport in models of neuropathic and inflammatory pain. Pain. 2006;121(1–2):105–14.

Chapter 4
The Pathophysiology of Neuropathic Pain

Colin Chun Wai Chong and Ashutosh Joshi

Abbreviations

CT Computed tomography
MRI Magnetic resonance imaging
NA Neuralgic amyotrophy

Introduction

The pathology of neuropathic pain is complex and very different from nociceptive pain. A variety of phenomenon occurring at peripheral, spinal and supraspinal levels have been implicated in the generation of neuropathic pain. It is possible that one or a combination of these phenomena contribute to symptoms in the patient. Here we provide an overview of these postulated mechanisms in the generation of neuropathic pain.

C. C. W. Chong (✉)
School of Medicine, University of Wollongong, Wollongong, NSW, Australia

Department of Radiology, Macquarie University Hospital, Sydney, NSW, Australia

Department of Radiology, Royal Brisbane and Women's Hospital, Brisbane, QLD, Australia

A. Joshi
Department of Radiology, Royal Brisbane and Women's Hospital, Brisbane, QLD, Australia

Department of Anaesthesia, Khoo Teck Puat Hospital, Singapore, Singapore
e-mail: ashutosh.joshi@ktph.com.sg

© The Author(s), under exclusive license to Springer Nature Switzerland AG 2022

J. de Castro, Y. El Miedany (eds.), *Advances in Chronic and Neuropathic Pain*, Contemporary Rheumatology, https://doi.org/10.1007/978-3-031-10687-3_4

Peripheral Mechanisms

Peripheral Sensitization

Following injury, inflammation and reparatory processes ensue, leading to a hyperexcitable state known as peripheral sensitization. In most patients, this state resolves as healing occurs and inflammation subsides. However, when nociception persists because of repeated stimulation from ongoing injury or disease (for example, in diabetes), the changes in primary afferent neurons may persist.

Peripheral sensitization can be attributed to multiple factors. Inflammatory mediators such as calcitonin gene related peptide and substance P, which are released from nociceptive terminals, increase vascular permeability. This leads to localized edema and the by-products of injury, such as prostaglandins, bradykinin, growth factors, and cytokines can escape. These substances result in lowered firing threshold and ectopic discharges leading to sensitization/excitation of nociceptors. Multiple substances can sensitize nociceptors and this may partly explain why no drug is universally effective and there is a ceiling effect for antagonists that work at only one receptor.

Ectopic discharges from the dorsal root ganglion, points along the injured nerve and sometimes adjacent fibers can present as spontaneous pain [1]. Such "cross talk" exhibited by adjacent uninjured nerve fibers where they become excited is called ephaptic transmission. Allodynia refers to pain produced by a normally non-painful stimulus, and it may result from decreased stimulation thresholds. Hyperalgesia refers to exaggerated pain perception as a result of damaged peripheral pain fibers. In part, this may be caused by ephaptic transmission or the expansion of receptive fields of injured nerves (or both). A clinical example of hyperalgesia might be an amputee who is unable to use a prosthesis because of tenderness overlying the stump.

Expression of Ion Channels

One contributor to spontaneous firing of nerve fibers after injury is the increased expression of sodium channels in dorsal root ganglia and around the terminal injury site (neuroma) of injured axons [2]. After nerve injury, the expression of some of these channels increases de novo, the expression of others diminishes, and some translocate into different cellular compartments [3]. The proliferation of heterotopic sodium channels may lower the stimulation threshold and provoke ectopic discharge, resulting in spontaneous pain. In addition, the spread of sodium channels may trigger central sensitization, leading to allodynia. Several adjuvant drugs, such as carbamazepine, act through the blockade of sodium channels. Yet, because none of these drugs is selective for channel subtypes involved in pain, all have low therapeutic indices and many side effects.

Certain types of calcium channels (N-type, T-type, and L-type), and to a lesser extent potassium channels, also play a role in neuropathic pain. After nerve injury, the expression of α2δ calcium channels increases in and around the dorsal root ganglia, increasing excitability [4]. These voltage gated calcium channels are the primary site of action for gabapentinoids, a first-line treatment for neuropathic pain [5], which have been shown in preclinical studies to reduce hyperalgesia and spontaneous pain [6].

Phenotypic Switch

After nerve injury, hundreds of genes that affect nerve function are upregulated or downregulated, and this can affect excitability, as well as transduction and transmission properties. Because gene expression affects cellular characteristics, this can result in a change in the phenotype of the nerve fiber, such that neuromodulators usually expressed in C fibers (such as calcitonin gene related peptide, substance P) are now expressed in other fibers [7]. This may theoretically result in stimuli that are usually innocuous being perceived as painful.

Sensory Denervation and Sprouting of Collateral Nerve Fibers

Following injury to a sensory nerve, atrophic changes (Wallerian degeneration) cause a decrease in the size of the cell body and the axon diameter, and eventually neuronal death. This leads to a decreased density of intraepidermal nociceptors. This may cause loss of sensation or, paradoxically, hyperalgesia and increased pain (deafferentation pain) [8]. One example of deafferentation pain is phantom limb pain after amputation. In response to local release of nerve growth factor, collateral sprouting may follow neuronal loss.

Sympathetically Maintained Pain

Sympathetically maintained pain is pain that is enhanced or maintained by an abnormality in the sympathetic nervous system. The concept of sympathetically maintained pain is most commonly linked to complex regional pain syndrome, although the same principles apply to other pain conditions, such as post-herpetic neuralgia [9]. There is a complex interaction between the anatomically distinct autonomic and somatosensory systems but probably includes the expression of α-adrenoceptors on primary afferent sensory fibers, sympathetic sprouting into dorsal root ganglia, and impaired oxygenation and nutrition in response to sympathetically mediated vasoconstriction [10]. Clinically, sympathetically maintained pain may manifest as temperature or color changes (or both) in an affected extremity, swelling or atrophy, and pain worsened by cold weather or stress, which enhances sympathetic outflow.

Spinal Mechanisms

Spinal Glutamatergic Regulation

Peripheral nerve injury increases neuronal excitability in the spinal cord by activating excitatory glutamate receptors [11]. Nerve injury also induces down-regulation of spinal glutamate transporters responsible for maintaining synaptic glutamate homeostasis. Increased regional glutamate availability secondary to loss of glutamate transporters can result in persistent and enhanced activation of both ionotropic (for example, NMDA and AMPA) and metabotropic glutamate receptors, leading to lower activation thresholds and increased neuronal excitability and neurotoxicity [12].

The term "windup" refers to the progressive increase in the frequency and magnitude of firing of dorsal horn neurons produced by repetitive activation of C fibers, a phenomenon that requires glutamatergic NMDA receptor activity. Spinal glutamatergic activity initiates intracellular signalling cascades, including activation of protein kinase C, that result in long-lasting neuroplastic changes in the spinal cord [13]. Because of its primary role in neuroplasticity and excitotoxicity, the NMDA receptor has been implicated in such diverse areas as memory, opioid tolerance, and opioid induced hyperalgesia—the phenomenon whereby opioid use paradoxically increases pain sensitivity [14]. The long-term use of these drugs to treat chronic neuropathic pain has also had mixed results, and their use may be limited by side effects, particularly psychomimetic ones, which seem to increase in proportion to potency. The use of ketamine infusions as a treatment for refractory neuropathic pain has generated intense interest, although studies are limited by methodological flaws and lack of long-term follow-up [15]. The rationale behind these infusions is that high doses may "reset" the nervous system back to its preinjury state, in essence reversing central sensitization.

Glial Activation and Proinflammatory Cytokines

Proinflammatory cytokines including interleukin-1β, IL-6, and tumor necrosis factor α (TNF-α) are produced peripherally and centrally in response to nerve injury [16]. These proinflammatory cytokines play a crucial role in inflammatory responses after nerve injury through intracellular mediators such as protein kinase C and 3′,5′-cAMP [17]. Proinflammatory cytokines also play an important role in sensitization of the CNS and may contribute to allodynia, hyperalgesia and neuroma formation [18].

Glial cells comprise about 70% of the central nervous system and play an important role in maintenance and homeostasis. Microglia are activated within 24 h of nerve injury, and astrocytes follow shortly thereafter, with activation persisting for up to 12 weeks. Glial cells undergo structural and functional transformation after injury, with astrocytes releasing a host of different proprioceptive factors, such as prostaglandins, excitatory amino acids and cytokines [19].

Microglial cells comprise less than 20% of spinal glial cells under normal conditions but proliferate rapidly at the dorsal root ganglia and spinal cord after nerve injury [19]. On activation, microglial cells stimulate the complement component of the immune system and release cytokines, chemokines, and cytotoxic substances such as nitric oxide and free radicals [19]. This proinflammatory milieu begins at synaptic sites in the brain stem and the site of nerve injury but spreads to more distant sites. The ensuing release of cytokines from astrocytes and microglia induces an array of cellular responses such as upregulation of glucocorticoid and glutamate receptors, leading to spinal excitation and neuroplastic changes [20]. IL-1β also enhances conditioned "fear memory" (conditioned fear related memories associated with behavioural responses) through glucocorticoids, suggesting that proinflammatory cytokines may participate in the affective experience of pain [21].

Supraspinal Mechanisms

Nociceptive signals can also be altered at supraspinal levels. The brains of patients with chronic pain are different from those without pain, with variations in metabolism and regional concentrations of neurotransmitters occurring in areas such as the thalamus and cingulate cortex [22]. In patients with neuropathic pain, cortical reorganization occurs after injury, and the extent of the changes seems to correlate with the degree of pain. For example, in upper extremity amputees with phantom limb pain, because of the close proximity of their somatotopic representations, the area of the brain responsible for moving the lips transgresses into the hand movement area of the motor cortex; this phenomenon does not occur in amputees without phantom limb pain [23]. The observation that these changes occur after injury suggests that disinhibition may not only be a consequence of nerve injury, but may render patients susceptible to chronic pain [24].

Changes that occur in supraspinal regions may explain the strong association between neuropathic pain and mood disorders. Investigators recently found that altered corticotropin releasing factor signalling in the limbic system, an area involved in emotions, may play a role in the development of neuropathic pain [25].

Disinhibition

Spinal Cord Level

Pain attenuating inhibitory neurons are activated once a nociceptive stimulus is transmitted to higher cortical centres. At the spinal cord level, there is increased release of GABA and glycine from primary afferent terminals. Also, there is enhanced activity in inhibitory GABAergic and glycinergic dorsal horn interneurons.

After nerve injury, a loss of inhibitory currents occurs as a result of dysfunctional GABA production and release mechanisms; impaired intracellular homeostasis from reduced activity of K^+Cl cotransporter or increased activity of Na^+K^- Cl cotransporter (or both), leading to increased Cl levels; and apoptosis of spinal inhibitory interneurons [26]. Loss of inhibitory control has been shown to provoke tactile allodynia and hyperalgesia [27], and to facilitate structural changes that increase transmission from Aβ fibers that normally transmit non-painful stimuli to nociceptive specific secondary order neurons in the dorsal horn [28].

Dorsal root ganglia exhibit decreased expression of μ opioid receptors after nerve injury and secondary spinal neurons become less responsive to opioids [29]. This may explain why patients with chronic neuropathic pain require higher doses of opioids than those with acute and chronic nociceptive pain [30].

Expectations and context also play a role in descending modulation. In one randomized study [31], 20 healthy subjects were subjected to painful electrical stimulation of the sural nerve after immersion of an arm in cold water. Half the subjects were told that the immersion would decrease the pain, whereas the other half were told that it would exacerbate the pain. Normally, exposure to a spatially distinct noxious stimulus should decrease the response to pain, a concept known as "descending (or diffuse) noxious inhibitory control." The study found that the analgesia expectancy group experienced a 77% decrease in pain intensity during immersion compared with no significant reduction in pain in the group that anticipated hyperalgesia. These findings agree with other studies that have found that a host of psychosocial factors such as emotions, expectations, and attention affect our intrinsic ability to inhibit pain [32]. This may explain why positive expectations tend to result in better treatment outcomes and a higher placebo response rate, and why we are less likely to perceive pain when an injury occurs while we are preoccupied (for example, during a sports game rather than at bedtime) [33].

Supraspinal Level

Transmission of nociceptive signals is modulated by descending pain pathways that originate in the periaqueductal gray, locus coeruleus, anterior cingulate gyrus, amygdala, and hypothalamus. The descending pain pathways are relayed through brainstem nuclei in the periaqueductal gray and medulla to the spinal cord. The inhibitory transmitters involved in these pathways include norepinephrine, 5-hydroxytryptamine, dopamine, and endogenous opioids. After nerve injury, several processes take place that mitigate the normal pain attenuating pathways. These include a diminution in tonic noradrenergic inhibition and a shift from a predominantly inhibitory role to a facilitative function for descending serotonergic modulation [34]. These neurotransmitters also affect mood and sleep and may partially explain the high association between neuropathic pain, depression, anxiety and sleep disturbances [35]. Commonly prescribed monoamine reuptake inhibitors such as tricyclic antidepressants are not only effective for neuropathic pain and depression but also alleviate anxiety and improve sleep [36].

Clinical Neuropathic Pain Syndromes

The International Association for the Study of Pain (IASP) announced the revision of the definition of pain following internal consultation as an "unpleasant sensory and emotional experience associated with, or resembling that associated with, actual or potential tissue damage" [37]. This definition addresses criticisms of the old definition that explicitly associate pain with tissue damage. By contrast, patients who experience neuropathic pain often experience pain in parts of the body that otherwise appear normal [38].

Lesions or disease affecting the somatosensory system either centrally or in the periphery can result in neuropathic pain. The putative pathophysiology and clinical pathogenesis of common and important neuropathic pain syndromes such as herniated intervertebral disc resulting in lumbar and cervical radiculopathy, post-herpetic neuralgia, complex regional pain syndrome and postsurgical neuropathic pain are outlined in this section.

Spinal radiculopathy can result in a piercing or stabbing pain that radiates into the arms or legs, depending on the level of involvement (Figs. 4.1, 4.2 and 4.3). Lumbosacral radicular syndrome is likely the most frequent neuropathic pain syndrome. Up until recently, mechanical compression of spinal roots mainly by disc protrusions, is thought to account for the majority of lumbar and to a lesser extent cervical and thoracic radiculopathy. In recent years, molecular biology and immunohistochemistry studies show that herniated disc tissue is not an inert material but biologically active with the ability to express inflammatory mediators including interleukin-1, interleukin-6, interleukin-8 and tumor necrosis factor [39]. The extruded nucleus pulposus releases bioactive substances resulting in chemical irritation in combination with immunological autoimmune response against itself result in an inflammatory cascade. Aside from disc protrusion, synovial cysts and spinal canal stenosis due to combination of disc bulges, thickening of ligamentum flavum and facet arthrosis can contribute to radiculopathy.

Compression of the nerve alters nerve root conduction and impairs nutritional support of spinal nerve roots through intrinsic and extrinsic vascularity and cerebral spinal fluid percolation [40]. Intraneural oedema leading to nerve injury or fibrosis

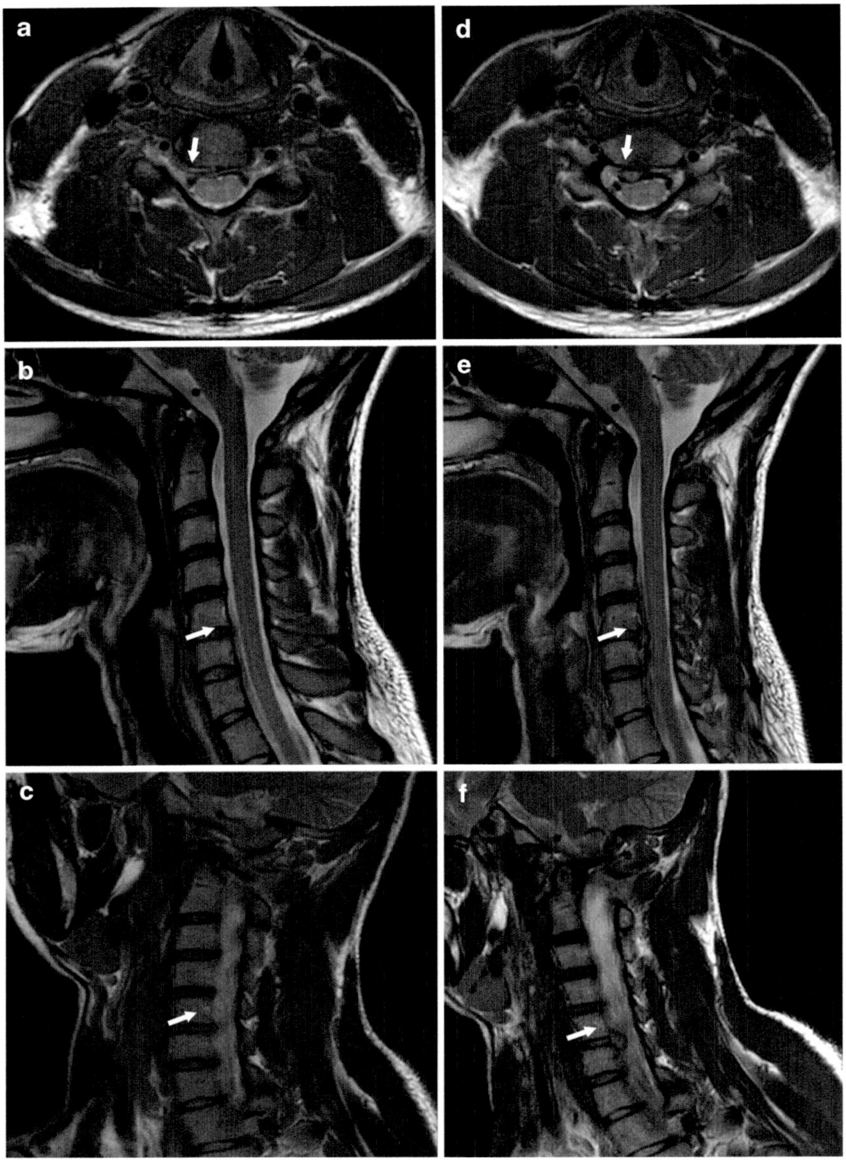

Fig. 4.1 Clinical case. A 28-year-old female mixed martial artist presents initially with intermittent upper limb radicular symptoms in the C7 dermatome from a left lateral hyperextension injury. T2 weighted MRI sequences on axial (panel **a**, white arrow), sagittal (panel **b**, white arrow) and sagittal oblique (panel **c**, white arrow) shows mild right sided disc protrusion at the C5/C6 level, and she was managed conservatively. Six months later, she experiences increasing severity and frequency of pain. T2 weighted MRI sequences on axial (panel **d**, white arrow), sagittal (panel **e**, white arrow) and sagittal oblique (panel **f**, white arrow) show impingement of the right C6 nerve root entry zone by a moderate focal right paracentral disc protrusion. Coronal T2 DIXON turbo spin (panel **g**, white arrow) and axial T2 weighted (panel **h**, white arrow) MRI sequences show oedema in the right serratus anterior muscle, which is innervated by the long thoracic nerve that arises from the roots of the C5, C6 and C6 nerves

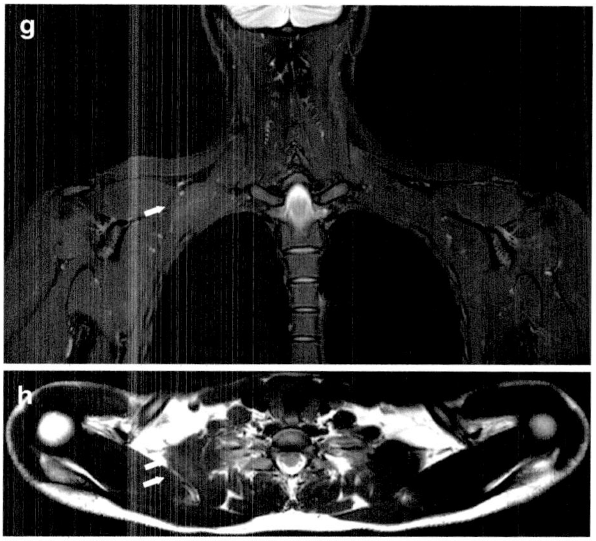

Fig. 4.1 (continued)

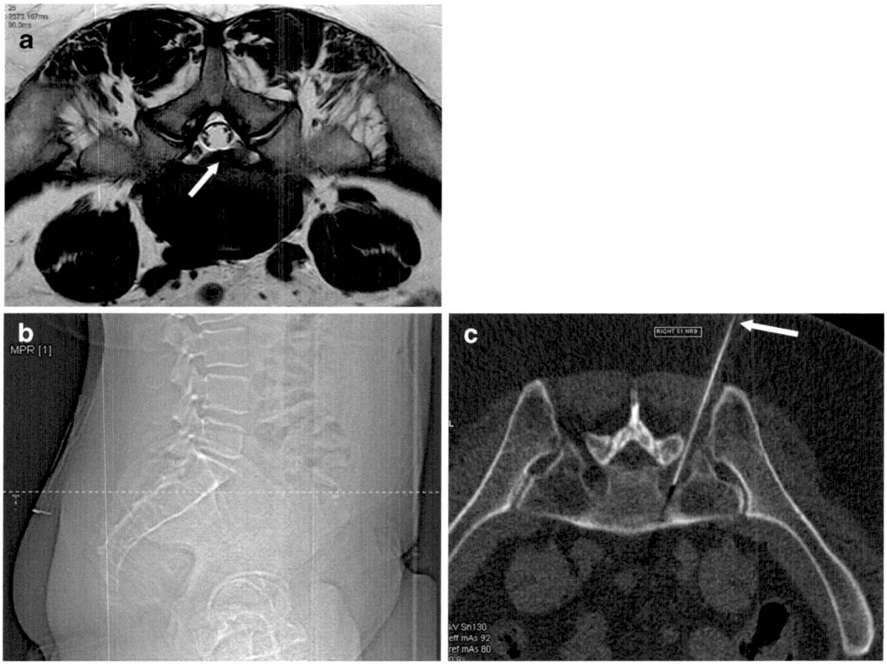

Fig. 4.2 Clinical case. A 35-year-old female presents with numbness and pain that corresponds to the right S1 dermatome. Axial T2 weighted Turbo Spin Echo MRI sequence (panel **a**, white arrow) shows impingement of the right S1 nerve by a focal right sided paracentral disc protrusion. Sagittal CT scout image (panel **b**) shows the level of injection of corticosteroid and where axial image (panel **c**) was obtained for CT guided injection of right S1 nerve (panel **c**, white arrow)

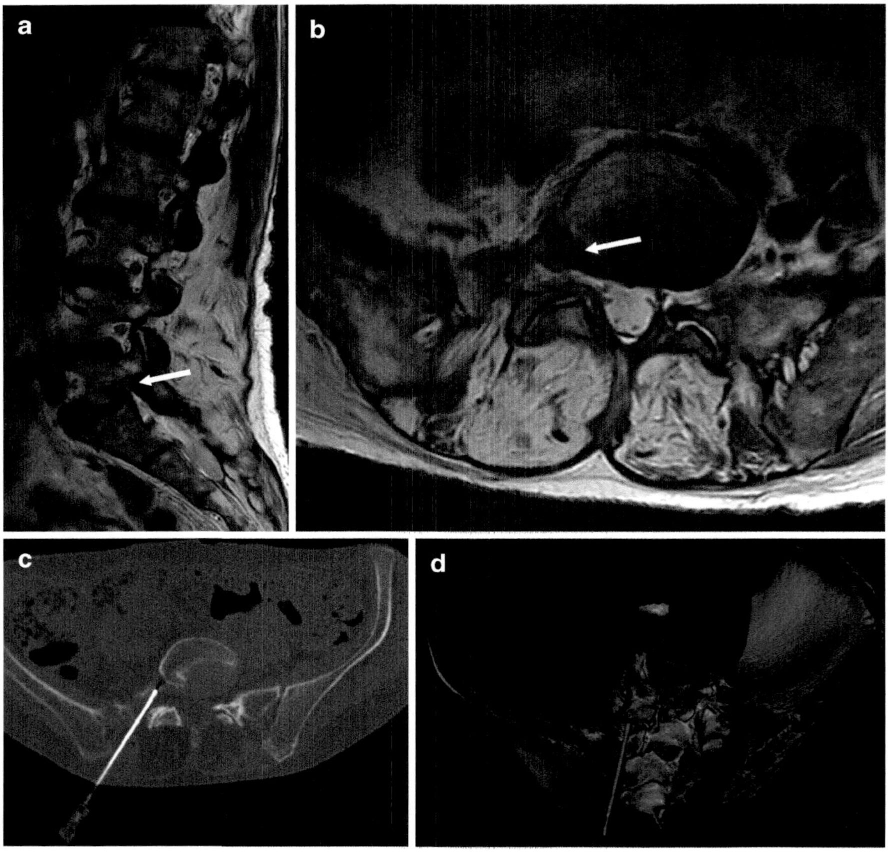

Fig. 4.3 Clinical case. A 55-year-old female presents with right L5 radiculopathy. Sagittal T2 MRI (panel **a**) and axial T2 weighted (panel **b**) shows moderate right sided foraminal stenosis due to combination of disc protrusion (panels **a**, **b**, white arrows), thickened ligamentum flavum and capsular hypertrophy from facet arthropathy. CT-guided pulsed radiofrequency ablation of the right L5 nerve was performed (panels **c**, **d**)

or intraneural "compartment syndrome" as pressures in the spinal nerve exceeds perfusion pressures resulting in ischaemia are contributory pathophysiological mechanisms. The spinal nerve lacks a perineurium, has poorly developed epineurium with more tenuous blood supply compared to peripheral nerve, and is therefore more vulnerable to compression. Tethering also contributes to high tensile forces on the spinal nerve [41].

The dorsal root ganglion (DRG) has an essential role in the pathophysiology of spinal radiculopathy pain [42, 43] as shown by the emergence of interventional therapy such as pulsed radiofrequency (PRF) treatment adjacent to the dorsal root ganglion, particularly in the cervical and lumbar spine (Fig. 4.3) [44, 45]. PRF involves the application of an electrode that uses intermittent administration of high frequency current to maintain the temperature at the electrode tip at 42 °C. The available data suggests the interference of PRF with the normal cell function at the DRG, via changes in myelin and intracellular axonal components of the pain afferents [46]. It is thought the electrical fields reversibly disrupt impulse transmission across small unmyelinated fibers. Increased c-Fos expression at central spinal levels in the dorsal horn and has also been shown to affect descending pain inhibitory pathways. PRF has been shown to induce an increased in ATF3 in the DRG. PRF applied to the L5 and L6 DRG of rabbits suggest PRF adjacent to the DRG may reduce neuropathic pain with significant effect on heat and mechanical hyperalgesia [47]. It is unclear to what extent these neuropathic pain models reflect the complex pathophysiology of spinal neuropathic pain or radicular pain. Spinal neuropathic or radicular pain is likely a complex phenomenon with divergence of the afferent nociceptive signal, leading to sensitization of DRG and probably dorsal horns at more than one level [48].

The complex divergence of pain signalling in radicular pain suggest multilevel excitation. Animal research on afferent signalling suggests multiple spinal segmental involvement [49, 50]. It is possible the pathophysiology of spinal neuropathic pain associated with spinal radiculopathy may differ from other types of neuropathic pain.

The high prevalence of lumbosacral radicular pain with an annual prevalence between 9.9% and 25% and a life-time prevalence of 1.2–43% [51] are consistent with the clinical experience of the authors that lumbosacral radicular pain is the most commonly occurring form of neuropathic pain. Although lumbosacral radicular pain is reported to be at least ten times higher than cervical radicular pain, major complications including embolic infarct have been reported with treatment for cervical radiculopathy [52] including corticosteroids via epidural administration which relies on the anti-inflammatory response of phospholipase A2 [53]. For these reasons, further research into understanding the complex pathophysiology of spinal neuropathic pain is required to optimise current treatment and develop new and better therapies for patients with these debilitating conditions.

Neuralgic amyotrophy (NA) is an acute and painful neuropathy involving upper brachial plexus (idiopathic brachial plexus neuritis), cervical plexus and lumbosacral plexus. Parsonage-Turner syndrome is a subset of neuralgic amyotrophy. NA is less common than spinal radiculopathy but not rare with an incidence of 1 per 1000 individuals. Recent reports suggest the incidence is much higher than previously assumed and the majority of patients never assumed full recovery [54]. Despite this, the diagnosis is often missed [55] with frequent recurrences. Both idiopathic and hereditary forms exist. Its pathophysiology remains unclear although an inflammatory and presumably autoimmune pathophysiology is assumed with infectious or mechanical precipitating conditions.

The presence of serum antibodies and the efficacy of immunotherapy support an immune-mediated pathogenesis [56]. More than 50% of patients with NA show a history of an event that triggered the immune system including infection, vaccination, surgery, pregnancy and mental stress. Ten percent of patients with NA have concomitant hepatitis E infection. Epineural perivascular T-cell infiltrates are

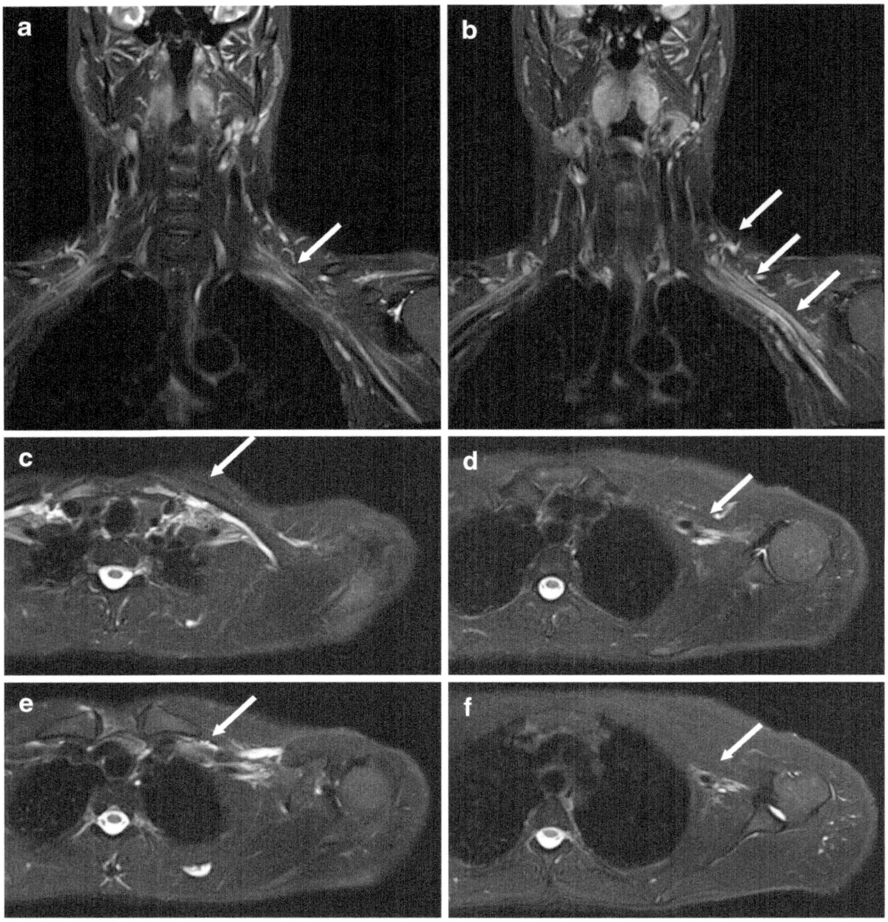

Fig. 4.4 Clinical case. A 41-year-old female presents with progressively worse pin, muscle weakness and numbness thought clinically to correlate to brachial plexopathy. Coronal DIXON T2 weighted MRI sequences (panels **a**, **b**, white arrows), and axial DIXON T2 weighted images (panels **c**–**f** from cranial to caudad, white arrows) shows diffusely increased T2 signal consistent with brachial neuritis

present in peripheral nerve biopsies. CD8+ T-lymphocytes, CD68+ macrophages and CD20+ B-lymphocytes surround the epithelial and endothelial vessels in involved peripheral nerves. Hyperintensity of peripheral nerve on T2-weighted MRI in acute phase of NA (Fig. 4.4) supports the hypothesis that immunological factors are involved in NA [57].

Participation in sports or heavy labour, strenuous upper extremity exercise supports the hypothesis that mechanical factors contribute to NA. The shoulder joint is the most mobile joint that is designed to allow wide range of movements. Wear and tear of blood-nerve barriers around the brachial plexus and weakened blood-nerve barrier may allow immune factors or cells to come in contact with the brachial plexus.

Mutations in the SEPT9 gene on chromosome 17q25 characterise the less common autosomal dominant hereditary form of neuralgic amyotrophy [58]. Overall, an underlying genetic predisposition, susceptibility to mechanical injury of the brachial plexus (possibly representing disturbance of the epineural blood-brain barrier) and an immune or autoimmune trigger for the attacks are implicated in NA [59].

Post-herpetic neuralgia (Fig. 4.5) is a neuropathic pain syndrome characterised by pain that persists for months to years after resolution of a herpes zoster rash, also known as shingles caused by reactivation of latent varicella zoster virus following initial infection. Damage to peripheral and central neurons may result from an immune or inflammatory response [60]. Dorsal horn atrophy and cell, axon and

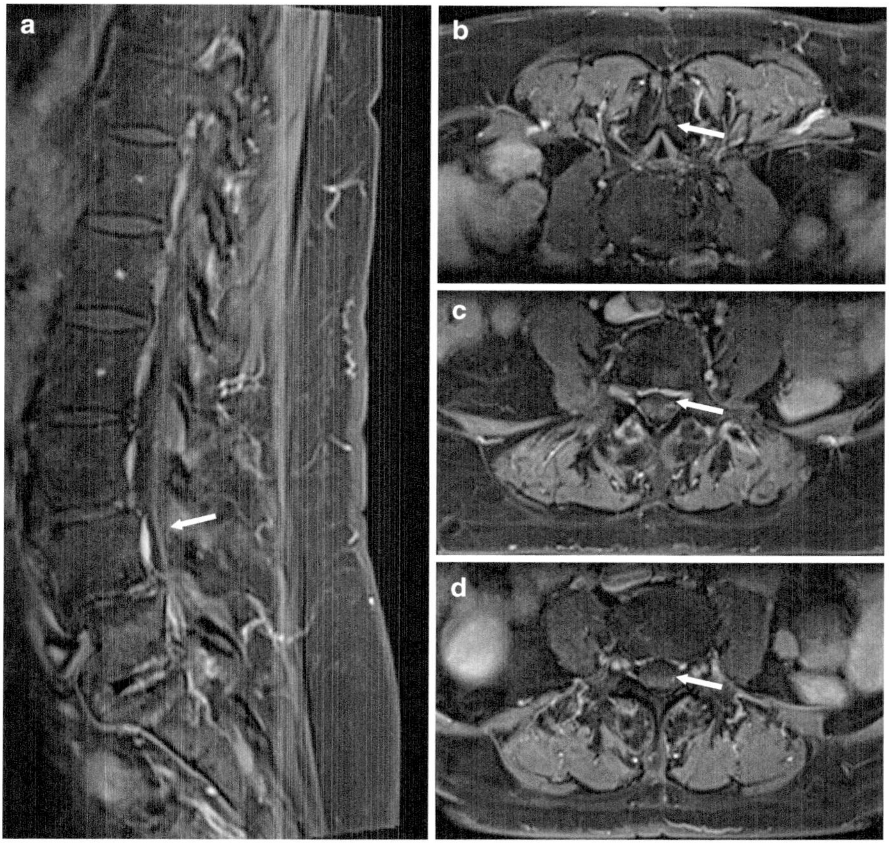

Fig. 4.5 Clinical case. A 76-year-old female presents with shingles in left lower limb, left foot drop and sciatica in left S1 distribution. Sagittal (panel **a**) and axial (panels **b**–**d**) T1 fat suppressed DIXON MRI sequence with intravenous contrast (panel **a**, white arrow) shows contrast enhancement of the left S1 nerve (panels **a**–**d**, white arrows)

myelin loss with fibrosis in the sensory ganglion were found in post-mortem studies [61]. Marked loss of myelin and axons in the nerve and sensory roots were present. Sensitization of unmyelinated cutaneous nociceptors can occur. Damaged peripheral and central nerve fibers develop a lower threshold for action potentials, spontaneously discharge and show disproportionate responses to stimuli. This leads to peripheral sensitization and pain without painful stimuli or allodynia. In acute phases of peripheral nerve injury, abnormal tonic impulse discharge from primary nociceptive afferent neurons induce slow temporal summation. This "wind-up" phenomenon lead to continuous partial depolarisation of second-order neurons with increased spontaneous impulse discharge and expanded receptive fields within the dorsal horn nociceptive neurons. The abnormal central processing involves the activation of *N*-methyl-D-aspartate (NMDA) receptors resulting in neuropathic pain, characterized by spontaneous pain, hyperalgesia and allodynia which is typical of post-herpetic neuralgia. In addition, tonic input from non-nociceptive AB afferent neurons, maintained by sympathetic efferent activity, contribute to the development and maintenance of neuropathic pain in general, and a burning sensation in particular [62].

Complex regional pain syndrome (CRPS) occurs acutely in about 7% of patients with limb fractures, limb surgery and other injuries [63] and is a multifactorial poorly understood chronic pain condition characterised by autonomic and inflammatory features (Fig. 4.6). Peripheral and central sensitization are the most strongly implicated processes. Changes on the spinal and supraspinal level directly linked to clinical signs of CRPS involve central sensitization, whereby spinal nociceptive neurons become hyper-responsive to peripheral input and increase nociceptive signalling to the cortex even in the absence of such input. Aberrant inflammatory response to tissue trauma can lead to sensitization of peripheral and spinal nociceptive fibers, neuro-inflammation and dysfunction of peripheral blood circulation although peripheral mechanism do not fully account for the persistent of CRPS symptoms long after inflammatory responses resolved [64]. Maladaptive plastic changes in the nervous system have also been reported. Coupling of sympathetic neurons with injured sensory neuros at peripheral neuroma sites or dorsal root ganglion sites of injured afferent nerves can lead to development of noradrenergic sensitivity following nerve injury [38]. A shift from inhibition towards facilitation of nociceptive input was also found in the endogenous pain modulation system in CRPS. Peripheral and central mechanisms can interact to produce clinical signs of CRPS. Pain, allodynia, hyperalgesia, oedema, cutaneous blood flow and sweating occurs. Functional cortical reorganization of sensory and motor representations of the limbs in CRPS has been reported [65]. Genetic and psychological factors may play a role.

Diabetes mellitus characterised by hyperglycaemia, hyperlipidaemia, hyperinsulinemia, altered insulin signalling result lead to several pathological changes in neuronal, immune and vascular cells. Nerve ischaemia due to microvascular changes, oxidative stress, inflammation and mitochondrial dysfunction resulting from hyperactivity of several pathways including the polyol, hexosamine, protein kinase C and advanced glycation product result in structural and functional alterations of the nervous system including progressive demyelination and axonal loss. Diabetic

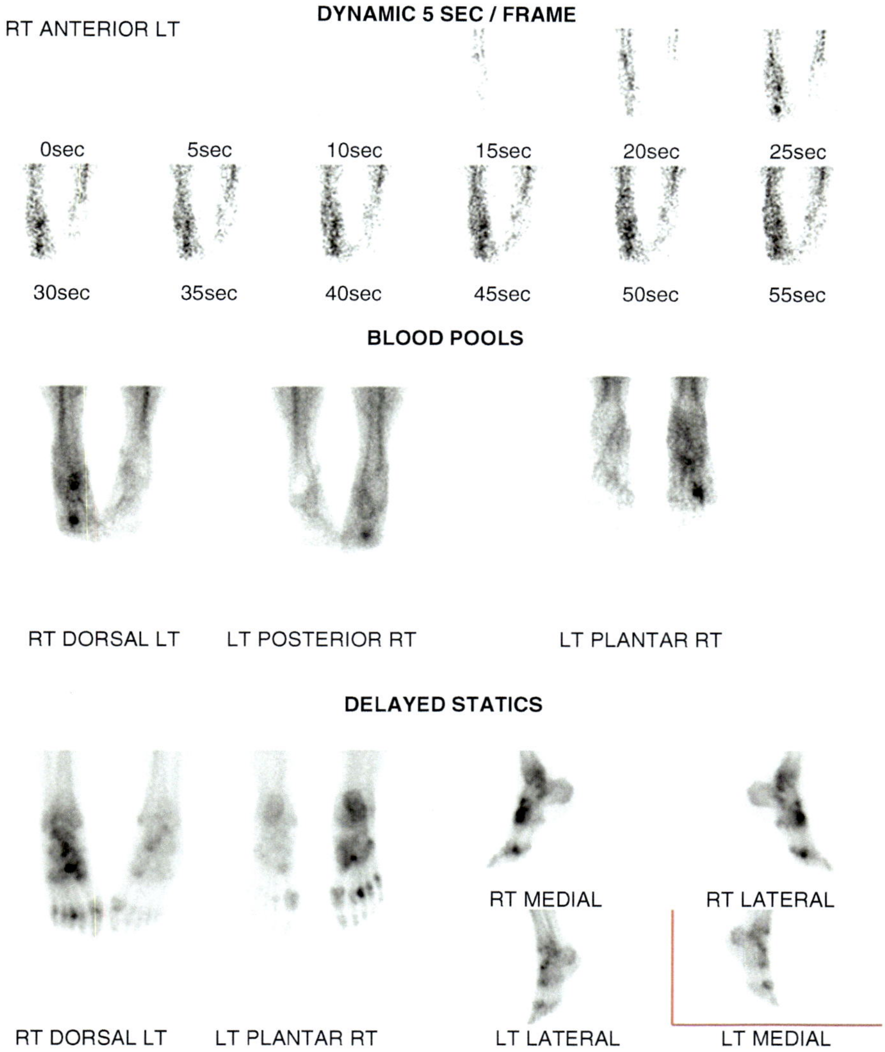

Fig. 4.6 Clinical case. A 64-year-old male presents with burning pain in her right foot for 2 weeks and complains of the right foot being warmer than the left foot. A triple phase nuclear scintigraphy was performed using Tc-HDP. The blood pool and the blood flow images show increased blood flow to the right foot and ankle with increased soft tissue uptake. Delayed bone images show marked focal activity involving the metatarsophalangeal joint of the third toe and generalised increased activity in the tarsal bones. There is slightly increased activity at the base of the first metatarsal. This is consistent with complex regional pain syndrome or reflex sympathetic dystrophy

neuropathy can be painless or painful (Fig. 4.7). Several factors contribute to the development of neuropathic pain in diabetic neuropathy including metabolic factors such as glycemic burden and obesity, as well as female gender, increasing age and ethnicity [66].

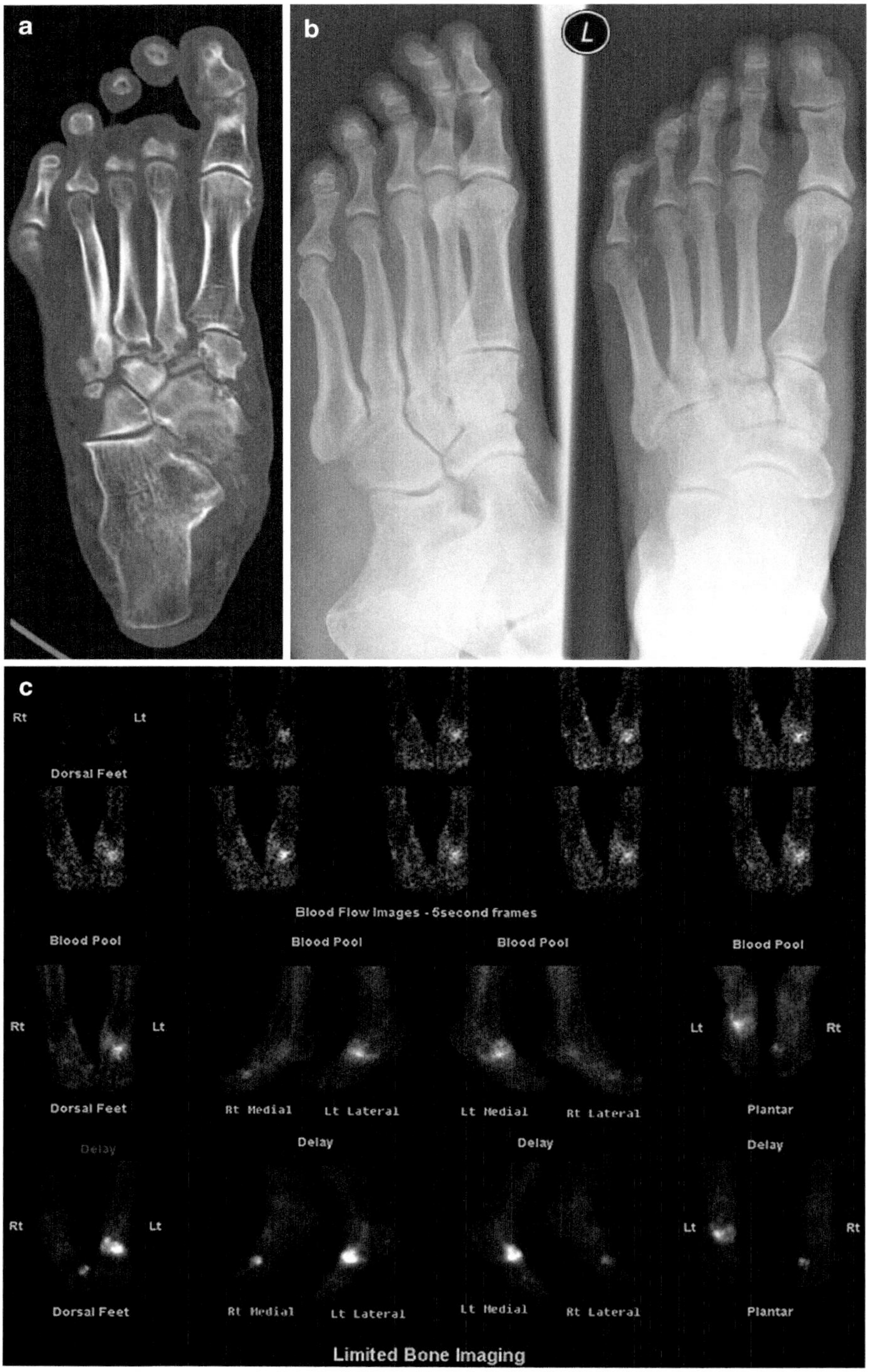
a
b
L
c
Rt
Lt
Dorsal Feet
Blood Flow Images - 5second frames
Blood Pool
Blood Pool
Blood Pool
Blood Pool
Rt
Lt
Dorsal Feet
Rt Medial
Lt Lateral
Lt Medial
Rt Lateral
Lt
Rt
Plantar
Delay
Delay
Delay
Delay
Rt
Lt
Dorsal Feet
Rt Medial
Lt Lateral
Lt Medial
Rt Lateral
Lt
Rt
Plantar
Limited Bone Imaging

Peripheral mechanisms of painful diabetic neuropathy are due to structural and functional abnormalities of the vasa nervorum and dysregulation of peripheral blood flow. Central mechanisms of painful diabetic neuropathy may be related to alterations in the spinal, somatomotor, limbic, thalamic, ascending and descending modulatory systems. Cortical atrophy within the somatomotor cortex and insula, abnormal cortical interactions within the somatomotor network and increased cerebral blood flow in the anterior cingulate cortex are changes in higher brain centres associated with neuropathic pain.

Border nerves comprising the ilioinguinal, iliohypogastric and genitofemoral nerves supply the skin in the borders between the thigh and anterior abdominal wall. Chronic neuropathic pain of the border nerves can result in chronic pelvic and genital pain, with significant psychosocial burden and impact on quality of life. Due to the path of these nerves through the border zone, lower abdominal surgeries can result in nerve injuries, particularly surgical incisions below the level of the anterior superior iliac spine or ASIS. Persistent postoperative pain following inguinal mesh surgery (Fig. 4.8) is not uncommon, occurring in 11% of patients [67]. More than a quarter of these patients have moderate to severe pain, mostly with a neuropathic origin. The proposed mechanisms of postoperative neuralgia include direct nerve entrapment within scar tissue, fibrous adhesions or mesh or pelvic slings resulting in nociceptive pain and paraesthesia along the distribution of the nerves, accident from fixation devices such as sutures and tacks, or ligation of the nerve with painful neuroma formation [68]. Non-surgical causes of neuropathic pain of the border nerves are less common (Fig. 4.9) including trauma with traction, extrinsic pelvic mass compression, and bicycle riding and compression by tight clothing [69].

Intercostal neuralgia (Figs. 4.10 and 4.11) is characterised by neuropathic pain along the distribution of the intercostal nerves [70]. Pain radiates in a back-to-front distribution and is associated with hyperalgesia of the overlying skin. Intercostal neuralgia has been reported after trauma, breast or abdominal surgery, thoracotomy, nerve entrapment, traumatic or iatrogenic neuromas. It may be related to herpes zoster infection, diabetic polyneuropathy, vertebral facet joint osteoarthrosis and dislocation of the costovertebral joint. Direct invasion of the intercostal nerves by

Fig. 4.7 Clinical case. A 71-year-old male presents with left midfoot pain and swelling. Axial CT (panel **a**) shows significant destruction of the tarsometatarsal joints with subchondral cyst formation and joint space narrowing, with mid-foot arthropathy involving the second and third tarsometatarsal joints. X-ray of the same foot 5 years ago (panel **b**) shows arthropathy involving the second and third tarsometatarsal joint. On the bone scan performed 5 years ago (panel **c**), flow studies and blood pool images show markedly increased vascularity in the mid left tarsometatarsal region with mild hyperemia at the right first metatarsophalangeal joint and sesamoids. Delayed images of both feet in four projections show markedly increased uptake on both sides of the left second and third tarsometatarsal joint, consistent with severe inflammation. Mild changes are seen in the other tarsometatarsal joints and the naviculo-medial cuneiform joint. Overall the bone scan shows inflammatory arthropathy involving the second and third tarsometatarsal joints

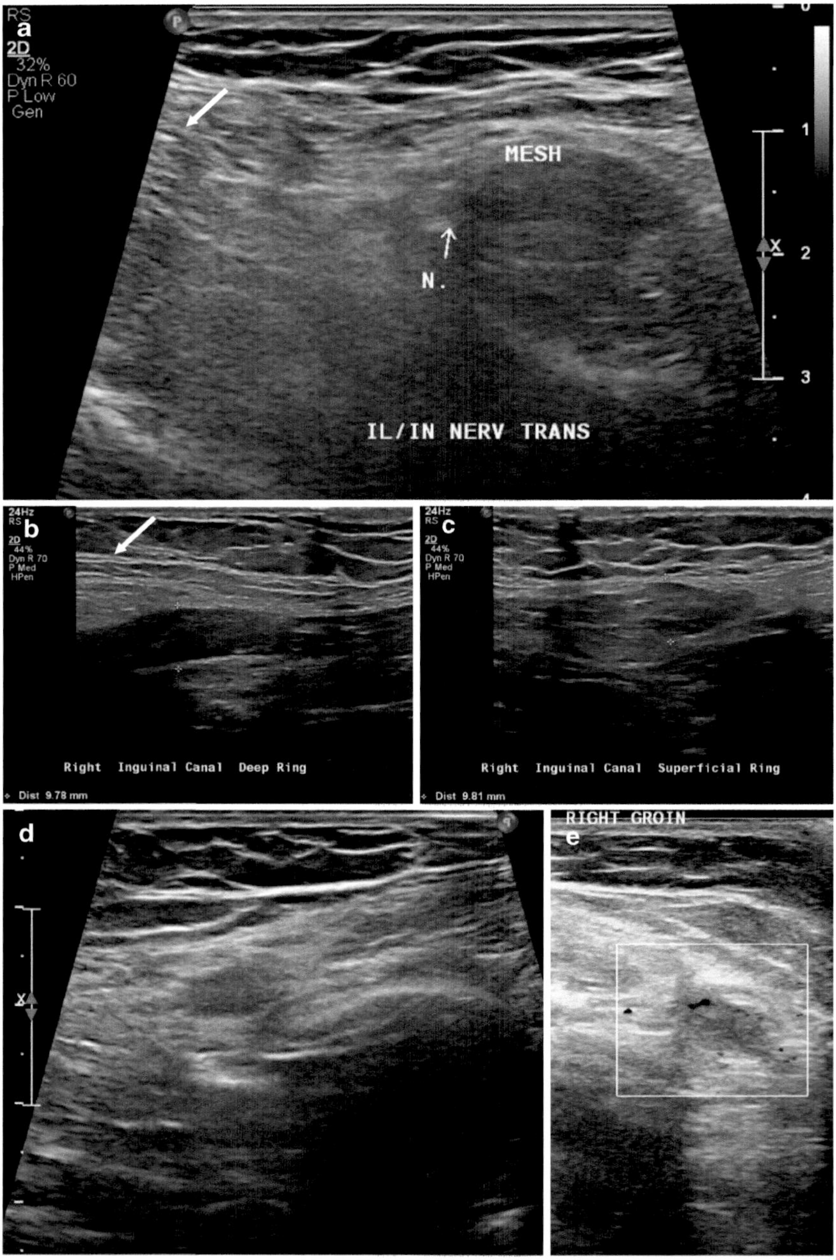

Fig. 4.8 Clinical case. A 64-year-old male presents with right groin pain after 4 months repair of right indirect inguinal hernia (Panels **a**, **b**, white arrows). On ultrasound (panel **c**), the mesh abuts the inguinal canal and is focally tender. The mesh lies close to and probably abuts the right ilioinguinal nerve (labelled "n"). Several months later, ultrasound (panels **d**) shows a 13 × 10 × 7 mm hypoechoic and vascular region in the superior-medial of the inguinal mesh (white arrow), possibly scar tissue or granulation tissue, which is new compared to the previous study. Internal vascularity on Doppler colour imaging is present (panel **e**)

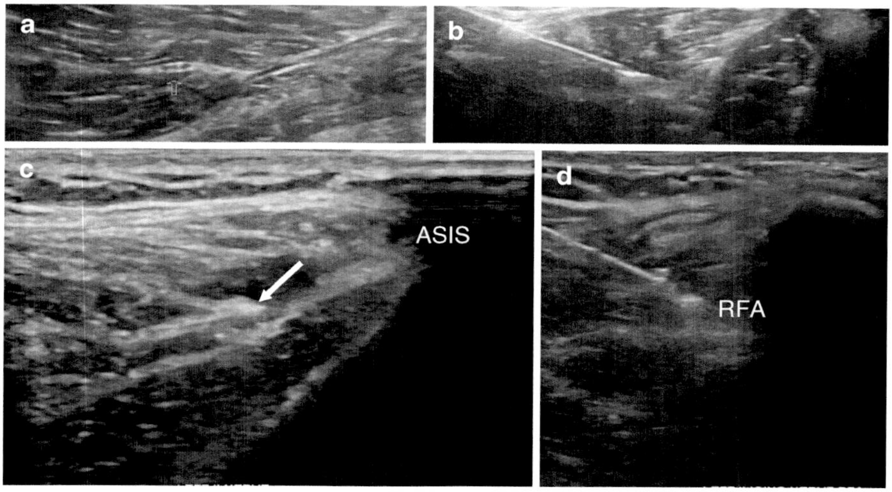

Fig. 4.9 Clinical case. A 35-year-old male presents with burning pain and numbness over the lower abdomen that radiates to the left inner thigh and genitalia. He was diagnosed with iliohypogastric and ilioinguinal neuralgia. Ultrasound image (panel **a**, black arrow) shows the iliohypogastric nerve was treated with pulsed radiofrequency treatment (panel **b**). Ultrasound image (panel **c**, white arrow) shows the ilioinguinal nerve at the level of the anterior superior iliac spine (ASIS). This nerve was also treated at the same time with pulsed radiofrequency (panel **d**)

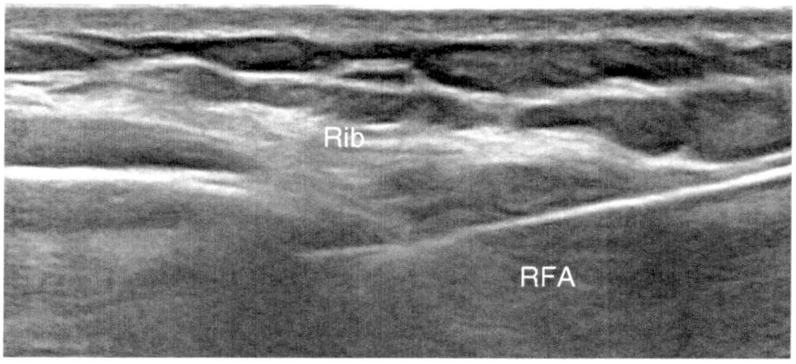

Fig. 4.10 Clinical case. A 35-year-old male presents with left T11 intercostal neuralgia post trauma. Pulsed radiofrequency electrode is placed next to the intercostal nerve

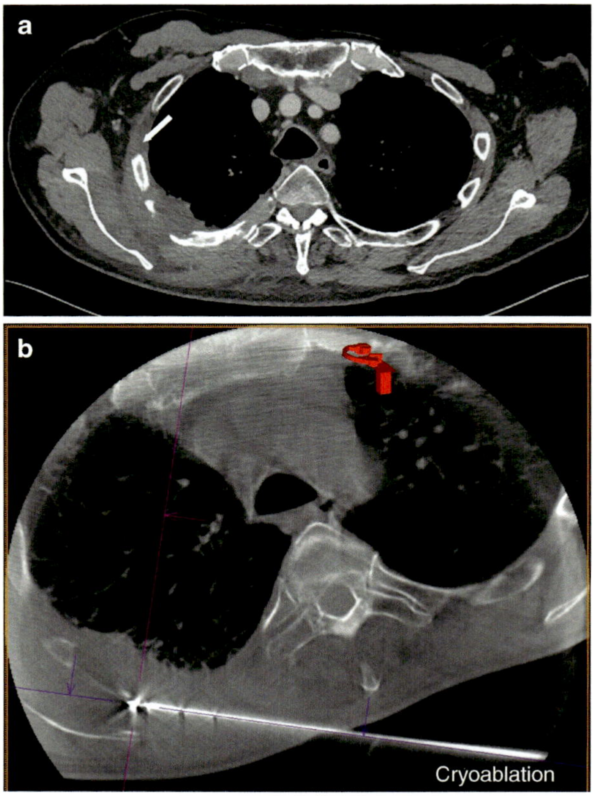

Fig. 4.11 Clinical case. A 83-year-old male with squamous cell carcinoma involving the right upper lobe presents with right sided unremitting right thoracic neuropathic pain in the distribution of the right T3 to T6 dermatomes. Axial CT scan (panel **a**, white arrow) shows invasion of the right T3 to T5 ribs and axial cone beam CT (panel **b**) show cryoablation of the metastatic tumor

tumor especially metastatic tumors can occur with mediastinal, paravertebral or costal lesions [71]. Inflammatory cytokines produced by certain tumors without direct compression of nerve root has also been reported. Inflammatory cytokines causing intercostal neuralgia has been reported in auto inflammatory disease and interleukin-1 is thought to be important in neuropathic pain. Other types of neuropathic pain due to damage, injury or dysfunction of nerves including trigeminal, occipital, pudendal and cluneal neuralgia (Fig. 4.12).

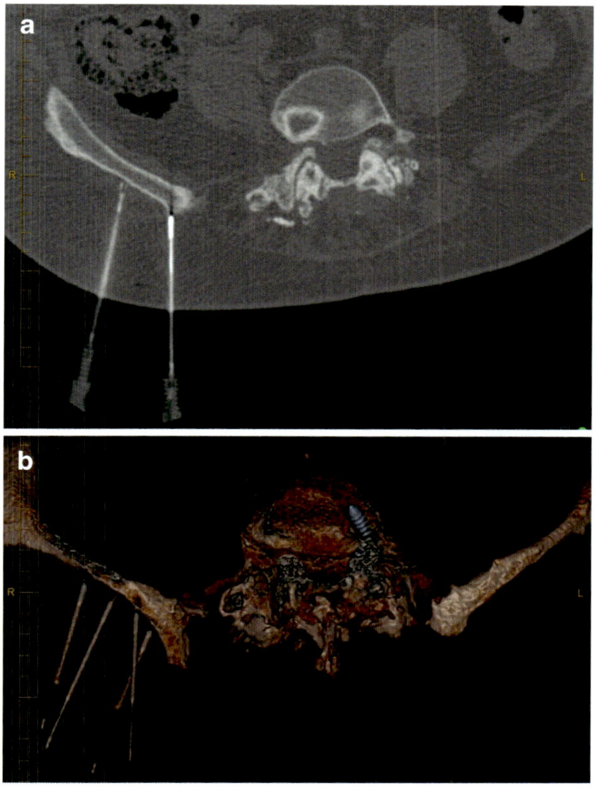

Fig. 4.12 Clinical case. A 83-year-old male presents with right sided cluneal neuralgia. Axial CT (panel **a**) and 3D CT reconstruction (panel **b**) shows pulsed radiofrequency treatment of the cluneal nerves

Conclusion

Most patients with neuropathic pain report spontaneous ongoing or shooting intermittent pain including burning and pricking pain. Evoked amplified pain responses following noxious or non-noxious stimuli can also occur. Evoked pain may spread to neighbouring areas and the underlying pathophysiology comprises of central and peripheral sensitization. Ectopic activity in compressed nerves or nerve roots, dorsal root ganglia or nerve-end neuroma may in different conditions underlie spontaneous pain. The sensitization of nociceptive pathways is characterised by maladaptive structural changes and cell-cell interactions and molecular signalling including changes in ion channels, activation of immune cells, glial-derived mediators and epigenetic regulation. Pharmaceutical therapy includes drugs acting on calcium channels, sodium channels and descending modulatory pathways [72].

The chronicity, severity and resistance of neuropathic pain to analgesia poses a tremendous burden to the health-care system, with significant debilitation to the patients. Multidisciplinary and interdisciplinary approach to managing neuropathic pain is crucial. Basic research driving the understanding the pathophysiology of

neuropathic pain can lead to a more specific mechanism-based treatment approach.DeclarationThis manuscript was not supported by any funding.
The authors declare they have no relevant conflicts of interest.

References

1. Wall PD, Devor M. Sensory afferent impulses originate from dorsal root ganglia as well as from the periphery in normal and nerve injured rats. Pain. 1983;17:321–39.
2. Devor M, Keller CH, Deerinck TJ, Levinson SR, Ellisman MH. Na^+ channel accumulation on axolemma of afferent endings in nerve end neuromas in Apteronotus. Neurosci Lett. 1989;102:149–54.
3. Levinson SR, Luo S, Henry MA. The role of sodium channels in chronic pain. Muscle Nerve. 2012;46:155–65.
4. Luo ZD, Chaplan SR, Higuera ES, Sorkin LS, Stauderman KA, Williams ME, et al. Upregulation of dorsal root ganglion (alpha) 2(delta) calcium channel subunit and its correlation with allodynia in spinal nerve-injured rats. J Neurosci. 2001;21:1868–75.
5. Attal N, Cruccu G, Baron R, Haanpää M, Hansson P, Jensen TS, et al. EFNS guidelines on the pharmacological treatment of neuropathic pain: 2010 revision. Eur J Neurol. 2010;17:1113-e88.
6. Field MJ, McCleary S, Hughes J, Singh L. Gabapentin and pregabalin, but not morphine and amitriptyline, block both static and dynamic components of mechanical allodynia induced by streptozocin in the rat. Pain. 1999;80:391–8.
7. Ueda H. Molecular mechanisms of neuropathic pain-phenotypic switch and initiation mechanisms. Pharmacol Ther. 2006;109:57–77.
8. Schüning J, Scherens A, Haussleiter IS, Schwenkreis P, Krumova EK, Richter H, et al. Sensory changes and loss of intraepidermal nerve fibers in painful unilateral nerve injury. Clin J Pain. 2009;25:683–90.
9. Cohen SP, Kapoor SG, Rathmell JP. Intravenous infusion tests have limited utility for selecting long-term drug therapy in patients with chronic pain: a systematic review. Anesthesiology. 2009;111:416–31.
10. Nickel FT, Seifert F, Lanz S, Maihofner C. Mechanisms of neuropathic pain. Eur J Neuropsychopharmacol. 2012;22:81–91.
11. Guo W, Zou S, Guan Y, Ikeda T, Tal M, Dubner R, et al. Tyrosine phosphorylation of the NR2B subunit of the NMDA receptor in the spinal cord during the development and maintenance of inflammatory hyperalgesia. J Neurosci. 2002;22:6208–17.
12. Miller KE, Hoffman EM, Sutharshan M, Schechter R. Glutamate pharmacology and metabolism in peripheral primary afferents: physiological and pathophysiological mechanisms. Pharmacol Ther. 2011;130:283–309.
13. Malmberg AB, Chen C, Tonegawa S, Basbaum AI. Preserved acute pain and reduced neuropathic pain in mice lacking PKC gamma. Science. 1997;278:279–83.
14. Mao J, Sung B, Ji RR, Lim G. Chronic morphine induces downregulation of spinal glutamate transporters: implications in morphine tolerance and abnormal pain sensitivity. J Neurosci. 2002;22:8312–23.
15. Cohen SP, Liao W, Gupta A, Plunkett A. Ketamine in pain management. Adv Psychosom Med. 2011;30:139–61.
16. Vallejo R, Tilley DM, Vogel L, Benyamin R. The role of glia and the immune system in the development and maintenance of neuropathic pain. Pain Pract. 2010;10:167–84.
17. Barkhudaryan N, Dunn AJ. Molecular mechanisms of actions of interleukin-6 on the brain, with special reference to serotonin and the hypothalamo-pituitary-adrenocortical axis. Neurochem Res. 1999;24:1169–80.

18. Leung L, Cahill CM. TNF-alpha and neuropathic pain—a review. J Neuroinflammation. 2010;7:27.
19. Mika J, Zychowska M, Popiolek-Barczyk K, Rojewska E, Przewlocka B. Importance of glial activation in neuropathic pain. Eur J Pharmacol. 2013;716(1–3):106–19.
20. Wang S, Lim G, Zeng Q, Yang L, Sung B, Mao J. Central glucocorticoid receptors modulate the expression and function of spinal NMDA receptors after peripheral nerve injury. J Neurosci. 2005;25:488–95.
21. Song C, Phillips AG, Leonard B. Interleukin 1 beta enhances conditioned fear memory in rats: possible involvement of glucocorticoids. Eur J Neurosci. 2003;18:1739–43.
22. Apkarian AV, Baliki MN, Geha PY. Towards a theory of chronic pain. Prog Neurobiol. 2009;87:81–97.
23. Lotze M, Grodd W, Birbaumer N, Erb M, Huse E, Flor H. Does use of a myoelectric prosthesis prevent cortical reorganization and phantom limb pain? Nat Neurosci. 1999;2:501–2.
24. Moseley GL, Flor H. Targeting cortical representations in the treatment of chronic pain: a review. Neurorehabil Neural Repair. 2012;26:646–52.
25. Rouwette T, Vanelderen P, Roubos EW, Kozicz T, Vissers K. The amygdala, a relay station for switching on and off pain. Eur J Pain. 2012;16:782–92.
26. Moore KA, Kohno T, Karchewski LA, Scholz J, Baba H, Woolf CJ. Partial peripheral nerve injury promotes a selective loss of GABAergic inhibition in the superficial dorsal horn of the spinal cord. J Neurosci. 2002;22:6724–31.
27. Drew GM, Siddall PJ, Duggan AW. Mechanical allodynia following contusion injury of the rat spinal cord is associated with loss of GABAergic inhibition in the dorsal horn. Pain. 2004;109:379–88.
28. Miraucourt LS, Dallel R, Voisin DL. Glycine inhibitory dysfunction turns touch into pain through PKC gamma interneurons. PLoS One. 2007;2:e1116.
29. Kohno T, Ji RR, Ito N, Allchorne AJ, Befort K, Karchewski LA, et al. Peripheral axonal injury results in reduced mu opioid receptor pre- and post-synaptic action in the spinal cord. Pain. 2005;117:77–87.
30. Benedetti F, Vighetti S, Amanzio M, Casadio C, Oliaro A, Bergamasco B, et al. Dose-response relationship of opioids in nociceptive and neuropathic postoperative pain. Pain. 1998;74:205–11.
31. Goffaux P, Redmond WJ, Rainville P, Marchand S. Descending analgesia—when the spine echoes what the brain expects. Pain. 2007;130:137–43.
32. Wager TD, Rilling JK, Smith EE, Sokolik A, Casey KL, Davidson RJ, et al. Placebo-induced changes in fMRI in the anticipation and experience of pain. Science. 2004;303:1162–7.
33. Enck P, Benedetti F, Schedlowski M. New insights into the placebo and nocebo responses. Neuron. 2008;59:195–206.
34. Wei F, Dubner R, Zou S, Ren K, Bai G, Wei D, et al. Molecular depletion of descending serotonin unmasks its novel facilitatory role in the development of persistent pain. J Neurosci. 2010;30:8624–36.
35. Bannister K, Bee LA, Dickenson AH. Preclinical and early clinical investigations related to monoaminergic pain modulation. Neurotherapeutics. 2009;6:703–12.
36. McCleane G. Antidepressants as analgesics. CNS Drugs. 2008;22:139–56.
37. Pain Australia [Internet]. [cited 2021 Oct 10]. https://www.painaustralia.org.au/media-document/blog-1/blog-2020/blog-july-2020/the-new-definition-of-pain.
38. Gilron IC, Watson PN, Cahill CM, Moulin DE. Neuropathic pain: a practical guide for the clinician. CMAJ. 2006;175(3):265–75.
39. Cosamalón-Gan I, Cosamalón-Gan T, Mattos-Piaggio G, Villar-Suárez V, García-Cosamalón J, Vega-Álvarez JA. Inflammation in the intervertebral disc herniation. Neurocirugia (Astur: Engl Ed). 2021;32(1):21–35.
40. Garfin SR, Rydevik B, Lind B, Massie J. Spinal nerve root compression. Spine (Phila Pa 1976). 1995;20(16):1810–20.

41. PM&R knowledge now [Internet]. [cited 2021 Oct 10]. https://now.aapmr.org/lumbar-radiculopathy/.
42. Van Zundert J, Harney D, Joosten EA, et al. The role of the dorsal root ganglion in cervical radicular pain: diagnosis, pathophysiology, and rationale for treatment. Reg Anesth Pain Med. 2006;31(2):152–67.
43. Abram SE. Pain mechanisms in lumbar radiculopathy. Anesth Analg. 1988;67(12):1135–7.
44. Yoon YM, Han SR, Lee SJ, Choi CY, Sohn MJ, Lee CH. The efficacy of pulsed radiofrequency treatment of cervical radicular patients. Korean J Spine. 2014;11(3):109–12.
45. Van Boxem K, van Bilsen J, de Meij N, Herrler A, Kessels F, Van Zundert J, van Kleef M. Pulsed radiofrequency treatment adjacent to the lumbar dorsal root ganglion for the management of lumbosacral radicular syndrome: a clinical audit. Pain Med. 2011;12(9):1322–30.
46. Erdine S, Bilir A, Cosman ER, Cosman ER Jr. Ultrastructural changes in axons following exposure to pulsed radiofrequency fields. Pain Pract. 2009;9:407–17.
47. Perret DM, Kim DS, Li KW, et al. Application of pulsed radiofrequency currents to rat dorsal root ganglia modulates nerve injury-induced tactile allodynia. Anesth Analg. 2011;113:610–6.
48. van Boxem K, Joosten EA, van Kleef M, Patijn J, van Zundert J. Pulsed radiofrequency treatment for radicular pain: where do we stand and where to go? Pain Med. 2012;13(3):351–4.
49. Wall PD, Lidierth M, Hillman P. Brief and prolonged effects of Lissauer tract stimulation on dorsal horn cells. Pain. 1999;83(3):579–89.
50. Lidierth M. Long-range projections of a delta primary afferents in the Lissauer tract of the rat. Neurosci Lett. 2007;425(2):126–30.
51. Konstantinou K, Dunn KM. Sciatica: review of epidemiological studies and prevalence estimates. Spine. 2008;33(22):2464–72.
52. Schneider BJ, Maybin S, Sturos E. Safety and complications of cervical epidural steroid injections. Phys Med Rehabil Clin N Am. 2018;29(1):155–69.
53. Van Zundert J, Huntoon M, Patijn J, Lataster A, Mekhail N, van Kleef M. 4. Cervical radicular pain. Pain Pract. 2010;10(1):1–17.
54. Gstoettner C, Mayer JA, Rassam S, Hruby LA, Salminger S, Sturma A, Aman M, Harhaus L, Platzgummer H, Aszmann OC. Neuralgic amyotrophy: a paradigm shift in diagnosis and treatment. J Neurol Neurosurg Psychiatry. 2020;91(8):879–88.
55. Van Eijk JJ, Groothuis JT, Van Alfen N. Neuralgic amyotrophy: an update on diagnosis, pathophysiology, and treatment. Muscle Nerve. 2016;53(3):337–50.
56. Moriguchi K, Miyamoto K, Takada K, et al. Four cases of anti-ganglioside antibody-positive neuralgic amyotrophy with good response to intravenous immunoglobulin infusion therapy. J Neuroimmunol. 2011;238:107–9.
57. Kim TU, Chang MC. Neuralgic amyotrophy: an under recognized entity. J Int Med Res. 2021;49(4):3000605211006542.
58. Kuhlenbaumer G, Hannibal MC, Nelis E, et al. Mutations in SEPT9 cause hereditary neuralgic amyotrophy. Nat Genet. 2005;37:1044–6.
59. van Alfen N. Clinical and pathophysiological concepts of neuralgic amyotrophy. Nat Rev Neurol. 2011;7(6):315–22.
60. Mallick-Searle T, Snodgrass B, Brant JM. Postherpetic neuralgia: epidemiology, pathophysiology, and pain management pharmacology. J Multidiscip Healthc. 2016;9:447–54.
61. Watson CPN, Deck JH, Morshead C, Van der Kooy D, Evans RJ. Post-herpetic neuralgia: further post-mortem studies of cases with and without pain. Pain. 1991;44(2):105–17.
62. Feller L, Jadwat Y, Bouckaert M. Herpes zoster post-herpetic neuralgia. SADJ. 2005;60(10):432. 436-7
63. Bruehl S. Complex regional pain syndrome. BMJ. 2015;351:h2730.
64. Halicka M, Vittersø AD, Proulx MJ, Bultitude JH. Neuropsychological changes in complex regional pain syndrome (CRPS). Behav Neurol. 2020;2020:4561831.
65. Di Pietro F, McAuley J, Parkitny L, et al. Primary motor cortex function in complex regional pain syndrome: a systematic review and meta-analysis. J Pain. 2013;14(11):1270–88.

66. Rosenberger DC, Blechschmidt V, Timmerman H, Wolff A, Treede RD. Challenges of neuropathic pain: focus on diabetic neuropathy. J Neural Transm (Vienna). 2020;127(4):589–624.
67. Nienhuijs S, Staal E, Strobbe L, Rosman C, Groenewoud H, Bleichrodt R. Chronic pain after mesh repair of inguinal hernia: a systematic review. Am J Surg. 2007;194(3):394–400.
68. Poh F, Xi Y, Rozen SM, Scott KM, Hlis R, Chhabra A. Role of MR neurography in groin and genital pain: ilioinguinal, iliohypogastric, and genitofemoral neuralgia. AJR Am J Roentgenol. 2019;212(3):632–43.
69. Cesmebasi A, Yadav A, Gielecki J, Tubbs RS, Loukas M. Genitofemoral neuralgia: a review. Clin Anat. 2015;28(1):128–35.
70. Abd-Elsayed A, Lee S, Jackson M. Radiofrequency ablation for treating resistant intercostal neuralgia. Ochsner J. 2018;18(1):91–3.
71. Kobayashi H, Shinoda Y, Ohki T, Kawano H. Intercostal neuralgia as a symptom of an osteoblastoma in thoracic spine. BMJ Case Rep. 2015;2015:bcr2015210720.
72. Finnerup NB, Kuner R, Jensen TS. Neuropathic pain: from mechanisms to treatment. Physiol Rev. 2021;101(1):259–301.

Part III
Age and Pain

Chapter 5
Neuropathic Pain in Children

Dessy Rakhmawati Emril and Jufitriany Ismy

Introduction

Based on International Association for the Study of Pain (IASP) definition, neuropathic pain is a pain caused by a lesion or disease of the somatosensory nervous system [1]. Somatosensory nerves could be found in the skin, muscles, joints, and fascia with distinct thermoreceptors, mechanoreceptors, chemoreceptors, pruriceptors, and nociceptors that allows the perception of touch, pressure, pain, temperature, position, movement, and vibration. Lesions or diseases of the somatosensory nervous system can lead to altered and disordered transmission of sensory signals into the spinal cord and brain. The common conditions associated with neuropathic pain include postherpatic neuralgia, trigeminal neuralgia, painful radiculopathy, diabetic neuropathy, HIV infection, leprosy, amputation, peripheral nerve injury pain, and stroke (in the form of central post-stroke pain) [2]. In children, neuropathic pain include genetic conditions that affect sensory nerve function such as Fabry's disease and erythromelalgia (EM) [3].

Neuropathic pain affects millions of people worldwide, with prevalence in general population in Europe estimated between 6.9 and 10% [4]. Report of neuropathic pain in children is not unclear. Studies about neuropathic pain in infant, children, and adolescents is very rare. One of the factors is because the most common neuropathic pain condition seen in adults are rare in children [5].

D. R. Emril (✉)
Neurologi Department, Medical Faculty of Universitas Syiah Kuala,
Banda Aceh, Aceh, Indonesia
e-mail: dessyemril@unsyiah.ac.id

J. Ismy
Pediatric Department, Medical Faculty of Universitas Syiah Kuala,
Banda Aceh, Aceh, Indonesia

© The Author(s), under exclusive license to Springer Nature
Switzerland AG 2022

J. de Castro, Y. El Miedany (eds.), *Advances in Chronic and Neuropathic Pain*,
Contemporary Rheumatology, https://doi.org/10.1007/978-3-031-10687-3_5

Pathophysiology

Neuropathic pain is defined as a primary lesion or disease of the somatosensory nervous systems. Neuropathic pain is the result of a series of different pathological mechanisms. Usually, the pathological mechanisms described is based on the anatomic localization. Neuropathic pain has a broad range of clinical conditions that can be categorized anatomically (e.g. central vs peripheral) and etiologically (e.g. degenerative, traumatic, infectious, metabolic, and toxic) [6]. The causes of neuropathic pain in children differ from adults [7] (Table 5.1).

Neuropathic pain is due to pathological changes in the functioning of nociceptors and nociceptive pathways causing abnormal pain signals leading to persistent and characteristic symptoms and signs. Neuropathic pain is complex because of the different types of damages that can possibly alter the neural tissue leading to neuropathic pain. Neuropathic pain is the result of a series of different pathological mechanisms. The pathological mechanisms described are based on the anatomic localization and the pathophysiological states. The onset of neuropathic pain may occur in all patients with the same injury or disease. However, the intensity of pain and degree of pain-related functional impairment vary considerably between individuals [8].

The mechanisms underlying neuropathic pain are not fully known, but may involve plastic changes in afferent nociceptive fibers from peripheral nerves and central spinal sensory relays, mainly leading to neuronal hyperexcitability.

Table 5.1 Etiology

Classification	Examples
Trauma	Post-surgery
	Phantom limb pain
	Brachial plexus injury
	Peripheral nerve injury
	Spinal cord injury
Complex regional pain syndrome	Following trauma/fracture
	No precipitating cause
Neurological and neuromuscular disease	Guillain-Barré disease
	Trigeminal neuralgia
	Multiple sclerosis
Metabolic disease	Fabry's disease
Neuropathy following infection	HIV/AIDS
	Post-herpathic neuralgia
Tumor	Nervous system tumour (neurofibromatosis)
	Invasion/compression by tumour
	Effect of treatment (e.g. post-surgery, chemotherapy)
Genetic	Erythromelalgia
	Paroxysmal extreme pain disorder

Central neuropathic pain is due to a lesion or disease of the spinal cord and/or brain. Cerebrovascular disease can affect the central somatosensory pathways. Similarly, neurodegenerative diseases are brain disorders that may also cause central neuropathic pain.

Diagnosis and Assessment

There is no standard consensus or criteria for diagnosis with regards to chronic pediatric pain. Experimental neurophysiology examination has not shown any findings after neurological injury in children because of the altered microglial response during development in childhood. However, peripheral nerve injury in children only presents itself as NP during adolescence. Nevertheless, exceptional cases of NP have been reported in very young children due to metabolic disorders, cancer, chemotherapy, neuromuscular disease, surgical operations, or traumatic injuries. Neuropathic pain in children can be difficult to diagnose, especially in younger children who might find it difficult to express the character of their pain [9].

History remains the mainstay of diagnosis; children may use qualitative descriptions that are indicative of NP, such as burning, shooting, radiating, burning, electricity-shock, stabbing, pricking, tingling, pins and needles, and pinching. Young children may be unable to clearly describe their pain using these terms but nevertheless, a history of pain should include the following parameters: evaluation of intensity; quality (sensory descriptors); temporal aspects of pain (frequency, spontaneous/paroxysmal or continuous, aggravating and relieving factors); and response to treatment. Pain intensity should be evaluated using a validated scale; unfortunately, observational scales have mostly been designed for use in acute pain settings and may not be reliable [8].

Physical examination is performed to find lesions in the somatosensory system and to find associated neurological signs. Sensory abnormalities are more difficult to spot in infants and younger children. Newer techniques, such as quantitative sensory testing (QST) evaluate the changing patterns of relationships between children with NP and adults. The QST requires cooperation and a level of cognitive function which currently is limited to research purposes in a limited pediatric population [8].

Patients typically experience a distinct set of symptoms, such as burning, electrical-like sensation, and pain resulting from non-painful stimulations (such as light touching); the symptoms may persist and have a tendency to become chronic. They also respond poorly to pain medication. Sleep disturbances, anxiety, and depression in patient with neuropathic pain is frequent and severe [2]. Electroneuromyography, microneurography, functional brain imaging and skin biopsy may be indicated although again their use is mostly limited to research. Assessment of pain-related disability is important. The quality of life, sleep, mood, and functional role of the child should be included in the standard assessment for all long-term pain including NP. In adults, chronic pain with NP is associated with a greater disease burden, impacting the quality of life, sleep, anxiety/depression, and use of healthcare and specialist services [8].

Diseases associated with neuropathic pain in childhood are rare, although they have a particular impact on treatment and genetic counseling which is needed to be recognized or ruled out. Alteration in the sodium (Na) channels can produce severe symptoms and can trigger pain. Erythromelalgia is associated with mutations in the SCN9A function and increased activation of the Nav1.7 channel that results in severe episodic pain and redness in children, usually in the feet, hands and in some cases the ears. Pain is exacerbated by ambient temperature and relieved by cold air, to the extent that prolonged immersion in ice water for relief may result in local tissue injury or hypothermia [7].

Genotype and specific amino acid substitution influence the degree of shift in Nav1.7 channel hyperpolarization, symptom severity, age of onset, and in some cases can predict relative response to non-specific sodium channel agents (mexiletine or carbamazepine). Extreme paroxysmal pain disorder, associated with distinct SCN9A mutations and an altered pattern of Nav1.7 kinetics are associated with pain and erythema in the buttocks and legs in early infancy and mandibular pain in older age. This can be triggered by mechanical stimuli, but respond favorably to Carbamazepine. Fabry disease is another multisystem disorder that can cause neuropathic pain. This is due to a variant in the GLA gene [7].

Lysosomal alpha-galactosidase A (AGAL-A) deficiency results in the accumulation of globotriaosylceramide (Gb3) and globotriaosylsphingosine (LysoGb3) in lysosomes in almost all cell types, including the nervous system. Neuropathic pain in the feet and hands (most commonly the soles of the feet, palms, and fingertips) in children may be the first symptom of Fabry disease. It begins at a younger age (median 7 years) and present with more severe symptoms in boys. Male due to X-linked inheritance [8].

The typical description include burning and tingling sensations, initial episodic pain, and is triggered by exercise, heat, and fever. A good relationship with a metabolic physician who can monitor the ongoing effects of the disease in other organ systems (e.g. renal, cardiac gastrointestinal) and consideration of enzyme replacement therapy are essential to optimize the management and improve outcomes [7].

There is no specific laboratory test for neuropathic pain in this age group. The diagnosis is made based on the clinical indicators. History taking remains the mainstay of diagnosis. Children may use qualitative description that are considered indicative of neuropathic disorder, such as burning, shooting, radiating, burning, electricity-shock (dysaesthesias), stabbing, pricking, tingling, pins and needles, and pinching. Young children may be unable to clearly describe their pain using these terms but nevertheless, pain history should include: evaluation of intensity, quality (sensory descriptors); temporal aspect of pain; and response to treatment [3] (Table 5.2).

Diagnosis and treatment of neuropathic pain in children and adolescents is very challenging for various reasons. First, the diagnostic criteria for neuropathic pain advised by IASP such as specific diagnostic tools like questionnaires, qualitative sensory testing, and electromyography (EMG) have not been validated or cannot be easily applied to children because the underlying pathology is often different from that in adults [9].

Table 5.2 Pain-assessment tools for nonverbal children with neurologic impairment [10]

r-FLACC-18

- Revised from the FLACC to include pain behaviors specific to children with cognitive impairment
- Like the FLACC, a 5-item pain assessment tool with a score ranging from 0 to 10
- Allows parents to individualize by adding behaviors specific to their child
- Option of indicating individualized behaviors can be beneficial for children with atypical pain behaviors and lack of other typical features, which may result in a false low score on other tools

INRS-19

- A personalized pain-assessment tool for nonverbal children with intellectual disability, based on the parent's knowledge of the child, developed for use in the hospital
- Parents and caregivers identify behaviors that indicate no pain to the worst possible pain on a scale ranging from 0 to 10
- Moderate to strong correlation between INRS ratings and NCCPC-PV (see below) total scores
- Option of indicating individualized behaviors can be beneficial for children with atypical pain behaviors and lack of other typical features, which may result in a false low score on other tools

NCCPC-PV-20

- 27-item pain-assessment tool for children with severe cognitive impairment
- Moderate to severe pain determined at a cutoff of ≥11 of 81
- In Breau et al.,20 this cutoff provided a sensitivity of 0.88 and specificity of 0.81
- Available for download for clinical use or use in research funded by not-for-profit agencies at http://pediatric-pain.ca/resources/our-measures/

NCCPC-R-21

- 30-item pain-assessment tool designed for nonverbal children ages 3–18 y with severe cognitive impairment
- Moderate to severe pain determined at a cutoff of ≥7 of 90
- In Breau et al.,21 this cutoff provided a sensitivity of 0.84 and specificity of 0.77
- Revised from the NCCPC-PV (postoperative version)
- Available for download for clinical use or use in research funded by not-for-profit agencies at http://pediatric-pain.ca/resources/our-measures/

PPP-10

- A 20-item pain-assessment tool for children with severe to profound cognitive impairment
- Scores of ≥14 were generally associated, by observers, with moderate or severe pain
- A cutoff of 14 provided a sensitivity of 1.0 and specificity of 0.91
- The tool is arranged to provide different scores to indicate a rating for "on a good day," "most troublesome pain," "second-most troublesome pain," etc.
- • available to download from the web, after registration at www.ppprofile.org.uk

Current guidelines for assessment and diagnosis of neuropathic pain are designed for adults, but these guidelines are often extrapolated to older children or adolescents. Screening questionnaires have been developed to identify neuropathic pain such as Leeds Assessment of Neuropathic Symptoms and Signs (LANSS), Douleur Neuropathique en 4 questions (DN4), Neuropathic Pain Questionnaire (NPQ), painDETECT, and identify Pain (ID-Pain). However, these questionnaires have not yet been validated in children [3]. Most of these questionnaires compromise questions about burning, pain, paraesthesias, pain attacks, mechanical and thermal hypersensitivity, and numbness [11].

Management

In general, management for neuropathic pain for adult focuses on treating symptoms because the causes of the pain can be rarely treated. Generally, patient with neuropathic pain do not respond to analgesics such as acetaminophen, NSAIDs, or weak opioids such as codeine [2].

Neuropathic pain in children can be severe, persist for many years, and is difficult to manage [3]. For pediatric pain, Lancet Child Adolescent Health Commission calls on clinicians, researchers, funding bodies, healthcare providers, and policy makers to achieve four transformative goals: 'make pain visible'; 'make pain understood'; and 'make pain better' [5].

Pharmacology

Pharmacological management is extrapolated from evidence-based guidelines for adults with neuropathic pain with very few controlled trials have been performed on children.

The first-line therapy for children with neuropathic pain include the use gabapentinoid anti-convulsant (Gabapentin and Pregabalin) and tricyclic anti-depressant (Amitriptyline and Notriptyline), but the benefit is limited. An initial therapeutic trial allows gradual titration to minimise sedation. Serotonin-selective reuptake inhibitor anti-depressant medications may be given among adolescents [3].

For class Gabapentinoids, Gabapentin can be used with starting dose of 2 mg/kg QHS, and slowly titrated up to an initial target dose of 6 mg/kg/dose TID (max. 300 mg/dose TID). The maximum dose escalation is 24 mg/kg/dose TID (max. 1200 mg/dose TID). The dosage for infant <1 year is 4.5 mg/kg/dose Q6H, and titrated to a maximum dose of 18 mg/kg/dose Q6H per oral. For Pregabalin, the starting dose is 0.3 mg/kg QHS, slowly titrated up to the initial target dose of 1.5 mg/kg/dose BID (max. 75 mg/dose BID). The maximum dose escalation is 6 mg/dose BID (Max/ 300 mg/dose BID) per oral [12].

Tricyclic anti-depressants are given once daily in the evening to improve sleep as well as pain. The dosage for Amitriptyline is 0.1 mg/kg QHS. This is slowly titrated up to 0.5 mg/kg (max. 20–25 mg) per oral. The dosage for Nortriptyline can start at 0.1 mg/kg QHS, and is usually titrated up to 0.5 mg/kg (max/ 20–25 mg) per oral [12].

Non-pharmacology

Physical therapy, exercise and movement representation techniques are suggested. Other treatments include mirror therapy, motor imagery, and imagination of normal pain-free movement. Psychological therapies and cognitive behavioral therapy

(CBT) can be added as treatments. Psychological interventions are designed to promote the management of pain and to reduce its adverse consequences [2].

References

1. Finnerup NB, Haroutounian S, Kamerman P, Baron R, Bennett DLH, Bouhassira D, et al. Neuropathic pain: an updated grading system for research and clinical practice. Pain. 2016;157(8):1599–606.
2. Colloca L, Ludman T, Bouhassira D, Baron R, Dickenson AH, Yarnitsky D, et al. Neuropathic pain. Nat Rev Dis Prim. 2017;3:17002.
3. Walker SM. Neuropathic pain in children: steps towards improved recognition and management. EBioMedicine. 2020;62:103124.
4. Bernetti A, Agostini F, de Sire A, Mangone M, Tognolo L, Di Cesare A, et al. Neuropathic pain and rehabilitation: a systematic review of international guidelines. Diagnostics. 2021;11(1):1–10.
5. Walco GA, Dworkin RH, Krane EJ, LeBel AA, Treede RD. Neuropathic pain in children: special considerations. Mayo Clin Proc. 2010;85(3 SUPPL):33–41.
6. Gilron I, Baron R, Jensen T. Neuropathic pain: principles of diagnosis and treatment. Mayo Clin Proc. 2015;90(4):532–45.
7. Walker SM. Neuropathic pain in children. In: Oxford textbook of paediatric pain. 1st ed. Oxford: Oxford University Press; 2014. hal. 205–14.
8. Howard RF, Wiener S, Walker SM. Neuropathic pain in children. Arch Dis Child. 2014;99(1):84–9.
9. de Leeuw T, der Zanden T, Ravera S, Felisi M, Bonifazi D, Tibboel D, et al. Diagnosis and treatment of chronic neuropathic and mixed pain in children and adolescents: results of a survey study amongst practitioners. Children. 2020;7(11):208.
10. Hauer J, Houtrow AJ. Pain assessment and treatment in children with significant impairment of the central nervous system. Am Acad Paediatr. 2017;139(6):1–29.
11. Baron R, Binder A, Wasner G. Neuropathic pain: diagnosis, pathophysiological mechanisms, and treatment. Lancet Neurol. 2010;9(8):807–19.
12. Friedrichsdorf SJ, Goubert L. Pediatric pain treatment and prevention for hospitalized children. Pain Rep. 2020;5(1):e804.

Chapter 6
Pain in Older Adults

Christopher W. Liu and Colin Chun Wai Chong

Abbreviations

AGS	American Geriatric Society
COX-2	Cyclooxygenase-2
NSAID	Non-steroidal anti-inflammatory drug
SNRI	Selective and norepinephrine inhibitors or SNRI
TCA	Tricyclic antidepressant

Introduction

Chronic pain is more common in old age compared to young adulthood [1]. As a conservative estimate, 25% of the older population living in the community suffer from chronic pain. And in residential facilities, up to 80% of the population may suffer from chronic pain [2, 3]. Apart from being a threat to quality-of-life and independence, a growing body of evidence has linked chronic pain to poor health

C. W. Liu
Department of Pain Medicine, Singapore General Hospital, Singapore, Singapore

Anesthesiology and Perioperative Sciences Academic Clinical Program, Duke-NUS, Singapore, Singapore
e-mail: christopher.liu.w.y@singhealth.com.sg

C. C. W. Chong (✉)
School of Medicine, University of Wollongong, Wollongong, NSW, Australia

Department of Radiology, Macquarie University Hospital, Sydney, NSW, Australia

Department of Radiology, Royal Brisbane and Women's Hospital, Brisbane, QLD, Australia

© The Author(s), under exclusive license to Springer Nature Switzerland AG 2022

J. de Castro, Y. El Miedany (eds.), *Advances in Chronic and Neuropathic Pain*, Contemporary Rheumatology, https://doi.org/10.1007/978-3-031-10687-3_6

outcomes including falls, frailty, cognitive decline, dementia, sleep disturbances and emotional distress [1, 4–6].

There are several differences between chronic pain in the older person and in the general population that makes it deserving a topic of its own. Compared to the general population, older people are more likely to have chronic pain. They also experience different types of pain—for example, postherpetic neuralgia and spinal stenosis are of concern to the older person but seldom of concern to the young. Also, older people perceive pain differently, have more medical comorbidities, have less physiological reserves and are often on multiple medications. All these factors should be taken into account when treating an older person.

Epidemiology of Chronic Pain

In the geriatric patient, the most common causes of chronic pain are musculoskeletal disorders, peripheral vascular disease, cancer pain and neuropathic pain [7]. A more detailed breakdown of these causes may be found in Table 6.1. It should be acknowledged there are very few good quality studies that have specifically examined this topic. Of the studies that have examined this topic, indirect methods, such as matching patients who are on analgesics with their diagnosis were used. Such techniques may lead to under-representation of certain pain disorders such as fibromyalgia.

The risk factors for chronic pain development include advanced age, female gender, ethnicity (blacks), lower socioeconomic status, increased pain severity, multiple sites of pain, genetics as well as smoking [8–10]. Apart from these risk factors, there are also psychopathologies that are associated with chronic pain such as anxiety, depression and catastrophizing behavior [8, 9]. However, the direction of the relationship between chronic pain and psychopathology is currently unclear.

Table 6.1 Most common diagnoses for chronic pain in older persons [7]

Diagnosis (% of population)
Osteoarthritis (21.9%)
Spinal disorders (19%)
Peripheral vascular disease (12.4%)
Osteoporosis (11.4%)
Malignancy (7.2%)
Gout (4.4%)
Headache (3.8%)
Diabetic neuropathy (1.7%)
Rheumatoid arthritis (1.6%)
Pressure ulcer (1.3%)
Herpes zoster (0.6%)

Changes in Pain Physiology

Pain transmission as well as perception are likely to be altered in the older person. However, the mechanisms that underlie these changes are poorly understood. Current evidence indicates that there are widespread changes that take place in the pain pathway during aging, involving both the peripheral and central nervous system.

In the peripheral nervous system, aging has been shown to be associated with neuronal loss, decreased nerve fiber density, decreased conduction velocity as well as changes in the neurochemistry [11]. In the central nervous system, similar changes are seen. For instance, neuronal loss and altered neurochemistry have been noted in the spine as well as in the brain, particularly in the areas that are involved in nociceptive processing [11]. Since the perception of pain is in part, contingent on the balance between the excitatory and inhibitory pathways of pain, it is likely that these anatomical and physiological alterations of the nervous system can affect pain perception in the older person.

Psychophysical experiments have been performed to determine if the older patients feel more or less pain. Generally, the threshold for pain is more likely to be increased in older people when the stimuli are brief, of lesser spatial extent and are at peripheral cutaneous / visceral sites. Extrapolating this, the older person is likely to have a slightly decreased ability to sense acute pain which therefore places one at a higher risk of injuries [11]. In contradistinction to brief stimuli, it has been found that older patients exposed to a more intense stimulus for a longer period [12], tend to have an increased pain perception as well as a longer period of hyperalgesia [11]. While the significance of this is unclear, it raises the possibility that older patients may experience more pain in certain circumstances.

Challenges and Barriers to Chronic Pain Treatment

Pain management in the geriatric population can be challenging for several reasons. The first reason is that chronic pain in likely to be under-diagnosed. From the cultural standpoint, an older person is likely to be more stoic than a young person leading to under-reporting of pain. The reason for their stoicism is not well understood but it has been postulated that it may be generational in nature—for example, the older person is likely to have gone through war, famine and lived in a society where it was considered inappropriate to complain [12]. Some older patients may also have misconceptions about pain—For example, they may wrongly attribute pain to "normal aging" or feel that pain may represent death / loss of autonomy / the need for further testing. From the biological standpoint, older patients may have sensory loss (for example, hearing impairment), speech as well as cognitive impairment. Together, these factors may result in the under-reporting of pain.

The healthcare system may also be contributing to the under-diagnosis of chronic pain. Some healthcare practitioners have misconceptions about chronic pain in the older person. Such misconceptions include the false belief that "aging" is synonymous with "pain" or that older people have less pain than the young [13]. Alongside this, physicians may also face the time pressure of working in a busy clinic and lack the time to screen patients for pain or have the tendency to brush off complaints about pain.

From the treatment standpoint, the older person is also more difficult to treat than the young patient. Stoicism, opioid-phobia and the fear of taking medications may lead to the unnecessary rejecting of treatments for a treatable condition. Apart from that, the older person may have multiple medical comorbidities, be on multiple medications, have organ impairment (for example renal impairment) and are more sensitive to the adverse effects of medications. As such, the older person is more likely to have drug-interactions or be intolerant to medications, leading to a reduced number of interventions that can be offered to the patient.

Assessment of Pain

Pain assessment in the elderly is not straightforward. Advancing age is associated with cognitive impairment, dementia as well as communication problems (for example, speech and hearing impairment). Furthermore, it has been observed that many older patients who deny pain, respond positively when asked about pain in other terms—for example soreness, aching or discomfort [14]. Considering these factors, the assessment of pain in the elderly should take into account both patient self-reported pain as well as input from caregivers and other healthcare professionals involved in the care of the patient.

Assessment of Pain in the Elderly

The goals of pain assessment in the elderly are summarized in Table 6.2.

Table 6.2 Goals of pain assessment in the elderly

Goals of pain assessment in the elderly
1. Obtain diagnosis—If possible
2. Pain severity
3. Impact of pain on quality of life
4. Impact of pain on function
5. Identify attitudes and beliefs about pain, treatment goals and expectations
6. Reviewing comorbidities and drugs

Obtain Diagnosis

Obtaining the diagnosis is an important aspect of pain assessment. In patients with secondary chronic pain conditions *(see section on causes of pain in older people)*, an accurate diagnosis can lead to a specific treatment (such as total knee replacement for knee osteoarthritis) or a pain intervention other than pain medications [15]. However, some patients may have a primary chronic pain condition (such as fibromyalgia), in which a specific treatment or pain intervention may be lacking. Other than obtaining a reasonable diagnosis for the patient's pain, it is also important to rule out life-limiting or serious conditions such as infections or cancer.

Assessing Pain Severity

As earlier noted, patients may deny the presence of pain but yet report the presence of "soreness", "aching" or "discomfort". Therefore, in a patient who denies having pain, it may be fruitful to rephrase the pain history to confirm the lack of pain—for example, "Do you hurt anywhere" or "What is stopping you from walking" [14].

With regards to pain severity, patient self-report is the gold standard even in the older patient. Pain scales such as the numerical rating scale and categorical pain scale are widely used in both clinical practice and in the research setting. Both scales have been shown to be responsive in both acute and chronic pain [14]. However, patients will differ in their abilities to use these scales.

A number of trials have been conducted to determine if patients with cognitive impairment are able to use self-assessment scales. In those with mild to moderate cognitive impairment, good comprehension of the pain scales was noted in 80% of the patients. In those with severe cognitive impairment, there was a slight decline to 60% of the patients [16]. In those showing good comprehension, the pain scales were found to have good inter- and intra-rater reliability [16]. These studies provide the basis for concluding that patient self-report as gold standard holds true, even for the majority of patients with cognitive impairment.

However, while self-report is the gold standard for patients who can comprehend the pain scale, it is inappropriate for those who cannot understand the pain scale or are non-verbal. In these patients, a behavioral pain assessment tool is a more appropriate technique for the assessment of pain severity. Multiple behavioral pain scales have been described for these patients. Of these, the most commonly used scales are the Pain in Advanced Dementia (PAINAD), Abbey and Doloplus scores [14].

Assessing the Impact of Pain

Chronic pain can significantly affect a person's quality of life. It has also been shown to affect the physical and emotional functioning of patients of all ages - including the older person. Consequently, the assessment of physical, emotional and social functioning has been recommended in both in the clinical [17] and research setting [18].

Consequently, multidimensional pain assessment tools have been developed both for research purpose as well as for clinical use. These tools rely on patient self-reporting and capture information beyond the pain score—for example, the quality of pain, impact of pain on function such as walking and sleep. Table 6.3 lists some of the multidimensional pain assessment tools that have been evaluated to be appropriate for the older person [17]. In a busy clinic, the use of these tools may not always be practical. In such cases, even asking the patients briefly about the impact of their pain on their ability to walk, perform housework, mood and sleep can yield useful information about the severity of the pain and the impact of their pain treatment.

It should be noted that these multidimensional pain assessment tools may not be appropriate in patients with cognitive impairment. In such patients, it is important to obtain a caregiver history as well as observe the patient for behavior suggestive of pain. Example of behavioral changes associated with pain includes changes in facial expression (frowning, grimacing), vocalization (sighing, moaning, verbal abuse), body movement (rigid, tense, restlessness, inactivity), changes in interpersonal interactions (disruptive, withdrawn), changes in activity patterns (appetite change, sleep changes, cessation of usual routines) as well as mental status changes (crying, distress, confusion, irritability) [19]. While there have been several attempts to create an observational tool for cognitively impaired patients, these tools have not been shown to be suitable for clinical use [17].

The development of validated scales can be very beneficial if used in an appropriate manner—for example, choosing a scale that is easy to use, has validated translations for the non-English speaking patient, written in appropriate font size etc. Nevertheless, it should be remembered that patient assessment cannot be

Table 6.3 Multidimensional pain assessment tools [17]

Multidimensional pain assessment tools
SF-MPQ
Functional pain scale
Pain disability index
Brief pain inventory
Geriatric pain measure (GPM)
Multidimensional pain inventory (MPI)
Structured pain interview (SPI)
Western Ontario and McMaster universities osteoarthritis index (WOMAC)
Arthritis impact measurement scale (AIMS)

reduced to the filling up of scales. The older patient should also be invited to talk about his or her pain experiences though the asking of open-ended questions.

Attitudes and Beliefs

Multiple attitudes and beliefs among pose as barriers to the effective treatment of persistent pain in the older person. These include—normalization of pain as part of aging, increased stoicism, reluctance to be a burden to others and concerns about use of analgesia (fear of tolerance, addiction and side effects) [20]. It is therefore, important to be mindful of these attitudes and beliefs, which may have to be addressed in order to optimize the quality of lives of these older persons.

Approach to the Treatment of Pain

The multimodal approach to pain should be emphasized as key to the effective treatment of pain in the older person. This approach involves the use of physical and psychological rehabilitation to restore function in patients with chronic pain. A large body of evidence suggests that physical therapy and psychological interventions are useful for the general population with chronic pain. In recognition that medications can have a decreased therapeutic index in the older patient, these treatment strategies are valuable for the management of chronic pain in the older person. However, in this chapter, the focus will be on the considerations when using medications and interventional pain strategies for the management of the older person.

Prescribing for Older People

General Principles of Pharmacological Management

Older persons with impaired quality of life or function are candidates for pharmacotherapy. Prescriptions must be individualized, taking into account the benefits and risks of the medication to the individual. Medications are usually trialed in young and healthy patients. Therefore, drug manufacturers seldom include a dosing strategy specific to the elderly patient and more importantly, the frail and unwell elderly patient. Consequently, a good working knowledge of physiological changes in the elderly, pharmacology of analgesics and good understanding of disease is required for the appropriate prescribing of analgesics to the older person.

These patients are at a higher risk of developing adverse effects. This is because aging is associated with decreased organ function, an increased number of diseases and polypharmacy. Consequently, in geriatric patients, additional consideration should be given to the physiological state of the patient as well as drug-drug interactions. Table 6.4 lists some of the important physiological changes that can affect the pharmacokinetics and pharmacodynamics of drugs.

Medications have a narrower therapeutic index in the older population. It is therefore important to "start low and go slow" and assess frequently for adverse effects when initiating and titrating analgesics for these patients. For patients with continuous pain, regular administration of pain medications helps to maintain a steady state analgesic plasma concentration, which is likely to result in a better outcome. On the other hand, for patients with episodic pain, an as-required dosing may be more appropriate [21].

Table 6.4 Physiological changes that can affect drug pharmacokinetics / pharmacodynamics

Organ system	Physiological changes	Implications
Body composition	Increased body fat Decreased body water / lean mass / albumin	Affects distribution of medications. Lower albumin / alpha glycoprotein can result in decreased binding of drugs (for example non-steroidal anti-inflammatory drugs NSAIDS or tricyclic antidepressants TCAs) Transdermal drug absorption may also be altered—For example, fentanyl serum concentrations are lower in cachectic patients on fentanyl patches
Central nervous system	Decreased brain volume Cognitive impairment	May be prone to adverse effects (for example sedation, falls and delirium). Anticholinergic drug in particular can increase the risk of delirium and constipation in these patients. Prescribers should therefore prefer medications lacking anticholinergic activity. Additionally, when prescribing medications that can potentially cause sedation or delirium, it is important to "start low, go slow" and regularly monitor patients for adverse effects to therapy
Gastrointestinal tract	Decreased gastric secretion and intestinal motility	Altered absorption of certain drugs Increased risk of constipation with use of opioids
Liver	Reduced hepatic volume and blood flow	Slight reduction in phase I metabolism and minimal changes in phase II metabolism. May predispose patients to adverse effects and drug-drug interactions.
Renal	Progressive nephrosclerosis Decrease renal blood flow Decline in GFR	May need to reduce dose of medications that are renally excreted or have active metabolites that are renally excreted for example gabapentin and morphine. May predispose patients to adverse effects (for example, renal failure with NSAID use).

Non-opioids

Paracetamol

Paracetamol is the most widely used analgesic among the older population. It is available over-the-counter, found in combination medications and is widely regarded as safer than other analgesics. Apart from these reasons, paracetamol is also mentioned as a first-line medication in several guidelines including one from the American Geriatrics Society [22, 23].

However, the use of paracetamol has come under more scrutiny recently as several meta-analyses have found a lack of clinically meaningful efficacy of paracetamol over placebo for several common pain conditions including osteoarthritis and low back pain [24, 25]. Nevertheless, paracetamol remains one of the safer analgesic medications in the market. At this juncture, it should be noted that the commonly held belief that paracetamol toxicity does not occur at the recommended dose of 1 g every 6 h may no longer hold true. There have been reported cases of liver toxicity with the use of normal doses of paracetamol in the elderly [26]. The exact pathophysiological mechanisms underlying this is unclear but may be related to low glutathione reserves (for example malnutrition, alcoholism), low weight or drug interactions [26].

Taken together, the dose of paracetamol should be decreased in the frail or small sized patient. If a trial of paracetamol demonstrates a lack of drug efficacy, paracetamol should also be weaned off promptly.

Non-steroidal Anti-Inflammatory Drugs (NSAIDS)

NSAIDS (Cyclooxygenase-II (COX-II) selective and non-selective NSAIDS) are widely used for the treatment of chronic musculoskeletal pain. In many countries, NSAIDS such as Ibuprofen may be bought without a prescription and an estimated 7.3% of patients above 60 years old filled at least one NSAID prescription each year.

As a class of medication, it is effective for a wide range of chronic musculoskeletal conditions. For example, a network meta-analysis found that NSAIDs (etoricoxib 60 mg/day and 90 mg/day, diclofenac 150 mg/day, Topical diclofenac) provide superior analgesia to opioids (tramadol 154—225 mg/day, tapentadol <316 mg/day, oxymorphone 80 mg/day and transdermal buprenorphine 0.36 mg/day) for the treatment of chronic knee and hip osteoarthritis [27].

Despite its efficacy, systemic NSAIDS have garnered a reputation because of their side effect profile. In the older patient, these adverse effects are magnified. The most common serious adverse effects include gastric ulceration, kidney injury and cardiovascular events [28]. NSAID use has also been associated with falls in the older patient [29]. However, it is difficult to prove causation since musculoskeletal pain itself can cause functional impairment and falls.

Gastrointestinal bleeding is the most common serious side effect of NSAID use in the elderly [28]. Studies have estimated that as a class, the use of NSAID in these patients is associated with a four-fold increase in gastrointestinal bleeding [30]. Additionally, the relative safety of NSAIDS have been studied. In terms of gastrointestinal bleeding, ibuprofen was associated with the lowest risk, followed by diclofenac, naproxen, indomethacin, ketoprofen and finally, meloxicam. Although the use of COX-II inhibitors can significantly reduce the risk of gastrointestinal bleeding [31], it does not eliminate this risk completely. Other strategies that can mitigate NSAID-related gastrointestinal bleeding includes coadministration of stomach acid suppressants such as proton-pump inhibitors and mistoprostol [28].

Renal impairment with NSAID use occurs due to the loss of prostaglandin-mediated renal vascular dilation. While it is relatively uncommon to see this side effect in younger patients, the risk for the older patient is higher since aging is associated with declining renal function and polypharmacy. This effect is not altered by the use of COX-II inhibitors [32]. Common drugs that interact with NSAIDS to precipitate renal failure in the elderly include diuretics and ACE inhibitors / angiotensin receptor antagonists [33].

Cardiovascular complications are a concern when prescribing NSAIDs. The withdrawal of rofecoxib was triggered after the APPROVE trial showed that the medication resulted in a significant increase in cardiovascular complications when compared to placebo [34]. Although this was initially attributed to the COX-II selectivity of rofecoxib, this adverse effect has now been demonstrated in both selective and non-selective NSAIDs. Considering that older patients are likely to have a higher baseline risk for cardiovascular events, this translates to a significantly larger increase in absolute risk for cardiovascular complications compared to the young patient. The literature is currently mixed with regards to which drug is the safest from the cardiovascular standpoint. In one network meta-analysis, the safest medications from the cardiovascular standpoint (in decreasing order) are naproxen, followed by rofecoxib[1], celecoxib, ibuprofen, diclofenac and lumiracoxib (see footnote 1) [35]. In contrast, two large multicenter randomized controlled trials showed that COX-II inhibitors (celecoxib and etoricoxib) were non-inferior to non-selective NSAIDS in terms of the risk of cardiovascular thrombotic outcomes [36, 37].

Topical NSAIDs are another group of commonly used medications. There is evidence supporting the short term use of topical NSAIDs but the long term data is lacking [27, 38]. Nevertheless, this route of NSAID administration appears to be safe, devoid of systemic side effects but may result in mild skin irritation in some patients.

Taken together, topical NSAIDs are preferred over systemic NSAIDS. Although systemic NSAIDs may be used in the older patient, it should be used with caution. Active peptic ulceration, impaired renal function / solitary kidney, heart failure and recent myocardial infarction are absolute contraindications for NSAID use. In patients with relative contraindications (such as hypertension, helicobacter pylori infection, history of peptic ulcer disease or concomitant use of steroids), systemic

[1] Rofecoxib and lumiracoxib have been taken off the market.

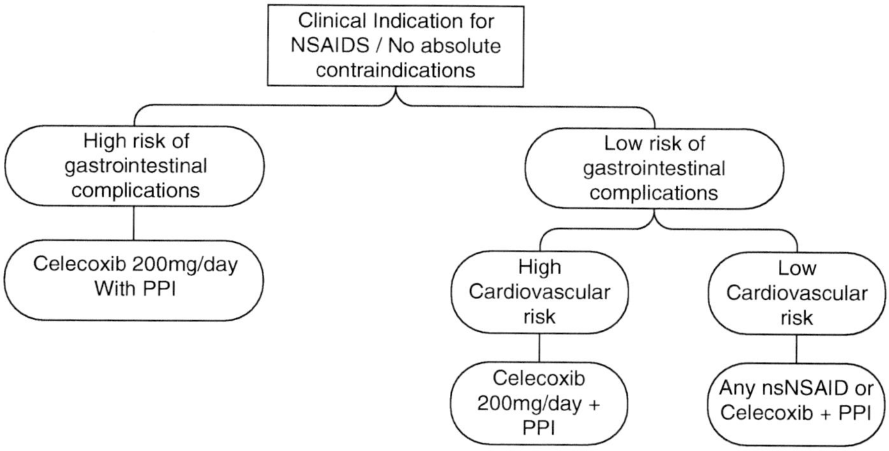

Fig. 6.1 Prescribing algorithm for NSAIDs based on risk profile. In the high cardiovascular risk population, celecoxib is recommended over etoricoxib as the PRECISION trial showed that celecoxib was non-inferior to Naproxen [36]. On the other hand, etoricoxib is has a more similar chemical structure to rofecoxib and was compared to Diclofenac in the MEDAL study [37] and Naproxen is likely to be a safer medication compared to Diclofenac based on one network meta-analysis [35]. Abbreviations: *nsNSAID* non-selective NSAID, *PPI* Proton pump inhibitor

NSAIDS should not be prescribed as a first-line medication. If used, appropriate risk mitigation strategies should be put in place. These include using it short-term for pain exacerbations, selecting the least toxic medication, using the lowest dose possible, peptic ulcer prophylaxis, considering drug-drug interactions as well as monitoring patients for potential adverse effects. See Fig. 6.1.

Adjuvants

Typical drugs used to treat somatic pain such as paracetamol and NSAIDS are unlikely to be beneficial for the treatment of neuropathic pain. The treatment of neuropathic pain in the general population is outlined in Fig. 6.2.

Although both gabapentinoids and tricyclic antidepressants are recommended as first-line treatment for neuropathic pain in the general population, this recommendation cannot be made for the older person. In this population group, a trial of topical lidocaine is likely to be associated with the least side effects and should be considered the first line drug for focal neuropathic pain (such as painful diabetic neuropathy) as it has been shown to be effective, well-tolerated and generally, devoid of systemic side effects [40].

If topical lidocaine is not suitable or ineffective, a gabapentinoid should be considered before the initiation of TCAs. Gabapentinoids can cause dizziness, somnolence, fatigue and weight changes. As such, it should be started at a lower dose in

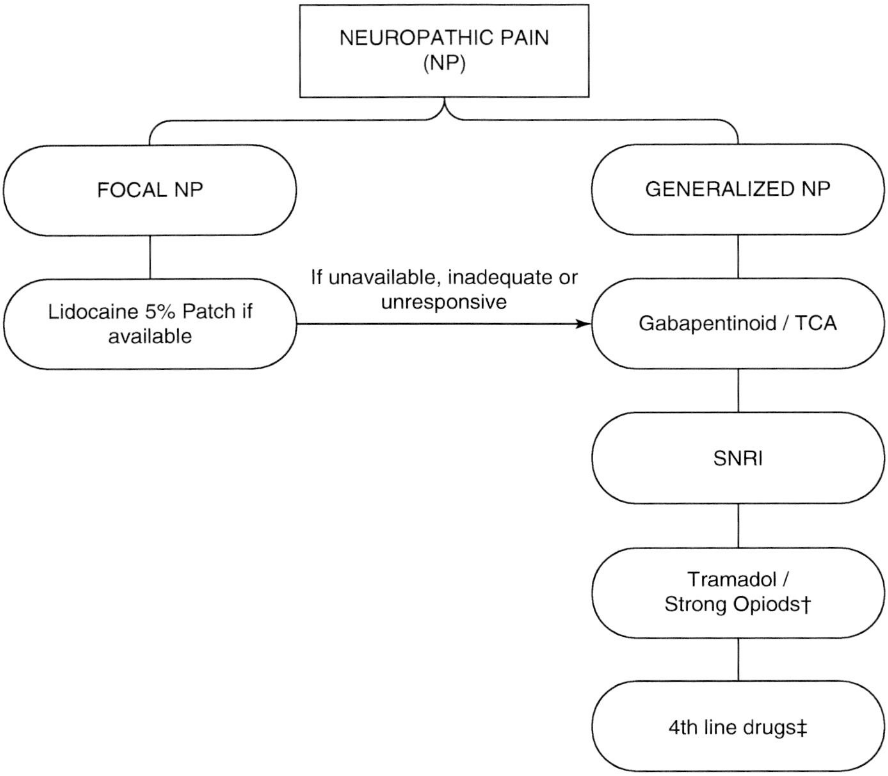

Fig. 6.2 Pharmacological treatment of neuropathic pain in the general population. († While opioids have been shown to have short-term benefits for the management of pain, there is a lack of evidence about its long term efficacy. As such, its use should be considered only when the risks outweigh its benefits. ‡ Fourth line drugs refer to medications which may be helpful from a pharmacodynamics standpoint but lack evidence. Examples include methadone, cannabinoids and other anticonvulsants (for example, Lamotrigine, topiramate and valproate [39])

the older person. Despite these side effects, it is considered to have a safer profile than other systemic anti-neuropathic drugs.

TCAs should not considered the first line antineuropathic medication in older people. This takes into consideration that TCAs are more prone to drug-interactions and are highly anticholinergic. Taken together, TCAs expose patients to an increased risk of serious adverse effects including QTc prolongation, sedation, confusion, orthostatic hypotension and sudden cardiac death (particularly when the dose of amitriptyline exceeds 100 mg/day) [41, 42]. Consequently, it is listed as a “potentially inappropriate drug” in the American Geriatric Society Beers Criteria [43] and a thorough risk-benefit analysis should be performed before initiating TCAs in the older person. If it is administered, the starting dose should be lowered and the patient should be frequently monitored for efficacy and adverse effects. Baseline and regular electrocardiogram have also been recommended [44].

Selective and noepinephrine inhibitors or SNRIs, in particular duloxetine and venlafaxine, are generally considered second line treatment for neuropathic pain.

Duloxetine has been shown to be beneficial for the treatment of diabetic neuropathy, fibromyalgia, chronic low back pain and knee osteoarthritis. In the older population, duloxetine is well-tolerated with minimal risk of severe or life-threatening side effects. Nevertheless, SNRIs may cause constipation, myalgia, palpitations and worsen hypertension which should be considered as significant side effects when dealing with the older population [45].

Carbamazepine and oxcarbazepine are the first line treatment for trigeminal neuralgia (TN) and glossopharyngeal neuralgia (GPN). In these patients, up to 90% will have an improvement in their symptoms at least in the short-to-intermediate term [46]. However, the plasma concentration of these medications are affected by albumin levels, the activity of the CYP3A4 enzymes and have serious side effects such as Steven Johnson's syndrome, leukopenia, hyponatremia, transaminitis and ataxia. In the older patient, there is a larger interindividual plasma concentration variation [47], more adverse effects (for example hyponatremia, ataxia leading to falls and osteoporosis [48] and a higher risk of drug-drug interaction due to polypharmacy. Considering these, both carbamazepine and oxcarbazepine are listed as "drugs to be used with caution" in the AGS Beer list [43]. However, due to the high level of efficacy of these medications when compared to the alternatives, they should still be considered first-line treatment for TN and GPN even in the elderly. However, a thorough risk-benefit analysis should be performed prior to recommending its use. In addition, patients should be closely monitored for adverse effects and have regular blood testing. If available, oxcarbazepine is preferred over carbamazepine due to its better side effect profile. The use of these medications should preferably be avoided in other neuropathic pain conditions.

Skeletal muscle relaxants can be classified as antispasmodics and antispastics. Antispasmodics are used for the treatment of spasms caused by local muscle injury or nerve compression. In contrast, antispastics are used to treat spasticity secondary to an upper motor neuron lesion. In general, there is little or no evidence to support the long-term use of skeletal muscle relaxants for low back pain and other spasms. In contrast, the use of antispasmodics in these patients can lead to dizziness, drowsiness and hypotension—leading to a two-fold increase in visits to the emergency room for falls and fractures [49]. Many antispasmodics (carisoprodol, chlorzoxazone, cyclobenzaprine, metaxalone, methocarbamol, orphenadrine and diazepam) have therefore been listed in the AGS Beer list and should be avoided [43]. Although baclofen is not listed in the AGS Beer list, it cannot be recommended as a first-line medication and caution should be taken when prescribing this.

Opioids

For the treatment of life-limiting conditions such as cancer pain, the use of opioids is recommended as the second and third steps of the World Health Organization's Pain Ladder [50]. However, the use of opioids for non-cancer pain has been called into question since the Opioid Crisis.

There is strong evidence that short term use of opioids can result in a small reduction in the pain score and function of patients with chronic pain, at the expense of a slightly higher rate of bothersome side effects (for example, nausea, constipation, somnolence) [51]. However, the evidence regarding the long term efficacy of opioids is limited and unlike the short-term use of opioids, chronic opioid consumption is associated with a dose-related increase in serious adverse effects such as all all-cause mortality, falls, myocardial infarction and erectile dysfunction. Consequently, opioids are not recommended as first-line therapy for chronic non-cancer pain [51]. Nevertheless, it is reasonable to give a trial of opioid therapy in selected patients where the expected benefit from opioids is estimated to outweigh its risk [52].

When prescribing opioids to the older patient, it is important to be well-versed with the physiological changes associated with aging, drug-drug interactions, as well as, the pharmacokinetic and pharmacodynamics profile of a wide range of opioid medications. The pharmacokinetic implications of aging have previously been summarized in Table 6.4. In terms of pharmacodynamics changes, older patients are more sensitive to the effects of opioid. Hence, it is important to initiate opioid therapy at a lower dose and escalate the dose slowly, all the while monitoring the patient for adverse effects. Table 6.5 outlines some of the strategies that have been recommended to reduce opioid related adverse effects.

Table 6.5 Strategies to reduce opioid related adverse effects

Assessment	• Detailed medical history and physical examination • Ensure that non-opioid therapies have been optimized • Assess risk of harm for example obstructive sleep apnea, sedatives, renal failure • Assess risk of addiction / misuse for example opioid risk tool(ORT) screening • Clear criteria for discontinuing opioid therapy
Prescribing	• Prescribe short acting opioids • Start low and go slow • Frequent reassessment of the patient. Initial reassessment should be within 1–4 weeks • Avoid co-prescribing with other sedatives such as benzodiazepines • If a patient's morphine milligram equivalent (MME) is ≥50 mg/day, consider offering naloxone
Monitoring	• Assess for the 4As of pain treatment outcomes: – Analgesia – Activities of daily living – Adverse effects – Aberrant drug taking • Consider pill counts, periodic urine drug screening especially in higher risk patients
Discontinuation	• Patients should be weaned if: – They engage in aberrant drug behavior – They have intolerable or serious opioid-related side effects • If a patient's MME is ≥90 mg/day and there is minimal treatment effect, consider discontinuing the opioid.
Specialist referral	• Specialist referral is indicated if: – Prescriber is unfamiliar with opioid prescribing – High risk for opioid related adverse effects including aberrant use – Daily MME exceeds 90 mg and there is no plan for discontinuation

Codeine is a weak opioid which is metabolized into morphine. It is associated with more nausea and constipation compared to other opioids [53]. Furthermore, it is dependent of CYP2D6. Consequently, it can result in unpredictable plasma concentrations in the slow and rapid-metabolizer.

Tramadol is a weak opioid. It derives its action from both mu receptor agonist as well as inhibition of serotonin and noradrenaline reuptake. It should be used with caution with patients on antidepressants due to the risk of serotonin syndrome. It should also be avoided in patients with cognitive impairment due to its ability to worsen it.

Buprenorphine is a partial agonist with a ceiling effect in terms of respiratory depression. For chronic pain, the transdermal route is the most common. Buprenorphine has a very high affinity of buprenorphine to the mu receptor agonist. Consequently, it may be difficult to reverse buprenorphine with conventional doses of naloxone. It may also result in decreased efficacy of other opioids with less mu-receptor affinity when used concomitantly with buprenorphine (for example, during surgery) [54].

Morphine is a strong opioid. It is metabolized to active metabolites (in particular, Morphine-6-Glucuronate) which are renally excreted. Consequently, it should be avoided in patients with significant renal impairment (GFR<30 ml/min).

Oxycodone is a strong opioid. Oxycodone is metabolized to noroxycodone via CYP3A4 and oxymorphone via CYP2D6. Although oxymorphone is an active metabolite, the plasma concentration of this is negligible and oxycodone is much more inactive compared to oxycodone. Taken together, it is considered safer to use oxycodone than morphine in patients with significant renal impairment [55].

Fentanyl is a strong opioid. For chronic pain, the transdermal route is most commonly utilized. It may be used in patients with renal and hepatic impairment and causes less constipation than morphine [56, 57]. In cachectic cancer patients, it has been observed that the absorption of drug may be impaired [57]. It is uncertain if the impact is similar in older patients with sarcopenia.

Methadone is both a mu-receptor agonist as well as an N-Methyl-D-Aspartate (NMDA) antagonist. It has complicated pharmacokinetics and pharmacodynamics and it should be restricted to specialists familiar with initiating and titrating methadone.

Interventional Strategies

Although many older persons can have effective treatment of their chronic pain with medications, some may develop dose-limiting adverse effects such as sedation and some fail to achieve adequate pain-relief despite being on therapeutic doses of analgesics. In these patients, interventional pain treatment is effective and safe. Despite their safety profile, there are some precautions necessary in the older person. Some of these precautions are listed in Table 6.6.

Table 6.6 Considerations for interventional pain procedures in the older person

Treatment type	Considerations
Steroid injection	Steroid injections are the most common types of interventional treatment options. Although generally safe, excessive use of steroids can cause side effects such as osteoporosis and worsening of pre-existing diabetes / hypertension. Strategies to minimize side effects from steroid injections include [58]: – Limit the number of steroid injections to 3 times a year – Avoid performing a series of injections separated by 1 week – Repeat injections only if patients had significant pain and functional benefits following the index injection – Avoid high-dose injections (>40 mg triamcinolone equivalent)
Botulinum toxin	Botulinum toxin is commonly used to treat spasticity. It has also been used to treat conditions such as muscle spasms and migraine headaches. The use of botulinum toxin can result in a medium term weakness of muscles. Complications such as ptosis or weakness in a lower limb muscle may increase the risk of falls. Consequently, physicians should be mindful of these complications and avoid causing them for example by ensuring accurate placement of the medications
Spinal cord stimulation	Spinal cord stimulation (SCS) is indicated for a number of conditions including failed back surgery syndrome, complex regional pain syndrome and peripheral neuropathy The older person is at a higher risk of complications due to changes in anatomy, concomitant use of antiplatelets and have lower immune function compared to the young [59]. Of note, there have been case reports of older patients developing spinal cord compression after the implantation of a spinal cord stimulation due to unrecognized thoracic spinal stenosis [60]. Considering that thoracic spinal stenosis can be found in 25% of patients with symptomatic lumbar spinal stenosis [61], routine preoperative magnetic resonance imaging is prudent for the older patient

Conclusions

Although there is some evidence that the geriatric patient may have a decreased noxious threshold for experiencing acute pain, there is also evidence that pain may be amplified when it is chronic. Therefore, the notion that older patients feel less pain should be considered obsolete. Chronic pain in this group of patients is common but is under-recognized and under-treated. To improve healthcare quality, it is imperative to increase our recognition of these key points. The management of these patients can be complicated as they are more likely to have cognitive impairment, a wide range of age-related or disease-related organ dysfunction and have significant drug interactions. Consequently, practitioners should be aware of how these factors will affect the management of these patients.

Funding This manuscript was not supported by any funding.

Conflict of Interest The authors declare they have no relevant conflicts of interest.

References

1. Gibson SJ, Lussier D. Prevalence and relevance of pain in older persons. Pain Med. 2012;13(Suppl 2):S23–6.
2. Blyth FM, March LM, Brnabic AJ, Jorm LR, Williamson M, Cousins MJ. Chronic pain in Australia: a prevalence study. Pain. 2001;89(2–3):127–34.
3. Stompor M, Grodzicki T, Stompor T, Wordliczek J, Dubiel M, Kurowska I. Prevalence of chronic pain, particularly with neuropathic component, and its effect on overall functioning of elderly patients. Med Sci Monit. 2019;25:2695–701.
4. Scudds RJ, Mc DRJ. Empirical evidence of the association between the presence of musculoskeletal pain and physical disability in community-dwelling senior citizens. Pain. 1998;75(2–3):229–35.
5. Duong BD, Kerns RD, Towle V, Reid MC. Identifying the activities affected by chronic nonmalignant pain in older veterans receiving primary care. J Am Geriatr Soc. 2005;53(4):687–94.
6. Welsh TP, Yang AE, Makris UE. Musculoskeletal pain in older adults: a clinical review. Med Clin North Am. 2020;104(5):855–72.
7. Huang YL, Tsay WI, Her SH, Ho CH, Tsai KT, Hsu CC, et al. Chronic pain and use of analgesics in the elderly: a nationwide population-based study. Arch Med Sci. 2020;16(3):627–34.
8. van Hecke O, Torrance N, Smith BH. Chronic pain epidemiology and its clinical relevance. Br J Anaesth. 2013;111(1):13–8.
9. Mills SEE, Nicolson KP, Smith BH. Chronic pain: a review of its epidemiology and associated factors in population-based studies. Br J Anaesth. 2019;123(2):e273–e83.
10. Larsson C, Hansson EE, Sundquist K, Jakobsson U. Chronic pain in older adults: prevalence, incidence, and risk factors. Scand J Rheumatol. 2017;46(4):317–25.
11. Gibson SJ, Farrell M. A review of age differences in the neurophysiology of nociception and the perceptual experience of pain. Clin J Pain. 2004;20(4):227–39.
12. Lane P, Smith D. Culture, Ageing and the Construction of Pain. Geriatrics (Basel). 2018;3(3):40.
13. Borsheski R, Johnson QL. Pain management in the geriatric population. Mo Med. 2014;111(6):508–11.
14. Schofield P. The Assessment of Pain in Older People: UK National Guidelines. Age Ageing. 2018;47(suppl_1):i1–i22.
15. Reid MC, Eccleston C, Pillemer K. Management of chronic pain in older adults. BMJ. 2015;350:h532.
16. Pautex S, Michon A, Guedira M, Emond H, Le Lous P, Samaras D, et al. Pain in severe dementia: self-assessment or observational scales? J Am Geriatr Soc. 2006;54(7):1040–5.
17. Hadjistavropoulos T, Herr K, Turk DC, Fine PG, Dworkin RH, Helme R, et al. An interdisciplinary expert consensus statement on assessment of pain in older persons. Clin J Pain. 2007;23(1 Suppl):S1–43.
18. Turk DC, Dworkin RH, Allen RR, Bellamy N, Brandenburg N, Carr DB, et al. Core outcome domains for chronic pain clinical trials: IMMPACT recommendations. Pain. 2003;106(3):337–45.
19. Snow AL, Shuster JL Jr. Assessment and treatment of persistent pain in persons with cognitive and communicative impairment. J Clin Psychol. 2006;62(11):1379–87.
20. Cousins MJ, Brennan F, Carr DB. Pain relief: a universal human right. Pain. 2004;112(1–2):1–4.
21. American Geriatrics Society Panel on Pharmacological Management of Persistent Pain in Older P. Pharmacological management of persistent pain in older persons. J Am Geriatr Soc. 2009;57(8):1331–46.
22. NICE. Osteoarthritis: care and management. National Institute for Health and Care Excellence: London; 2021.
23. Dunham M, Schofield P, Knaggs R. Evidence-based clinical practice guidelines on the management of pain in older people–a summary report. Br J Pain. 2020:2049463720976155.

24. Machado GC, Maher CG, Ferreira PH, Pinheiro MB, Lin CW, Day RO, et al. Efficacy and safety of paracetamol for spinal pain and osteoarthritis: systematic review and meta-analysis of randomised placebo controlled trials. BMJ. 2015;350:h1225.
25. Ennis ZN, Dideriksen D, Vaegter HB, Handberg G, Pottegard A. Acetaminophen for chronic pain: a systematic review on efficacy. Basic Clin Pharmacol Toxicol. 2016;118(3):184–9.
26. Ging P, Mikulich O, O'Reilly KMA. Unexpected paracetamol (acetaminophen) hepatotoxicity at standard dosage in two older patients: time to rethink 1 g four times daily? Age Ageing. 2016;45(4):566–7.
27. da Costa BR, Pereira TV, Saadat P, Rudnicki M, Iskander SM, Bodmer NS, et al. Effectiveness and safety of non-steroidal anti-inflammatory drugs and opioid treatment for knee and hip osteoarthritis: network meta-analysis. BMJ. 2021;375:n2321.
28. Wongrakpanich S, Wongrakpanich A, Melhado K, Rangaswami J. A comprehensive review of non-steroidal anti-inflammatory drug use in the elderly. Aging Dis. 2018;9(1):143–50.
29. Woolcott JC, Richardson KJ, Wiens MO, Patel B, Marin J, Khan KM, et al. Meta-analysis of the impact of 9 medication classes on falls in elderly persons. Arch Intern Med. 2009;169(21):1952–60.
30. Sabzwari SR, Qidwai W, Bhanji S. Polypharmacy in elderly: a cautious trail to tread. J Pak Med Assoc. 2013;63(5):624–7.
31. Walker C. Are all Oral COX-2 selective inhibitors the same? A consideration of celecoxib, Etoricoxib, and diclofenac. Int J Rheumatol. 2018;2018:1302835.
32. Ungprasert P, Kittanamongkolchai W, Price C, Ratanapo S, Leeaphorn N, Chongnarungsin D, et al. What is the "safest" non-steroidal anti-inflammatory drugs? Am Med J. 2012;3:115–23.
33. Loboz KK, Shenfield GM. Drug combinations and impaired renal function – the 'triple whammy'. Br J Clin Pharmacol. 2005;59(2):239–43.
34. Bresalier RS, Sandler RS, Quan H, Bolognese JA, Oxenius B, Horgan K, et al. Cardiovascular events associated with rofecoxib in a colorectal adenoma chemoprevention trial. N Engl J Med. 2005;352(11):1092–102.
35. Trelle S, Reichenbach S, Wandel S, Hildebrand P, Tschannen B, Villiger PM, et al. Cardiovascular safety of non-steroidal anti-inflammatory drugs: network meta-analysis. BMJ. 2011;342:c7086.
36. Nissen SE. Cardiovascular safety of celecoxib, naproxen, or ibuprofen for arthritis. N Engl J Med. 2017;376(14):1390.
37. Combe B, Swergold G, McLay J, McCarthy T, Zerbini C, Emery P, et al. Cardiovascular safety and gastrointestinal tolerability of etoricoxib vs diclofenac in a randomized controlled clinical trial (the MEDAL study). Rheumatology (Oxford). 2009;48(4):425–32.
38. Tugwell PS, Wells GA, Shainhouse JZ. Equivalence study of a topical diclofenac solution (pennsaid) compared with oral diclofenac in symptomatic treatment of osteoarthritis of the knee: a randomized controlled trial. J Rheumatol. 2004;31(10):2002–12.
39. Moulin D, Boulanger A, Clark AJ, Clarke H, Dao T, Finley GA, et al. Pharmacological management of chronic neuropathic pain: revised consensus statement from the Canadian Pain Society. Pain Res Manag. 2014;19(6):328–35.
40. Gammaitoni AR, Davis MW. Pharmacokinetics and tolerability of lidocaine patch 5% with extended dosing. Ann Pharmacother. 2002;36(2):236–40.
41. Attal N, Cruccu G, Haanpää M, Hansson P, Jensen TS, Nurmikko T, et al. EFNS guidelines on pharmacological treatment of neuropathic pain. Eur J Neurol. 2006;13(11):1153–69.
42. Ray WA, Meredith S, Thapa PB, Hall K, Murray KT. Cyclic antidepressants and the risk of sudden cardiac death. Clin Pharmacol Ther. 2004;75(3):234–41.
43. 2019 American Geriatrics Society Beers Criteria® Update Expert Panel, et al. American Geriatrics Society 2019 Updated AGS Beers Criteria® for Potentially Inappropriate Medication Use in Older Adults. J Am Geriatr Soc. 2019;67(4):674–94.
44. Dworkin RH, Backonja M, Rowbotham MC, Allen RR, Argoff CR, Bennett GJ, et al. Advances in neuropathic pain: diagnosis, mechanisms, and treatment recommendations. Arch Neurol. 2003;60(11):1524–34.

45. Abou-Raya S, Abou-Raya A, Helmii M. Duloxetine for the management of pain in older adults with knee osteoarthritis: randomised placebo-controlled trial. Age Ageing. 2012;41(5):646–52.
46. Cruccu G, Di Stefano G, Truini A. Trigeminal Neuralgia. N Engl J Med. 2020;383(8):754–62.
47. Battino D, Croci D, Rossini A, Messina S, Mamoli D, Perucca E. Serum carbamazepine concentrations in elderly patients: a case-matched pharmacokinetic evaluation based on therapeutic drug monitoring data. Epilepsia. 2003;44(7):923–9.
48. Suljic EM, Mehicevic A, Mahmutbegovic N. Effect of long-term carbamazepine therapy on bone health. Med Arch. 2018;72(4):262–6.
49. Alvarez CA, Mortensen EM, Makris UE, Berlowitz DR, Copeland LA, Good CB, et al. Association of skeletal muscle relaxers and antihistamines on mortality, hospitalizations, and emergency department visits in elderly patients: a nationwide retrospective cohort study. BMC Geriatr. 2015;15:2.
50. Liu WC, Zheng ZX, Tan KH, Meredith GJ. Multidimensional treatment of cancer pain. Curr Oncol Rep. 2017;19(2):10.
51. Chou R HD, Turner J, Blazina I, Chan B, Levander X, McDonagh M, Selph S, Fu R, Pappas M. Opioid Treatments for Chronic Pain. In: Quality AfHRa, editor. Rockville, MD: AHRQ Publication No. 20-EHC011; 2021.
52. Dowell D, Haegerich TM, Chou R. CDC guideline for prescribing opioids for chronic pain - United States, 2016. MMWR Recomm Rep. 2016;65(1):1–49.
53. Arnstein P. Balancing analgesic efficacy with safety concerns in the older patient. Pain Manag Nurs. 2010;11(2 Suppl):S11–22.
54. Kohan L, Potru S, Barreveld A, Sprintz M, Lane O, Aryal A, et al. Buprenorphine management in the perioperative period: educational review and recommendations from a multisociety expert panel. Reg Anesth Pain Med. 2021;46(10):840–59.
55. Dean M. Opioids in renal failure and dialysis patients. J Pain Symptom Manag. 2004;28(5):497–504.
56. Radbruch L, Sabatowski R, Loick G, Kulbe C, Kasper M, Grond S, et al. Constipation and the use of laxatives: a comparison between transdermal fentanyl and oral morphine. Palliat Med. 2000;14(2):111–9.
57. Heiskanen T, Mätzke S, Haakana S, Gergov M, Vuori E, Kalso E. Transdermal fentanyl in cachectic cancer patients. Pain. 2009;144(1):218–22.
58. Mattie R, Miller DC, Smith C. On behalf of the spine intervention society's patient safety C. annual maximum dose of epidural steroid injection. Pain Med. 2019;20(10):2069–70.
59. Dorshkind K, Swain S. Age-associated declines in immune system development and function: causes, consequences, and reversal. Curr Opin Immunol. 2009;21(4):404–7.
60. Wang D, Qureshi M, Smith J, Khetani N. Spinal cord compression related to spinal cord stimulator. Pain Med. 2018;19(1):212–4.
61. Park MS, Moon SH, Kim TH, Oh JK, Lyu HD, Lee JH, et al. Asymptomatic stenosis in the cervical and thoracic spines of patients with symptomatic lumbar stenosis. Global Spine J. 2015;5(5):366–71.

Part IV
Pain Processing Medical Problems

Chapter 7
Cancer Pain

Theresia C. T. Novy

Introduction

One of the most common symptoms in cancer patients is pain. At least 40% of cancer patients suffer from pain [1], although advanced cancer may be associated with a much higher prevalence [2].

The prevalence of pain in cancer patients is as high as 55% during treatment, 39.3% after curative treatment, and 66% in the late stage of the carcinoma. As high as 38% of cancer patients reported moderate to severe pain (numeric rating scale ≥5) [2, 3].

In 1986, the World Health Organization (WHO) developed guidelines for the pharmacologic management of patients with cancer pain, which was revised in 1997 [4]. The WHO concept of therapy has been validated by many studies. The guidelines are designed to improve pain relief in sick patients through the use of an "analgesic ladder". With the application of WHO guidelines, adequate analgesia is achieved in 75% to 90% of patients [4]. The remaining 10–25% require interventional pain procedures. Some patients with well-controlled pain may experience painful side effects from drug therapy. These patients may also benefit from intervention options. Therefore, the decision to do an intervention procedure is an individual decision, as the risks and benefits may vary from patient to patient [5].

T. C. T. Novy (✉)
Bandung Pain Rehab Center, Bandung, Jawa Barat, Indonesia

PainManagement.Network, Bandung, Jawa Barat, Indonesia

Bandung Adventist Hospital, Bandung, Jawa Barat, Indonesia

© The Author(s), under exclusive license to Springer Nature Switzerland AG 2022

J. de Castro, Y. El Miedany (eds.), *Advances in Chronic and Neuropathic Pain*, Contemporary Rheumatology, https://doi.org/10.1007/978-3-031-10687-3_7

Mechanism of Cancer Pain

Cancer treatment, aiming to eliminate the tumor tissue, can be a double-edged sword. Antineoplastic treatment (i.e. radiotherapy and chemotherapy), may result in peripheral nerve neurotoxicity and pain. When these adverse effects become severe, oncologists should modify the treatment. However, this adjustment may diminish the patient's survival rate and the prognosis of cancer.

When the cancerous tissue is inoperable or reoccurs, the stromal cells will release algogenic factors which then evoke pain. Nociceptor will be sensitized and activated by release of chemical agents such as cytokines (tumor necrosis necrosing factor-α(TNF-α) and interleukin-6(IL-6), granulocyte-macrophage colony stimulating factors (GMCSF), endothelins, nerve growth factor (NGF). The factors then will cause injury to the nerve fibers, then create nerve-sprouting, and finally, neuroma formation which will evoke breakthrough pain [6–8].

Dull, constant, and gradual over time are the most common descriptions of pain caused by cancerous tissue. A spontaneous extreme pain overlaying the constant pain is the nature of breakthrough pain, which may cause disability in patients [6, 9].

Assessment of Cancer Pain

Treatment of cancer pain interventions depends largely on the patient's condition. Physicians should receive a history of previous pain treatment and the patient's current medical history, with close attention to the details related to pain, including onset and duration (whether the pain is acute or chronic, ongoing or breakthrough), intensity (rated by visual analog scale, verbal rating scale, or numeric rating scale), location and distribution (whether the pain is focal, multifocal, or generalized; or a referred pain), and quality of the pain (whether it is sharp or aching. These signs and symptoms indicate a somatic nociceptive pain; while diffuse or gnawing pain, indicates a visceral nociceptive pain; Burning and tingling sensation however, indicates a neuropathic pain) Pain may take a toll on daily living such that it may affect sleep and appetite, social and professional life, and psychological status.

General medical and neurological examinations are important in pain investigation in order to establish the right diagnosis and choose the suitable treatment or intervention. Patient might show any sign of discomfort such as guarding painful areas, grimace, or heavy breathing. A change in gait and posture could be suggestive of the effects of pain in the patient.

Appropriate laboratory tests are also necessary. The most recent radiological assessment is very important. In addition to their diagnostic value, radiological examinations can be of great help to pain specialists in planning appropriate interventions. Contraindications to the interventional procedure include infection of an active injection site, ubiquitous infection, and coagulopathy. It is also important to assess the patient's emotional and psychological state prior to the procedure. This will guide the physician's decision as to whether the patient is fit for a procedure. Pain can be influenced by social, cultural, and psychological factors and all of these must be considered, as they may directly or indirectly influence the outcome of the intervention. Patient's expectations must be determined. It is important for the pain physician to determine whether the patient's expectations and what the procedure can achieve are reasonable. If the patient insists on unrealistic treatment, then it is wiser not to go through procedures.

Some questionnaires regarding pain in cancer patients have been developed. The Edmonton Classification System for Cancer Pain (ECS-CP) (Fig. 7.1), includes five domains of adequate pain control: pain mechanism, incidental pain, psychological distress, addictive behavior, and cognitive function. Based on score of the five domains, patients are classified as having good, intermediate, or poor pain control [1, 11].

The Cancer Pain Prognostic Scale (CPPS) was developed to predict pain relief in cancer patients with moderate to severe pain. The domains include: pain severity, emotional well-being, daily opioid dose, and pain characterization. The total score can be measured between 0 to 17, higher score means higher chance for pain relief [1, 11].

Screenings for neuropathic pain were also developed, although not mainly intended for cancer pain It includes LANSS, DN4, and pain DETECT [1].

Cancer Pain Syndrome

Cancer pain syndrome can be grouped into acute and chronic. Acute pain in cancer is mostly caused by invasive procedures such as during the diagnostic and surgical interventions, and during the administration of therapeutic agents. Chronic pain syndromes in cancer patients sets in when there is an involvement of bones, soft tissues, visceral organs, and nervous system.

Acute pain syndromes can be further categorized based on pain characteristics, nature of therapy leading to the pain, or specific involvement of tissue causing the pain [12].

Acute pain syndromes are based on pain characteristic:

1. Tumor-related nociceptive pain syndromes:
   When cancerous tissue invades the somatic or visceral organs, it leads to acute pain. Bone pain syndrome is seen most often among cancer patients, and may lead to neuropathic pain.
   Obstruction, infiltration, or compression can lead to visceral nociceptive pain.
2. Tumor-related neuropathic pain syndromes:
   Any infiltration or compression of peripheral nerve structures may lead to neuropathic pain. It may also result from the pharmacologic side effects of treatment characterize by nerve toxicity.

Edmonton Classification System for Cancer Pain

Patient Name: ______________________________

Patient ID No: ______________________________

For each of the following features, circle the response that is most appropriate, based on your clinical assessment of the patient

1. **Mechanism of Pain**

No	No pain syndrome
Nc	Any nociceptive combination of visceral and/or bone or soft tissue pain
Ne	Neuropathic pain syndrome with or without any combination of nociceptive pain
Nx	Insufficient information to calssify

2. **Incident Pain**

Io	No incident pain
Ii	Incident pain present
Ix	Insufficient information to classify

3. **Psychological Distress**

Po	No psychological distress
Pp	Psychological distress present
Px	Insufficient information to classify

4. **Addictive Behavior**

Ao	No addictive behavior
Aa	Addictive behavior present
Ax	Insufficient information to classify

5. **Cognitive Function**

Co	No impairment Patient able to provide accurate present and past pain history unimpaired
Ci	Partial impairment Sufficient impairment to affect patient's ability to provide accurate present and/or past pain history
Cu	Total impairment Patient unresponsive, delirious or demented to the stage of being unable to provide any present and past pain history
Cx	Insufficient information to classify

ECS-CP profile: N_I_P_A_C_ *(combination of the five responses, one for each category)*

Assessed by: ______________________ **Date:** ______________________

Fig. 7.1 Edmonton Classification System for Cancer Pain. Adapted from Fainsinger, R. L., & Nekolaichuk, C. L. (2008). A "TNM" classification system for cancer pain: The Edmonton Classification System for Cancer Pain (ECS-CP) [10]

Acute pain syndrome related to cancer treatment

1. Surgery-related pain syndromes
   The tissue damage post-surgery will lead to nociceptive pain, and any nerve injury will cause neuropathic pain. The severity of pain is based on the extent of the injury and the procedure, and the surgical site. Some interventions are related to post-surgical pain syndromes such as post thoracotomy, post mastectomy, post-radical neck surgery, post-amputation pain syndrome.

2. Chemotherapy and hormonal therapy-related pain syndromes
   Toxicity from chemotherapy and hormonal therapy may manifest as acute pain. Steroid may lead to bone necrosis and can possibly cause bone pain. Chemotherapy drugs such as taxane may cause myalgia and athralgia [13]. Hand-foot syndrome or palmar-plantar erythrodysesthesia syndrome is linked to administration of chemotherapy such us cytarabine, capecitabine, 5-fluorouracil, vinorelbine, docetaxel [14].
3. Radiation therapy associated pain syndromes
   Pain after radiation therapy is manifested as bone pain after radiotherapy for bone metastases, mucositis after head and neck radiation, and visceral inflammation after abdominal or pelvic radiation. Proctitis leads to painful tenesmus while cystitis manifests as dysuria and other urinary tract infection symptoms [14]. Neuropathy from radiation therapy is also reported such as seen in brachial plexopathy [12, 14].

Chronic pain in cancer can be directly caused by the cancer tissue compressing an adjacent structure. It could be the musculoskeletal or visceral structures (nociceptive pain) or neural structures (neuropathic pain) or it could arise secondary to the treatment of cancer.

The most common source of pain is bone metastases [15]. Multifocal bone pain from metastases is common in multiple myeloma and in breast, prostate, and lung cancer. Bone pain is caused by direct invasion of cancer cells in the bone, secondary pathologic fracture, or destruction to surrounding structures of bone. The pain is characterized as focal, aching, and increased with movement or weight bearing. Vertebral pain usually presents itself below the metastases site. The following are examples of such pain: Odontoid lesions affect the base of the neck, interscapular region pain is referred from C7 or T1 vertebra, and iliac crest or greater trochanter region pain is referred from T12 or L1. The pain from the hip or inguinal area are evoked by walking while the pain in the knee or thigh is characterized as a local aching, which might be induced by pelvic and hip metastases.

Cancer pain from visceral organ is associated with hepatic distension, peritoneal carcinoma, chronic obstruction of intestine, perineal and adrenal pain, ureteric obstruction, and leptomeningeal metastases.

Hepatic and adjacent organ metastases may cause dull discomfort and pain provoked by positional or deep inspiration, in the upper right abdominal region and right flanks or midback. Intestinal obstruction is characterized by a continuous and colicky pain pattern. It is associated with nausea, vomiting, and constipation. Perineal pain in the colon or rectum secondary to a malignant lesion, genitourinary tract in the male, reproduction system among females may appear as severe bladder contraction, tenesmus, and is increased with positional changes.

Neuropathic pain may emerge as cranial neuralgias, cervical, brachial or lumbosacral plexopathies, and radiculopathies. Cranial neuralgia may appear from the base of the skull, sinuses, leptomeningeal regions, and head and neck with soft tissue metastases. Brachial plexopathy is mostly caused by lung cancer, breast cancer, or lymphoma. Sacral plexus injury may manifest as perineal pain and dysfunction of bladder and bowel.

Chronic pain in some cancer treatment can emerge following radiation therapy, hormonal therapy, chemotherapy and post-surgery. Radiation therapy may cause chronic pain syndrome from injury of visceral organs, soft tissue, and nervous tissue. Pain is usually less apparent except for the prominent signs manifested as motor weakness, sensory changes, lymphedema, and skin changes.

WHO Pain Ladder

There are three fundamentals in pain relief [16, 17]:

1. Modify the pain source, using antineoplastic drugs and modalities for treating the cancerous tissue.
2. Alter the central perception of pain using pharmalogical management such as NSAIDs, opioids, and adjuvants which include antidepressants, anticonvulsants, corticosteroids; psychotherapy may be incorporated to address behavioral pain problems.
3. Block the pain transmission from the pain source to the central nervous system using interventional pain management by means of nerve blocks, central neural blocks with epidural infusion, and neurosurgical procedures such as cordotomy or myelotomy.

WHO proposed a cancer pain relief in 1986, including an analgesic ladder, which was then revised in 1996. WHO 3 step analgesic ladder is a simple and effective method, and can be easily understood even by non-pain physicians. Here we provide the modified version of Pain Ladder, which we usually use in our Clinic (Fig. 7.2). With this method 70–90% pain relief in cancer patients has been reported [17, 18].

WHO analgesic ladder depicts pain medication based on their pain scale. The lowest level is 0 for no pain. The first step or 1 is for mild pain where non-opioid with or without adjuvant is suggested; the second step or 2 is for moderate pain where weak opioid drugs with or without non-opioid medications, and with or

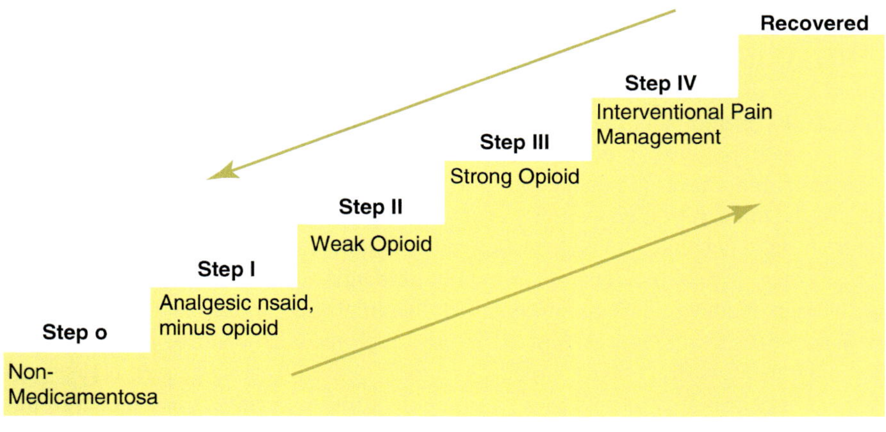

Fig. 7.2 Modified WHO cancer pain ladder. Adapted from World Health Organization. Cancer Pain Relief: With a guide to opioid availability, 1997 [4]

without adjuvant are suggested. Finally, the third step or 3 is for severe pain using strong opioid added with non-opioid and adjuvant agents. The fourth step is reserved for interventional Pain Management (IPM).

Principles in WHO analgesic ladder are as follows: by mouth, by the clock, by the ladder, for the individual, and with attention to detail [17, 18].

(a) By mouth means analgesics should be given orally when possible. To control the baseline pain, analgesic drugs should be given by the clock, meaning that the analgesic drugs should be given at fixed intervals of time rather than on demand, depending on the pharmacokinetics of the drug.
(b) Clinical examination is important in starting the medication; "by the ladder" principle aims for analgesic prescription according to subjective pain intensity of the patient.
(c) According to Bonica: the "right" dose is the dose that relieves the patient's pain with the minimum side effects, summarizing the individuality principle of the analgesic ladder.
(d) Attention to details means adequate treatment outcome and regularity of drug administration are important. Written and individual instruction are preferred to encourage and improve compliance of patients, families, and health workers with regards to the administration of the medications.

Although treated with the WHO Cancer Pain Analgesic Ladder, about 10–25% of cancer patients are reported to be non-responsive to the medications. This problem stimulates discussion among pain clinicians regarding the need to revisit the WHO Pain Ladder [18–20]. Recommendation to the WHO pain ladder includes adding the fourth step for interventional pain management or surgery, management for breakthrough pain, the inclusion for fixed-dosed drugs for step 2, and for clinicians to recognize the need for leapfrogging through the steps. Patients with severe to very severe pain, those unresponsive to conventional treatments, and those who presents with significant side effects from oral pain medications may benefit from this recommendation.

Pharmacologic Strategies

Non-opioid Drugs

Non-opioid drugs based on WHO Pain Ladder is used for the first step management of cancer pain. These drugs can be used independently, or together with opioid drugs to reduce the dose in order to achieve adequate pain relief.

Acetaminophen is an over the counter drug and widely used without prescription. Acetaminophen however, is highly associated with hepatotoxicity contributing to more than 50% of overdose-related acute liver failure, and about 20% of cases of liver transplant in the United States [21]. The recommended maximum dose is 4000 mg a day for patients with normal liver function [22, 23]. The dose for acetaminophen or acetylsalicylic is 650 mg every 4 h.

NSAIDS (Non-Steroidal Anti-Inflammatory Drugs) are a group of drugs used for fever, pain, and inflammation. The anti-inflammatory effect could also be achieved by blocking the cyclooxygenase (COX) enzyme which then inhibitis the synthesis of prostaglandin. COX-2 and prostaglandin cascades play significant roles in cancer inflammogenesis [24, 25]. Celecoxib is an example of COX-2 inhibitor drug and it can be consumed twice a day at 100 mg/tablet. NSAIDS drugs such as Ibuprofen can be consumed at 800 mg, four times a day while Diclofenac is given at 50 mg/tablet, four times a day.

Opioid Drugs

Opioid drugs achieve their analgesic effects by attaching to opioid receptors (mu, kappa, delta), both peripherally and centrally. The oral route is preferred in most patient due to its convenience and simplicity. Regular scheduling at sufficient dose should be prescribed for constant ongoing pain control. Prescribing it "as needed" or "pro re nata (prn)" may increase the patient's anxiety and required effective dose [4, 23].

Breakthrough pain can be provoked by movements or procedures. Extra short-acting doses of similar drugs can be given as needed. If a patient needs more than 2–4 breakthrough doses in 24 h, then the routine dosing should be increased [23].

There are some factors that should be considered in giving opioid prescription:

1. Previous opioid use
2. Pain severity and nature
3. Patient's age
4. Any metastases of cancer, particularly involving hepatic and renal
5. Coexisting diseases

Tramadol in oral form usually comes in 50 mg or 100 mg dose and can be consumed every 4–6 h, with a maximum dose of 400–600 mg a day. Dihydrocodeine in 60–120 mg can be consumed up to a maximum of 240 mg a day. Oral morphine usually starts with 10–20 mg four times a day, and can be increased as needed (no maximum dose). Pethidine in oral form can be consumed up to 500 mg a day [26].

Adjuvants in Cancer Pain

Adjuvant drugs in cancer pain management might be needed for any of these causes:

1. To treat any side effects of a given pain reliever (antiemetics or laxatives)
2. To increase pain relief effect (corticosteroid in nerve-compression pain)
3. To treat coexisting psychological problems, such as insomnia, anxiety, and depression

Nausea and vomiting in cancer patients could be induced by chemotherapy, [27, 28], radiotherapy, [28], and opioid [29]. Up to 70% patients with advanced cancer presents with nausea, with 10–30% of them practically vomiting [29]. Neuroleptic drugs is used for opioid-induced nausea. These include haloperidol given at 1-2 mg up to a maximum of 5 mg once a day, and Prochlorperazine given at 5 mg every 8 h up to a maximum of 10 mg every 4 h [4]. For opioid-induced nausea unresponsive to neuroleptics due to drug-induced delayed gastric emptying, metoclopromide is given at 10 mg every 8 h to a maximum of 20 mg every 4 h to replace the neuroleptic drugs [4].

Laxative should be prescribed when starting opioid medications. Oral preparation is preferred unless suppositories are indicated. Twice a day of two tablets standardized senna is chosen for the starting dose, and could be increased to two tablets every 4 h if necessary. Faecal softener such as 200 mg docusate 2–3 times a day might also be needed. Bisacodyl or enema as suppository laxatives could be used when patient is severely constipated [4].

Steroids are commonly used when there is an increased in intracranial pressure, acute spinal cord compression, superior vena cava syndrome, metastatic bone pain, neuropathic pain, symptomatic lymphedema, and hepatic capsular distension. Patients with advanced cancer who experienced pain may respond to steroids with relatively small doses, such as two times of 1-2 mg dexamethasone. A severely acute pain due to a neuropathic lesion can be given a short course of high dose IV steroid, such as 100 mg IV dexamethasone and can be tapered down the following day. A gradual decrease to the minimum effective dose should be applied following pain reduction [17].

Psychotropic drugs are needed in cancer pain for pain relief (tricyclic antidepressant and anticonvulsants for nerve injury pain). And should includ antiemetic (haloperidol for opioid-induced nausea), anxiolytic (clonazepam or alprazolam), night sedative, and antidepressant.

Epileptic drugs such as gabapentin can be consumed 100 mg a day to a maximum 4800 mg a day. Pregabalin 50 mg three times a day can be increased to 100 mg three times a day after a week up to a maximum dose of 600 mg a day. Pregabalin may cause sedation, ataxia, oedema and cognitive dysfunction. Carbamazepine should be started as low as 100 mg twice a day up to 400–1800 mg a day and then must be tapered off before discontinuing.

Antidepressants are used for cancer pain intervention, whose example include tricyclic antidepressants (imipramine, desipramine, amitriptyline) and Serotonin and Norepinephrine Reuptake Inhibitor (SNRI) such as venlafaxine, duloxetine, and milnacipran [30].

Technique Choice [31–37]

The life expectancy of cancer patients plays an important role in the choice of appropriate intervention techniques. Various techniques can provide analgesia from a few days to a few weeks. Others, such as neurolysis blocks can give analgesia for a few months, while some, such as implantable medicine supplies, can provide good pain relief only for a few years. Therefore, implanted devices are best suited for patients with a lifespan of at least 1–2 years. The benefits as well as the immediate and long-term risks of a planned procedure must be fully explained to the patient. The procedure which is likely to take immediate effect must be chosen. If there is more than one choice, choose the option with the fewest and least serious side effects, but has enough opportunity to reduce the pain. Regional painkillers such as neuropathic opioids and the administration of local anesthetics are generally considered. First, because they do not endanger neurological integrity. Ablative or neuro-destructive procedures that have a close risk-benefit relationship should be delayed provided that pain relief can be achieved through non-ablative categories. However, some procedures, such as celiac plexus block in patients with pancreatic cancer, may have favorable risk-benefit relationships that require early treatment with neurolysis. Diagnostic blocks using local anesthetics should be used to evaluate the effectiveness of the planned neurolysis procedure prior to the actual procedure. This block also serves to assess the impact of possible neurological deficits as a result of ablation. The advantages of neurolytic techniques include a shorter duration of time compared to regional painkiller techniques using continuous neurosis drug delivery and greater cost-effectiveness for patients with short lifespans. However, neurolysis can lead to complications such as permanent motor loss, paresthesia and dysesthesia. Other factors that may influence the choice of technique are patient expectations and the availability of local experts and trained staff. A properly chosen procedures can reduce the need for ubiquitous opioids and improve the quality of life.

Central Neural Block [31–33, 38]

Intrathecal opioids exert their analgesic effects by reducing the release of presynaptic neurotransmitters and inhibiting the transmission of pain by hyperpolarizing the membranes of postsynaptic neurons in the dorsal horn. Continuous administration of a neuropathic drug may be accomplished by intrathecal or epidural catheterization. Medication can be administered by an external injection pump or a system of whole implanted intrathecal drug delivery (ITDD). Medications are performed intrathecally in minutes and in the right amount, avoiding ubiquitous toxicity and side effects. In a randomized controlled trial, ITDD was associated with improved quality of life, decreased pain, and a 6-month survival (53% of patients in the ITDD group were still alive compared to 32% of patients in the conventional medical group). However, improving patient survival was not the main endpoint of the study and more work is needed to confirm or refute this hypothesis. Although there are no rules governing when choosing an epidural over intrathecal pathway or vice versa, it is important to understand the advantages and disadvantages of each before deciding. Important factors such as life expectancy and the supportive needs of the patient have to be considerate. Nurses are required to be considerate. It is also important to train family members who are involved in caring for the patients while receiving continuous infusions of neuropathic drugs.

Epidural Infusion Analgesia [32, 38, 39]

Continuous administration of neuropathic drugs to patients with cancer pain by the epidural route is very common. The use of epidural analgesia in this group of patients differs from the one used in acute pain such as postoperative pain or labor pain. Cancer patients often present with an abnormal coagulation profile and level, and have dysfunction of immune response which puts them at risk of bleeding and infection. Therefore, it warrants an absolute contraindication to approach with a normal epidural catheter placement. After careful consideration and discussion with the patient and family of the risks involve, the potential benefits of pain reduction, and the reduced need for opioids with fewer side effects provides a way to a better quality of life although with limited life expectancy. The main drugs are opioids, but the combination with local anesthetics increases their effectiveness. Other medications such as clonidine may be added to further increase its efficacy. The normal starting dose of opioids for an epidural infusion can be estimated by calculating the total dose of opioids (oral or parenteral) taken by the patient. This should include a dose for acute pain. This is then converted into an equivalent epidural dose of morphine. Most doctors use 10:1 parenteral to epidural morphine dose conversion. During epidural opioid titration, small doses of short-acting opioids may be given to treat severe pain. With this method, the side effects associated with high doses of oral or parenteral opioids can be avoided as long as they achieve much better analgesia. Because the volume of the infusion and the dose of drug administered by the epidural route are larger than that given by intrathecal route, an external injection pump should be used, as the reserve capacity of the implanted pump is limited. Filling the pump can increase the risk of infection. That's why it's important to watch out for signs of infection regularly. In patients with persistent cancer pain with a lifespan greater than 3 to 6 months, epidural analgesia can be used as a test to assess the effectiveness of pain relief prior to the placement of a permanent implant ITDD system. Epidural analgesia can be used for a longer time (up to months with a silastic catheter). Patients with epidural catheters are good enough to go home with an IV. Accidental removal or removal of the catheter is not a crisis. Pain can be treated conventionally with opioids while the catheter is repositioned at the right time.

Intrathecal Analgesia with ITDD System [34, 38, 40, 41]

ITDD system gives better pain control and fewer complications. Administration is with a catheter implanted with a medication pump, which can be external or internal (implanted). Intrathecal infusion uses a lower dose and volume than an epidural infusion. Most clinicians use a 10:1 conversion by epidural to intrathecal morphine dose. Therefore, when using a fully internalized pump system, there is a longer interval between pump fillers. Introducing a foreign body into the body carries the risk of infection, especially with an external pump system, as there is a connection between the skin and the central nervous system. Therefore, a fully implanted ITDD system can offer the advantage of a lower risk of infection. However, similar percentages of infection have been reported with intrathecal or epidural administration with antibiotic prophylaxis, but there is evidence that intrathecal catheters are safer when used for more than 3 weeks. If life expectancy is short (i.e., from a few days to a few weeks), using an external pump and epidural catheter may be more appropriate. Once an implanted ITDD pump has been inserted, appropriate precautions must be taken for ongoing maintenance (changing the pump program and charging session). The filling range also affects the stability of the selected mixture of active ingredients. Complications of intrathecal therapy can be broadly divided into catheter-related, pump-related, drug-related, and those associated with the catheter insertion procedure itself. Catheter-related complications include wound infection, meningitis, microfracture/damage, misinformation, migration, hygroma, fibrosis blockage, and intrathecal catheter tip granuloma, which causes neurological deficits. Failure problems with the pump include unexpected battery discharges, motor or component errors, and programming errors. There is a risk of post-puncture headache due to loss of cerebrospinal fluid during catheter insertion, contusion, and damage to surrounding structures. The infusion of local anesthetics can lead to neurotoxicity and persistent neurological damage. The formation of granulomas at the tip of the intrathecal catheter is a serious complication that can cause compression of the spinal cord and paralysis of the distal mass. The effect appears to be related to the morphine concentration (>25 mg/ml), the daily dose (>10 mg/day) and the duration of treatment. Cases were recorded within 1 month after therapy. Symptoms include lower back pain, motor or sensory deficits in lower extremities, and loss of bladder and bowel function. Analgesic failures can be high in cancer patients. Epidural metastases or spinal stenoses are common in patients who report failure or poor outcomes with a central neurosis drug. Intrathecal infusion analgesia has been shown to be less expensive than ubiquitous treatment after 3–6 months for cancer pain and after 11–22 months for non-cancer pain. An external pump system should be used when the patient's survival is less than 3 months, and an intrathecal catheter with an internal pump should be used for patients with a longer lifespan.

Intrathecal Neurolysis [32, 42, 43]

Intrathecal neurolysis plays an important role in the treatment of cancer pain. This involves the administration of a neurolysis agent such as alcohol or phenol into the subarachnoid space. The goal is to achieve purely sensory segment blocks, although this is rarely achieved even by skilled hands. This procedure can be fraught with potentially destructive complications such as disability. Therefore, the patient should be prepared to accept the possible problems that may arise from the procedure such as inadequate pain control with the development of tumor size, short-term effects, weakness of the muscles of lower extremities and dysfunction of the direct constrictor or bladder. It is also important for patients and their families to understand that these procedures are designed to relieve pain, and not to totally eliminate it, and reduce the need for pain medication. Candidates for intrathecal neurolysis should be those with a short lifespan (less than 1 year) with insurmountable and well-localized cancer pain. The best results are obtained when intrathecal neurolysis is used for somatic pain. One study showed that 78–84% of patients with somatic pain responded well to treatment. In contrast, only 19–24% of patients with visceral pain had good pain control after the procedure.

Sympathetic Blocks [33, 34, 44]

There are several sites of sympathetic block that can be used to treat cancerous pain of the visceral organs. The sympathetic chain in the right places levels can also be targeted and blocked for any painful complaints. Neurolysis is done in almost all sympathetic blocks because catheter placement is difficult and impractical. The celiac plexus can be used for pain associated with cancer in the upper stomach area. The upper hypogastric plexus can be blocked due to cancerous pain of the pelvic organs such as the ovaries, bladder, and prostate. Impar block ganglia are effective for anal or vaginal cancer pain (Fig. 7.3).

Celiac Plexus Block [44–47]

The celiac plexus is located retroperitoneal in the upper abdomen. It is located on the level of the vertebrae T12 and L1 in front of the column of the diaphragm. The celiac plexus surrounds the abdominal aorta and the superior mesenteric and celiac arteries. The autonomic nerves that supply the liver, pancreas, gallbladder, stomach, spleen, kidneys, intestines, and adrenal glands appear in the full juice. Several studies have looked at the effectiveness of celiac plexus neurolysis in treating gastric cancer pain. One study evaluated the effectiveness of three different approaches to celiac plexus neurolysis in pancreatic cancer. Of the 61 patients with pancreatic cancer, 48% had complete pain relief after neurolysis blockade. The remaining 52% require additional therapy. A second study compared the procedure with oral drug therapy in 20 patients and found that celiac plexus neurolysis resulted in the same reduction in pain scores as therapy with a combination of NSAIDs and opioids. However, opioid use was significantly lower in the group of patients who underwent neurolysis than in the group that received only oral drug therapy during the 7 weeks of the study. In addition, the incidence of side effects such as relief, nausea, vomiting, and constipation was higher in patients receiving oral drug therapy. A study on the efficacy and safety of celiac plexus block concluded that this procedure provided long-term relief for 70–90% of patients with pancreatic and other upper stomach cancers. However, celiac plexus block may not be fully effective in advanced and untraceable pancreatic cancer. Such patients probably have other components of pain, such as somatic and / or neuropathic, that may not fully respond to a neurolysis block. The success rate of this block also decreases significantly when there are signs of a non-pancreatic disease, such as: celiac disease or portal adenopathy.

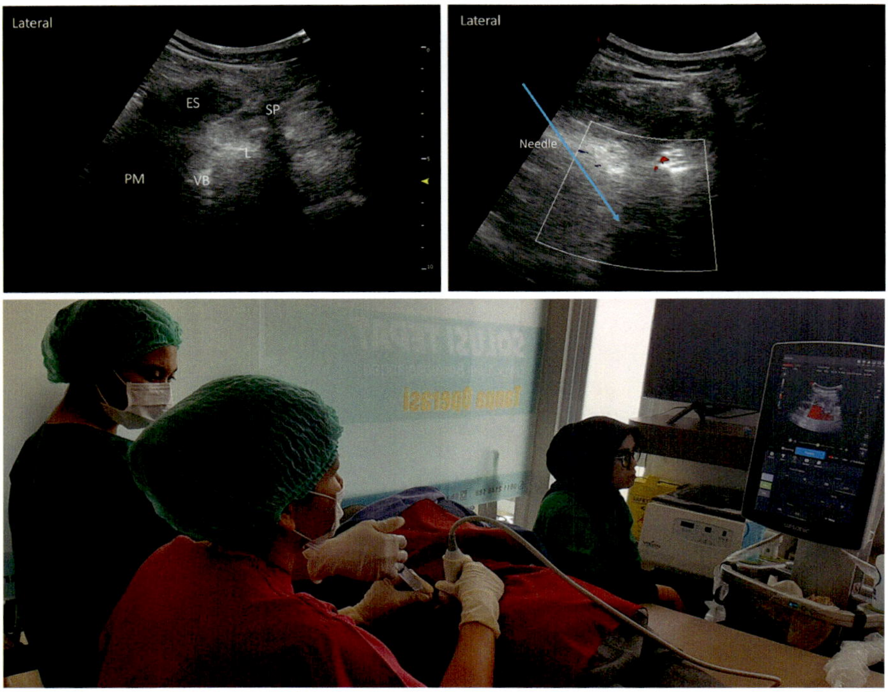

ES = Erector Spinae
L = Lamina
PM = Psoas Muscle
SP = Tip of Spinosus Process
VB = Vertebral Body
Blue arrow = Needle

Fig. 7.3 USG lumbar sympathetic block. Courtesy of Bandung Pain Rehab Center

Superior Hypogastric Block [44, 48, 49]

Cancer patients with a tumor spread to the pelvis may experience severe pain that does not respond to oral or parenteral opioids. Superior hypogastric block is effective for pain in the distal colon and rectum, as well as pain in the pelvic structures. This plexus is a retroperitoneal structure that extends on both sides of the lower third of the fifth lumbar vertebra to the upper third of the body of the first sacral vertebra. Several studies have shown the effectiveness of neurolysis block of the superior hypogastric plexus in the treatment of pelvic cancer pain. One study showed that this block has an effect on reducing pain scores in 18 of 26 patients (69%) with pelvic cancer pain. Another study looked at 159 patients with cancer-pelvic pain. Seventy-two percent (72%) had satisfactory pain relief after one or two neurolytic procedures. The average use of opioids decreased by 40% in all patients studied after 3 weeks of treatment.

Ganglion Impar Block [44, 50, 51]

The impar ganglion is an isolated retroperitoneal structure located at the level of the sacrococcygeal junction. This marks the end of two chains of the sympathetic nerve. Visceral pain in the perineal area can be effectively treated by neurolysis of the impar ganglion. Various approaches to ganglion control have been described in the literature and the clinical value of this block is well known. No serious complications of this block have been reported, although infection and fistula formation can be harmful and life-threatening in immunocompromised patients or those who have received radiation therapy to the perineum.

Peripheral Nerve Block [36, 52, 53]

Peripheral nerve or plexus blocks help when cancer pain occurs in one or more peripheral nerves. The role of peripheral nerve blocks as the sole or main method of pain relief in cancer patients may be limited, as most of these patients experience pain in a variety of situations, particularly those with advanced disease. However, when combined with other concomitant therapies such as chemotherapy and radiation, an element of the patient's general painful condition may be removed. Neurolytic agents such as alcohol or phenol have traditionally been used to block peripheral nerves. Alcohol can create a painful anesthetic when injected around the myelin nerves. Phenol is much more painful to inject and a better choice for peripheral nerve neurolysis. Other types of nerve destruction include radiofrequency ablation and cryo-ablation. In recent years there has been growing interest in the use of local anesthetic infusions to block peripheral nerves, aided by advances in catheter and infusion pump technology. The use of nerve stimulus or ultrasound to aid nerve identification and catheter placement facilitate nerve blocking procedures, achieving better pain relief results. Physicians can face many challenges when performing peripheral nerve blocks in cancer patients. The presence of open tissue edema in advanced malignancy may make it difficult or impossible to identify markers such as protrusions and peripheral impulses. Neuroanatomy can be distorted by tumor invasion or compression, as well as scarring and contracts of radiation therapy. This can be solved by placing the block and catheter using a real-time ultrasonic guide. Reported peripheral nerve blocks include femoral nerve block, sciatic nerve block, arm plexus block, suprascapular block, psoas compartment block, distal lumbar plexus block, erector spinae block (Fig. 7.4), paravertebral block, and interpleural block (Fig. 7.5), ilioinguinal nerve block (Fig. 7.6), sphenopalatine ganglion block (Fig. 7.7), trigeminal ganglion block (Fig. 7.8). Interpleural block has been used in the treatment of cancer pain due to metastatic bronchogenic carcinoma, which affects the pleural and thoracic wall, as well as chronic pain in patients with end-stage pancreatic, kidney cells, breast cancer and lymphoma.

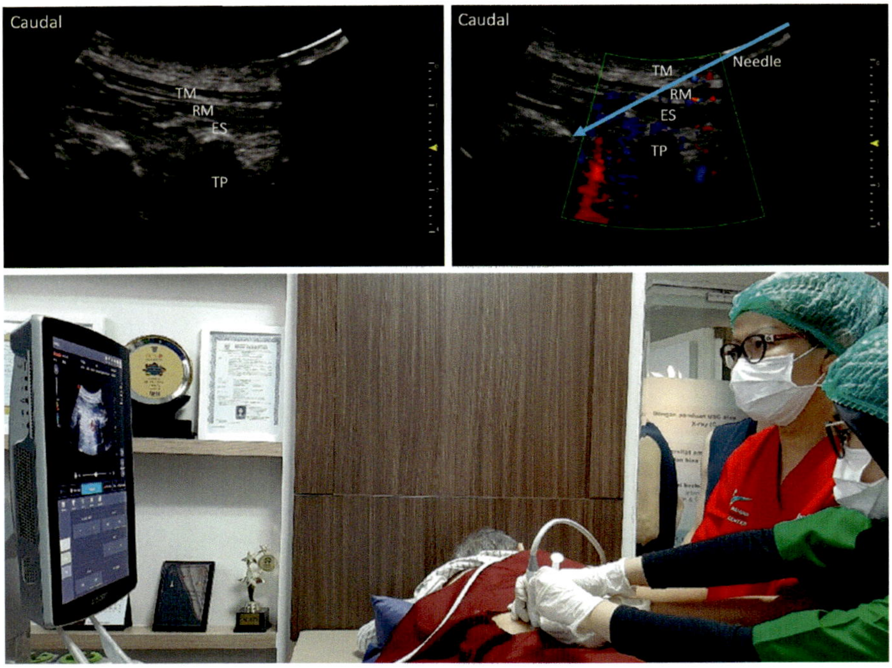

TM = Trapezius muscle
RM = Rhomboid muscle
ES = Erector spinae
TP = Transverse Process of T4
Blue arrow = needle
The needle is inserted in-plane from cranial to caudal with the linear probe placed longitudinally, 3 cm lateral to the midline.

Fig. 7.4 Erector spinae block. Courtesy of Bandung Pain Rehab Center

Neurostimulation [32, 34, 54]

Peripheral Nerve Stimulation

Peripheral Nerve Stimulation (PNS) is based on the "gate control theory of pain" by Melzack and Wall on 1965. The gates in the spinal cord dorsal horn laminae regulate nociceptive and non-nociceptive input. When the non-nociceptive input gates are activated (electrified), it close or override the gates for non-nociceptive input. This theory explains why when we rub a painful site on our body, the pain is reduced [55].

Some theories that explain the pain-relieving effect of PNS include: [1] failure of excitation in c-fiber nociceptors and dorsal horn activity suppression, [2] axon conduction propagation prevented by stimulation-induced blockade of cell membrane depolarization, and [3] dorsal horn neurons long-term potentiation and decreased

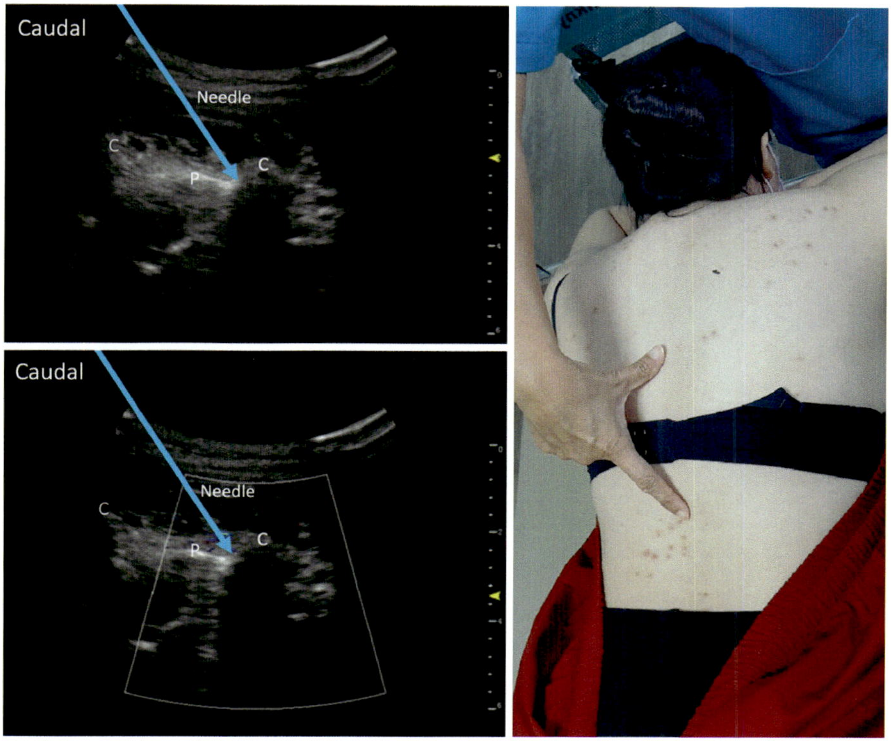

C = Costa
P = Pleura
Blue arrow = Needle

Fig. 7.5 Left 8th–9th Intercostal Nerve block in Lung Cancer patient metastasized to left Latissimus Dorsi Muscle. Courtesy of Bandung Pain Rehab Center

hyperexcitability, [4] excitatory amino acids depletion (aspartate, glutamate), and inhibitory transmitters release increase (GABA) [55].

PNS is recommended for chronic and severe pain, intractable pain despite conventional treatment and surgery. Criteria for PNS recipients are: [55].

1. Predominantly localized pain to one nerve
   Pain should correspond to the sensory distribution of a single peripheral nerve. Neuromodulation techniques such as PNS or Subcutaneous Peripheral Nerve Stimulation (SPNS) are effective for focal distributed pain [56].
2. Pain relieved by peripheral nerve block
   Primary pain and secondary hyperalgesia should be relieved by local anesthetic in the peripheral nerve.
3. No pathologies correctible by surgery
   Imaging for PNS screening is important to exclude any correctible pathology, such as osseous entrapment due to fracture, callus, or fibrous bands by plain film radiograph, MRI for identifying compressive mass.

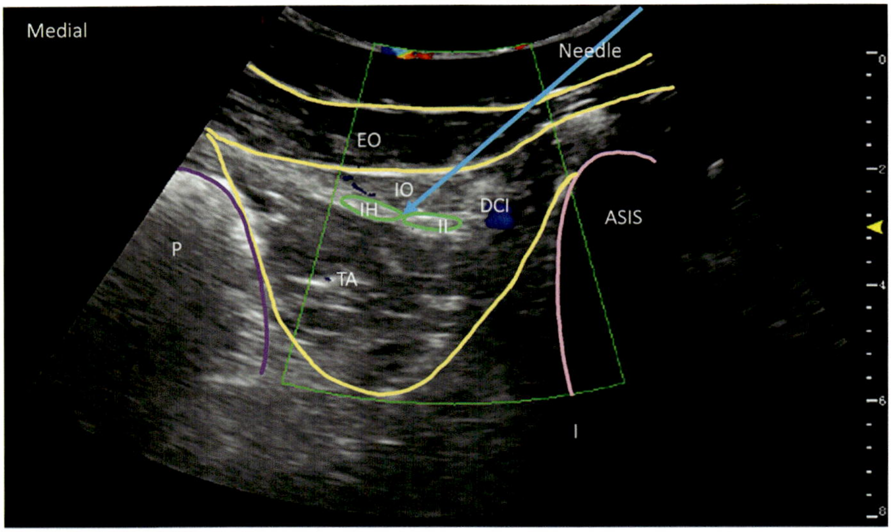

ASIS = Anterior Superior Iliac Spine
DCI = Deep Circumflex Iliac Artery
EO = External Oblique Muscle
II = Ilioingiunal Nerve
IH = Iliohypogastric Nerve
IO = Internal Oblique Muscle
P = Peritoneum
T = Transversus Abdominis Muscle
Blue arrow = Needle

Fig. 7.6 Ilioinguinal nerve block. Courtesy of Bandung Pain Rehab Center

4. Satisfactory results from psychological assessments
   Physicians should be aware of any psychological problem such as mood disorders, personality disorders, drug-seeking or manipulative behaviors, or any concern that will affect the stimulator use and outcome.

PNS and SPNS are valuable options for unresectable tumors where the neural elements are involved; such as head and neck tumors resulting chronic headaches or facial pain, abdominal or pelvic tumors leading to visceral pain, and extremity tumors causing neuropathic pain [56].

Typically, two-procedure set-up is done for PNS placement: first is the implantation of temporary electrode to test the adequacy of the treatment; and secondly, after 5–7 days when adequate pain relief is achieved to create a subcutaneous pocket for the receiver/battery [55, 57].

Successful benefits from PNS for cancer associated neuropathic pain are recorded in post-mastectomy pain syndrome, lumbar and cervical radiculopathy, and femoral nerve radiculopathy. PNS are implanted for 60 days in seven cases. The average pain score before PNS was 9.0, and can decrease to an average of 3.1 after extraction (on the 60th day and 1 on the 45th day for emergency MRI) [58].

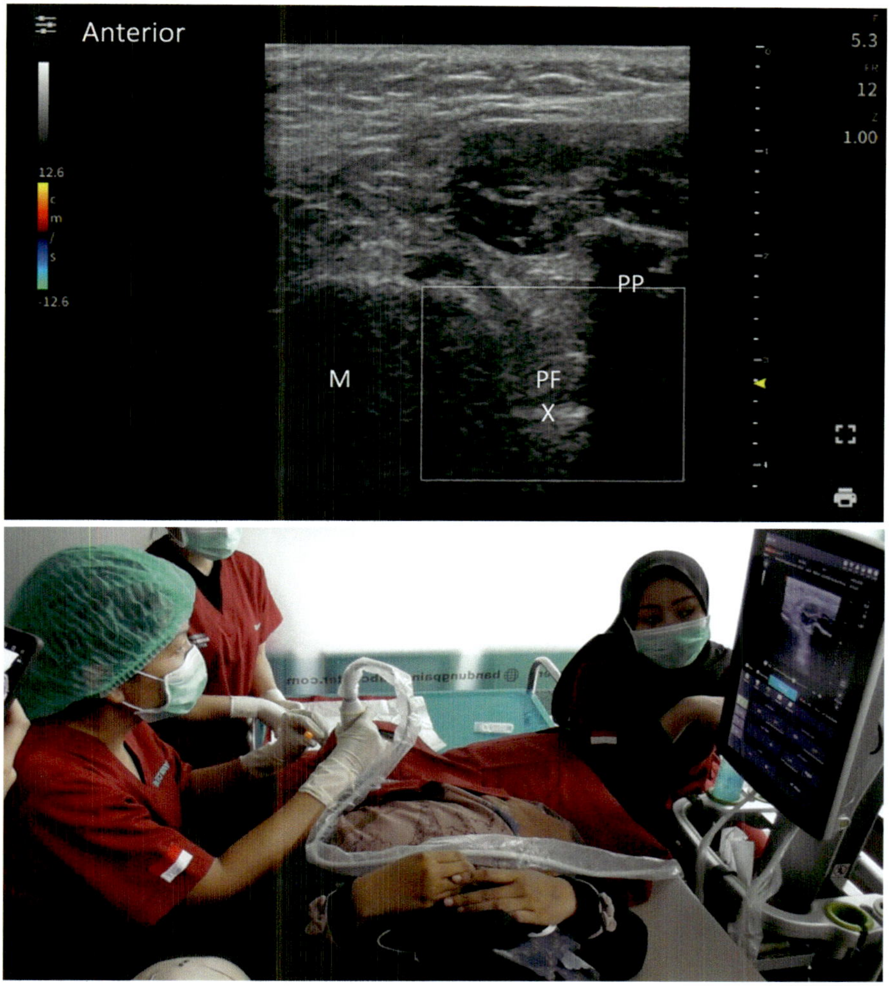

M = Maxilla
PF = Pterygoid fossa
PP = Pterygoid process of the sphenoid bone
X = Needle tip placement
The patient is positioned supine with the head facing the contralateral side of the needle position. The linear probe is positioned transversely anterior to the ear tragus.

Fig. 7.7 Sphenopalatine ganglion block. Courtesy of Bandung Pain Rehab Center

Spinal Cord Stimulation

Spinal Cord Stimulation (SCS), which came out as one of the clinical applications of gate control theory, has been used since 1970 to treat neuropathic and ischemic pain, with more than 30.000 SCS implantations each year [59].

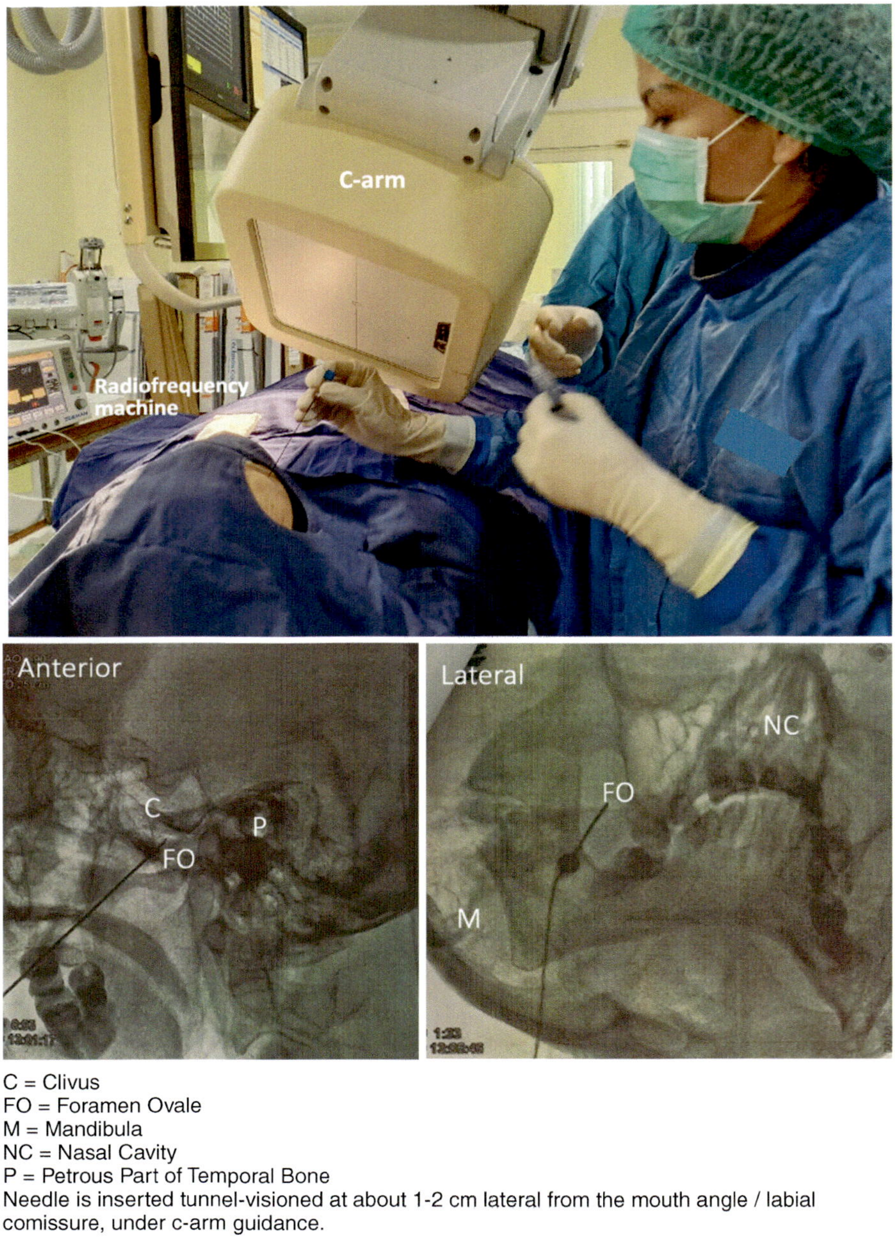

Fig. 7.8 Radiofrequency with CT scan guide in trigeminal ganglion. Courtesy of Bandung Pain Rehab Center

The goal of SCS implantation is to induce a comfortable level of paresthesia which will cover pain in cancer patients. The clinical goal in SCS treatment is to achieve at least 50% pain relief. Other benefits of SCS include: [1] decrease in medication and other health care needs, [2] improvement of activities of daily living, independence, quality of life, neurologic function, and decrease in signs of depression, [3] return to work if the only obstacle was uncontrollable chronic pain [59].

The implantation stages of SCS are as follows [54]:

1. Pain physician visit to evaluate the pain and to confirm whether patient is suitable for SCS
2. Psychological evaluation to understand the patient's needs and expectations from the therapy.
3. Trial stimulation to evaluate the pain improvement in quality of life (activities of daily living, psychological and social factors), the stimulation takes about 3 to 8 days.
4. Diagnostic imaging with MRI to ascertain whether the patient has an obstruction within high lumbar and thoracic spinal to consider any problem about safe lead placement. This stage can be done before trial stimulation. Imaging also will help the physicians to decide whether to refer the patient to a surgeon for implantation, or to decide the lead size suitable for the patient's condition.
5. Permanent implantation.

A study including 15 cancer patients with associated intractable chronic low back pain reported a significant pain relief (>50% reduction in Visual Analog Scale/VAS) in 12-month follow-up. Thirteen patients were able to decrease or discontinue their pain medications, while two patients still take oxycodone or morphine. Positive outcomes in their quality of life were also reported with gradual return to social and educational activities [60].

In another study including 14 lung cancer patients with intractable chronic chest pain, it was reported to show significant pain relief (≥50% reduction in VAS) after one-month follow up, and improvement in 12 month follow up. Four patients decreased their pain medication while the others discontinued. No complications were reported [61].

References

1. Caraceni A, Shkodra M. Cancer pain assessment and classification. Cancers (Basel). 2019;11(4):510.
2. Everdingen MHJVDB, De Rijke JM, Kessels AG, Schouten HC, Van Kleef M, Patijn J. Prevalence of pain in patients with cancer: a systematic review of the past 40 years. Ann Oncol. 2007;18(March):1437–49.
3. Bhaskar AK, Simpson KH. Interventional management of pain in cancer and palliative care key points. Medicine (Baltimore) [Internet]. 2019;48(1):9–13. https://doi.org/10.1016/j.mpmed.2019.10.014.
4. World Health Organization. Cancer pain relief: with a guide to opioid availability, vol. 34. 2nd ed; 1997. p. 172.

5. Tay W, Ho K. The role of interventional therapies in cancer pain management. Ann Acad Med Singapore. 2009;38(11):989–97.
6. Mantyh PW. Cancer pain: causes, consequences, and therapeutic opportunities. In: McMahon SB, Koltzenburg M, Tracey I, Turk D, editors. Wall and Melzack's textbook of pain. 6th ed. Philadelphia: Elsevier Saunders; 2013.
7. Zhu Z, Friess H, di Mola FF, Zimmermann A, Graber HU, Korc M, et al. Nerve growth factor expression correlates with perineural invasion and pain in human pancreatic cancer. J Clin Oncol Off J Am Soc Clin Oncol. 1999;17(8):2419–28.
8. Ye Y, Dang D, Zhang J, Viet CT, Lam DK, Dolan JC, et al. Nerve growth factor links oral cancer progression, pain, and cachexia. Mol Cancer Ther. 2011;10(9):1667–76.
9. Mercadante S, Ripamonti C, Fulfaro F. Malignant bone pain: pathophysiology and treatments. Curr Rev Pain. 2000;4(3):187–96.
10. Fainsinger RL, Nekolaichuk CL. A " TNM " classification system for cancer pain: the Edmonton classification system for cancer. Support Care Cancer. 2008;16:547–55.
11. Situ D, Wang J, Shao W, Zhu Z-H. Assessment and treatment of cancer pain: from Western to eastern. Ann Palliat Med. 2012;1(1):32–44.
12. Garg R. Acute pain syndromes in cancer, J Anesth Crit Care. 2016;4(3)
13. Fernandes R, Mazzarello S, Majeed H, Smith S, Shorr R, Hutton B, et al. Treatment of taxane acute pain syndrome (TAPS) in cancer patients receiving taxane-based chemotherapy—a systematic review. Support Care Cancer. 2016;24(4):1583–94.
14. Portenoy RK, Ahmed E. Cancer pain syndromes. Hematol Oncol Clin North Am [Internet]. 2018;32(3):371–86. https://doi.org/10.1016/j.hoc.2018.01.002.
15. Paice JA. Management of Pain at the end of life. In: Benzon HT, Fishman SM, Cohen SP, Hurley R, Malik K, Peng P, editors. Essentials of pain medicine. 4th ed. Philadelphia: Elsevier; 2017.
16. Sharma V, de Leon-Casasola O. Cancer pain. In: Benzon HT, Rathmell JP, Wu CL, Turk DC, Argoff CE, Hurley RW, editors. Practical management of pain. 5th ed. Philadelphia: Elsevier Mosby; 2014.
17. Fitzgibbon DR. Cancer pain: principles of management and pharmacology. In: Fishman SM, Ballantyne JC, Rathmell JP, editors. Bonica's management of pain. 4th ed. Lippincott William & Wilkins; 2010.
18. Vargas-Schaffer G. Is the WHO analgesic ladder still valid? Can Fam Physician [Internet]. 2010;56(6):514–7. e202-5. Available from: http://www.ncbi.nlm.nih.gov/pubmed/20547511%0A, http://www.pubmedcentral.nih.gov/articlerender.fcgi?artid=PMC2902929
19. Mcguire LS, Slavin K. Revisiting the WHO analgesic ladder for surgical management of pain. AMA J Ethics. 2020;22(8):E695–701.
20. Pergolizzi BJV, Raffa RB. The WHO pain ladder: do we need another step? Pract Pain Manag [Internet]. 2014;14(1):1–17. Available from: http://www.practicalpainmanagement.com/resources/who-pain-ladder-do-we-need-another-step
21. Yoon E, Babar A, Choudhary M, Kutner M, Pyrsopoulos N. Acetaminophen-induced hepatotoxicity: a comprehensive update. J Clin Transl Hepatol. 2016;4(2):131–42.
22. Herndon CM, Dankenbring DM. Patient perception and knowledge of acetaminophen in a large family medicine service. J Pain Palliat Care Pharmacother [Internet]. 2014;28(2):109–16. https://doi.org/10.3109/15360288.2014.908993.
23. Lookabaugh BL, Von Gunten CF. Approach to the Management of Cancer Pain. In: Benzon HT, Raja SN, Fishman SM, Liu SS, Cohen SP, Hurley R, et al., editors. Essentials of pain medicine. 4th ed. Philadelphia: Elsevier; 2017.
24. Wong RSY. Role of nonsteroidal anti-inflammatory drugs (NSAIDs) in cancer prevention and cancer promotion. Adv Pharmacol Sci. 2019;2019:3418975.
25. Liu B, Qu L, Yan S. Cyclooxygenase-2 promotes tumor growth and suppresses tumor immunity. Cancer Cell Int. 2015;15(1):2–7.

26. Paez Borda A, Fonteyne V, Papaioannou EG, Charnay-Sonnek F. Guidelines on pain management & palliative care. Eur Assoc Urol [Internet]. 2013;(March):261–81. Available from: https://uroweb.org/wp-content/uploads/25-%0APain-Management_LR.pdf
27. Kandasamy G, Sivanandy P, Khobrani M, Almaghaslah D, Almanasef M. Effectiveness of antiemetics in the management of chemotherapy-induced nausea and vomiting in cancer patients following chemotherapy guidelines. Indian J Pharml Sci. 2019;81(March):757–65.
28. Navari RM. Managing nausea and vomiting in patients with cancer: what works. Oncology (Williston Park). 2018;32(3):121–125,131,136.
29. Sykes NP. Cancer pain management, gastrointestinal dysfunction as opioid side effects. In: Schmidt RF, Willis WD, editors. Encyclopedia of Pain [Internet]. Berlin: Springer; 2007. p. 240–3. https://doi.org/10.1007/978-3-540-29805-2_528.
30. Murinson BB. The role of antidepressants in the treatment of chronic pain. In: Deer TR, Leong MS, Gordin V, editors. Treatment of chronic pain by medical approaches. Springer; 2015. p. 43–50.
31. Rathmell JP. Atlas of image-guided intervention. 2nd ed. Philadelphia: Lippincott William & Wilkins; 2012.
32. Waldman SD. In: Waldman SD, editor. Atlas of interventional pain management. 4th ed. Philadelphia: Elsevier Saunders; 2015.
33. Baheti DK, Bakshi S, Gupta S, Gehdoo RSP, editors. Interventional pain management: a practical approach. 2nd ed. New Delhi: Jaypee Brothers Medical Publishers; 2016.
34. Diwan S, Staats P, editors. Diwan-Staat's atlas of pain medicine procedure. New York: McGraw-Hill Education Medical; 2015.
35. Benzon HT. In: Benzon HT, Rathmell JP, Wu CL, Turk DC, Argoff C, Hurley RW, editors. Practical Management of Pain. 5th ed. Elsevier Mosby; 2014.
36. Hadzic A, Carrera A, Clark TB, Gadsden J, Karmakar MK, Sala-Blanch X, et al., editors. Hadzic's peripheral nerve blocks and anatomy for ultrasound-guided regional anesthesia. 2nd ed. New York: McGraw-Hill Medical; 2012.
37. Fishman SM, Ballantyne JC, Rathmell JP, editors. Bonica's management of pain. 4th ed. Philadelphia: Lippincott William & Wilkins; 2010.
38. Vissers KCP, Besse K, Wagemans M, Zuurmond W, Giezeman MJMM, Lataster A, et al. Pain in patients with cancer. In: van Zundert J, Patijn J, Hartrick CT, Lataster A, Huygen FJPM, Mekhail N, et al., editors. Evidence-based interventional pain medicine according to clinical diagnoses. West Sussex: Wiley-Blackwell; 2012.
39. Rathmell JP. Interlaminar epidural injection. In: Atlas of image-guided intervention in regional anesthesia and pain medicine. 2nd ed. Philadelphia: Lippincott William & Wilkins; 2012.
40. Datta S. Intrathecal Implantable Devices. In: Baheti DK, Bakshi S, Gupta S, Gehdoo RSP, editors. Interventional pain management: a practical approach. 2nd ed. New Delhi: Jaypee Brothers Medical Publisher (P) Ltd.; 2016.
41. Rathmell JP. Implantable spinal drug delivery system placement. In: Atlas of image-guided intervention in regional anesthesia and pain medicine. 2nd ed. Philadelphia: Lippincott William & Wilkins; 2012.
42. Doshi KM. Subarachnoid or intrathecal neurolysis. In: Baheti DK, Bakshi S, Gupta S, Gehdoo RSP, editors. Interventional pain management: a practical approach. 2nd ed. New Delhi: Jaypee Brothers Medical Publishers; 2016.
43. Candido KD, Knezevic NN. Neurolytic blocks. In: Diwan-Staat's atlas of pain medicine procedures. New York: McGraw-Hill Education Medical; 2015.
44. LoDico MJ, de Leon-Casasola O. Neurolysis of the symphatetic axis for cancer pain management. In: Benzon HT, Rathmell JP, Wu CL, Turk DC, Argoff CE, Hurley RW, editors. Practical management of pain. 5th ed. Philadelphia: Elsevier Mosby; 2014.
45. Candido KD, Knezevic NN. Celiac plexus block using CT guidance. In: Trescot A, editor. Diwan-Staat's atlas of pain medicine procedures. New York: McGraw-Hill Education Medical; 2015.

46. Candido KD, Staats PS, Hunter CW, Diwan S. Celiac plexus block using fluoroscopic guidance. In: Trescot A, editor. Diwan-Staat's atlas of pain medicine procedures. New York: McGraw-Hill Education Medical; 2015.
47. Jain S. Celiac Plexus Block. In: Baheti DK, Bakshi S, Gupta S, Gehdoo RSP, editors. Interventional pain management: a practical approach. 2nd ed. New Delhi: Jaypee Brothers Medical Publishers; 2016.
48. Jain S. Superior hypogastric plexus block. In: Baheti DK, Bakshi S, Gupta S, Gehdoo RSP, editors. Interventional pain management: a practical approach. 2nd ed. New Delhi: Jaypee Brothers Medical Publishers; 2016.
49. Stogicza A. Superior and inferior hypogastric plexus block. In: Trescot A, editor. Diwan-Staat's atlas of pain medicine procedures. New York: McGraw-Hill Education Medical; 2015.
50. Chien GCC, Singh H, Vrooman BM. Ganglion Impar block. In: Baheti DK, Bakshi S, Gupta S, Gehdoo RSP, editors. Interventional pain management: a practical approach. 2nd ed. New Delhi: Jaypee Brothers Medical Publishers; 2016.
51. Hunter CW, Diwan S. Ganglion Impar block. In: Trescot A, editor. Diwan-Staat's atlas of pain medicine procedures. New York: McGraw-Hill Education Medical; 2015.
52. Hadzic A, Vloka JD. Peripheral nerve blocks principles and practice. New York: McGraw-Hill Professional; 2004.
53. Hadzic A, editor. Hadzic's textbook of regional anesthesia and acute pain management. 2nd ed. New York: McGraw-Hill Education; 2017.
54. Hurley RW, Burton AW. Spinal cord and peripheral nerve stimulation. In: Benzon HT, Rathmell JP, Wu CL, Turk DC, Argoff CE, Hurley RW, editors. Practical management of pain. 5th ed. Philadelphia: Elsevier Mosby; 2014. p. 939–51.
55. Dorsi MJ, Belzberg AJ. Peripheral nerve stimulation. In: Fishman SM, Ballantyne JC, Rathmell JP, editors. Bonica's management of pain. 4th ed. Philadelphia: Wolters Kluwer Health/Lippincott Williams & Wilkins; 2010.
56. Sweet JA, Boulis NM. Peripheral nerve stimulation for the treatment of cancer. Pain. 2019;2019:255–9.
57. Nayak R, Banik RK. Current innovations in peripheral nerve stimulation. Pain Res Treat. 2018;2018(1):9091216.
58. Mainkar O, Sollo CA, Chen G, Legler A, Gulati A. Pilot study in temporary peripheral nerve stimulation in oncologic pain. Neuromodulation. 2020;23(6):819–26.
59. Linderoth B, Meyerson BA. Spinal cord and brain stimulation. In: McMahon SB, Koltzenburg M, Tracey I, Turk D, editors. Wall and Melzack's textbook of pain. 6th ed. Philadelphia: Elsevier Saunders; 2013.
60. Yakovlev AE, Resch BE. Spinal cord stimulation for cancer-related low Back pain. Am J Hosp Palliat Med. 2012;29(2):93–7.
61. Yakovlev AE, Resch BE, Karasev SA. Treatment of cancer-related chest wall pain using spinal cord stimulation. Am J Hosp Palliat Med. 2010;27(8):552–6.

Chapter 8
Neurodegenerative Diseases and Pain

Ernesto S. Cruz, Ian B. Maitin, Najaah Hussain, Joseph Lapenna, and Mia Song

Introduction

Many neurologic and neurodegenerative disorders are complicated by chronic and frequently debilitating pain. As our understanding of the physiology of pain evolves, the concept that the brain plays a pivotal role in the development and control of chronic aberrant pain signals has solidified. It is the current belief that pain may be a result of neurological disease and may often be considered a component of the disease. Multiple Sclerosis, Parkinson's disease, Syringomyelia and Stroke are a few of the neurologic disorders in which patients often experience some type of chronic pain which complicates their disease course and influences their quality of life. The degenerative diseases affecting the central nervous system are going to increase in parallel to the lengthening of survival. The management of Alzheimer's disease (AD) and other dementias, Parkinson's disease (PD) and PD-related disorders, and motor neuron diseases (MND), is mainly targeted to motor and cognitive impairment, with special care for vital functions such as breathing and activities of daily living. Focused treatment of pain in these conditions may have a positive impact on the global burden of these devastating diseases.

E. S. Cruz (✉) · I. B. Maitin · N. Hussain · J. Lapenna · M. Song
Department of Physical Medicine and Rehabilitation, Philadelphia, PA, USA

Lewis Katz School of Medicine at Temple University, Philadelphia, PA, USA

© The Author(s), under exclusive license to Springer Nature Switzerland AG 2022

J. de Castro, Y. El Miedany (eds.), *Advances in Chronic and Neuropathic Pain*, Contemporary Rheumatology, https://doi.org/10.1007/978-3-031-10687-3_8

Parkinson's Disease

Parkinson's Disease is a chronic neurodegenerative disorder, with many disabling motor ramifications, resulting from depletion of dopamine in the substantia nigra. The disease is frequently associated with tremors, rigidity, and postural instability with functional deficits. Less known is the prevalence of chronic pain among Parkinson patients [1]. This non-motor effect is under recognized and often untreated. Up to 60% of Parkinson patients experience significant pain which affects their quality of life [2]. Many patients fail to mention pain to their physician which they are experiencing. Some physicians do not recognize their patient is in pain, or do not prioritize treatment for pain, while other physicians are uncomfortable or unfamiliar with treating chronic pain. Lastly, some physicians regard chronic pain in some patients as psychogenic. Analgesic use has been found to be lower for Parkinson pain patients than non-Parkinson patients despite evidence of more severe pain and impairment of quality of life [3].

There are multiple sources of pain in this population, such as dystonia, musculoskeletal pain, central pain, and nerve pain [2]. Management of Parkinson pain should be initiated as early as possible. It is imperative to distinguish Parkinson pain from non-Parkinson, and to separate the types of Parkinson pain, as treatment varies with the type of pain.

Dystonia may cause sustained muscle twisting with forceful or painful contractions. Dystonia can cause joint pathology, such as frozen shoulder, which elicits pain. Focal dystonia, such as in the foot, is quite painful and can be addressed with toxin injection. More diffuse dystonia may respond to anticholinergics, amantadine, baclofen or deep brain stimulation [4].

Parkinson rigidity may cause joint or muscle pain which limits function and usually presents with aching, cramping and muscle and joint pain. This can be treated with NSAID's, opiates, antidepressants, and analgesics. Range of motion and stretching of the muscles is effective and transcranial magnetic stimulation has shown some effect. Mobility is helpful in the context of rigidity and stiffness.

Neuropathic pain in Parkinson patients may be due to central basal ganglia dysfunction and some patients get relief of pain with levodopa. There is evidence of abnormal somatosensory processing in the basal ganglia [2]. An irritated nerve root may distribute radicular pain, can be diagnosed with electrodiagnostics, and treated with therapy or decompressive surgery if severe.

Muscle cramping and dystonia are the most frequent pain complaints in Parkinson patients [4]. Opioids and cannabinoids have shown to be effective for treatment of pain in Parkinson patients, but safinamide has proven to be most effective [3]. Safinamide is a selective, reversible monoamine oxidase B inhibitor which decreases dopaminergic degradation and reuptake. The drug also inhibits voltage gated sodium channels in the inactivated state; thus the pain reduction may be due to dopaminergic and non-dopaminergic actions. Opioids are analgesic and inhibit neurotransmission, while cannabinoids control pain by way of cannabinoid receptor agonism. A comprehensive multidisciplinary approach to pain in the Parkinson patient has been shown to be effective, as have electrical therapy and Chinese therapies [3, 5].

Least effective in treating Parkinson pain are Dopa agonists, hydrotherapy, massage, mindfulness, and Pandoprunox, a partial Dopamine agonist used as an adjunct to Levodopa [3].

There is a known relationship between pain and depression, and such is true for Parkinson patients. They experience more severe depression, longer duration of depression, and lower mini-mental exam scores than other patients. The pain and depression decrease quality of life for Parkinson patients. Birgatta, et al. found that Parkinson patients felt a reduction in health-related quality of life, frequently related to pain [6].

There are no guidelines for the treatment of pain in Parkinson's Disease. There is a need for an algorithm or protocol to assist in treatment of this under recognized pathology which can affect function and quality of life.

Syringomyelia

Syringomyelia is a chronic spinal cord pathology in which a cavitation, or syrinx, develops within the spinal cord. It is rare (<1% of neurologic cases admitted) and most commonly associated with Chiari 1 malformation [5]. Pain is a common effect of the syrinx with 50–90% of syringomyelia patients experiencing chronic pain [7]. Frequently this presents with radicular pain, interscapular pain, or central spinal cord pain. 40% of patients' experience dysesthetic pain with burning, stinging, aching or pins and needles [7]. Symptoms are usually restricted to the upper limbs and thorax and can be aggravated by coughing or sneezing. There may be dermatomal pattern hypersensitivity. Skin symptoms may include hyperhidrosis, glossy skin, paleness, or coldness [7].

Animal studies have implemented substance P as a neurotransmitter having a role in pain modulation of spinal cord patients in which there is loss of spinal cord inhibition [7]. Some of the pain may be sympathetic-mediated, similar to causalgia peripherally. Studies have shown improvement with sympatholytic treatment such as stellate ganglion blocks and sympathectomy [7]. There appears to be a direct relationship between markers of spinal cord damage and central neuropathic pain [8].

Syringomyelia may alter neurotransmitter concentrations of gamma amino butyric acid, endorphins, enkephalins, cholesystokinins, neuropeptide Y, and others [7].

Cavitary lesions of the spinal cord can be defined with good resolution by MRI. Milhornt, et al. described dysesthetic pain in syringomyelia patients [9]. Fifty-one patients out of 131 reviewed experienced dysesthetic pain (37%). MRI revealed extension of the syrinx in the dorsolateral quadrant of the spinal cord ipsilateral to the pain in 43 of 51 patients (84%). Twenty-two of 37 (59%) improved with surgical treatment of the syringomyelia. Fifteen of 51 patients (41%) developed post-operative dysesthetic pain refractory to medical treatment. Some improved with time but six patients continued to have pain 2–6 years post operatively. One patient achieved pain relief with stellate gangliotomy and one got transient relief with regional sympathetic blocks. The study concluded that dysesthetic pain may be caused by disturbance of pain modulating content in the dorsolateral quadrant of the spinal cord and may cause a causalgia-like syndrome [9].

Analgesics and neuropathic pain medications such as antiepileptics, antispasmodics, and anti-inflammatories have had minimal effect on syringomyelia pain [7]. There is a need for standardized treatment protocols for pain due to syringomyelia to improve the quality of life for these patients.

Stroke

Post stroke pain is a well-recognized condition to be a persistent neuropathic pain of central origin, and that cannot be attributed to peripheral (nociceptive or neurogenic) origins. Shoulder pain is more common affecting up to 72% of post stroke survivors [10]. It is largely refractory to medical and surgical and thereby constitutes an unmet medical need.

It is well-documented that strokes, particularly the structures along the spinothalamocortical tract (spinothalamic tract, lateral thalamus, thalamic–parietal projections), produce central pain syndromes (central post-stroke pain) [10, 11]. The mechanisms underlying the severe, spontaneous, burning pain that occurs with thalamic stroke remain unclear. Several studies clearly showed that damage to specific regions of the brain produces central pain.

A pseudo thalamic syndrome, producing pain asymbolia (absent or inadequate emotional responses to painful stimuli) [12], results from a stroke producing damage to the posterior insula region [13, 14]. This is consistent with evidence indicating a significant role of the posterior insula in processing of thalamic pain.

Several findings related to central pain shed light on pain processing: (1) damage to the classic pain sensory systems (spinothalamic tract) seems to be pivotal in producing central pain syndromes resulting from stroke. Loss of grey matter in chronic pain has been well described and the altered connectivity resulting from either direct damage or indirect changes may contribute to a central pain syndrome [15]; (2) in thalamic pain, there is increased excitability of thalamic regions. Although there may be diminished activation in the thalamus at rest, hyperactivity (including bursting activity) is found in central post-stroke pain, suggesting derangement of an oscillatory pattern inside a sensory thalamocortical loop [16]; and (3) other changes including alterations in neural connectivity (deafferentation) [17], decreases in opioid receptor concentrations damage to lateral nociceptive thalamoparietal fibers, and altered chemistry are present in central pain. Functional imaging studies of a patient with thalamic pain suggest that the release of activity in anterior cingulate and posterior parietal regions is a plausible mechanism for central pain [18]. Current consensus about the pathogenesis of post stroke pain with various theories have been put forward, including hyperexcitability of thalamic neurons after interruption of ascending fibers in the spinothalamic pathway [19, 20], release of inhibition through a specific lesion to the lemniscal pathway or the spinothalamic tract [21], and release of inhibition through degeneration of corticothalamic neurons that project to the reticular nucleus and activate GABA-ergic inhibitory neurons which regulate neuronal excitability in the somatosensory relay nuclei of the thalamus [22, 23].

Treatment

It is not the intent of this section to provide details on pharmacological and nonpharmacological treatments of post stroke pain. Amitriptyline, a tricyclic antidepressant, is usually the drug of first choice [11, 20, 21]. However, its utility is limited by common adverse effects such as dry mouth, drowsiness, and constipation, as well as rarer instances of urinary retention, orthostatic hypotension and cardiac arrhythmia [20]. It is tempting to speculate that the apparent analgesic effect of amitriptyline may in fact stem from its mood-enhancing properties; however, it is not necessarily accompanied by a reduction in depressive symptoms [11].

Nonsteroidal anti-inflammatory drugs such as ibuprofen, acetylsalicylic acid and cyclo-oxygenase-2 inhibitors are not recommended. Antidepressants [12, 22, 23] such as amitriptyline and nortriptyline, as well as antiepileptics including lamotrigine, gabapentin, pregabalin and carbamazepine can be used as first-line treatments. For patients who are refractory to these treatments, opioids such as morphine [24] or levorphanol [25] may be prescribed, although no large studies have directly examined their efficacy for CPSP. Local anesthetics such as lidocaine [24], N-methyl-D-aspartate receptor antagonists including ketamine [26], cannabinoids, and botulinum toxin A are not recommended. In terms of combination therapy, gabapentin or pregabalin with amitriptyline is not effective. Gabapentin is relatively safe, with the most common side effects being dizziness and sedation. Lamotrigine is an anti-epileptic medication with non-NMDA anti-glutamatergic activity and is relatively well-tolerated, although there is documented potential for severe dermatologic adverse reactions such as Stevens-Johnson syndrome and toxic epidermal necrolysis.

Nonpharmacological interventions have also been used in the treatment of post stroke pain. For example, deep brain stimulation of the central grey matter was used years ago for intractable pain. Study showed that chronic epidural electrical stimulation of the motor cortex results in a reduction in pain [25–27]. Treatment of this condition can be frustrating and multi-modal approaches are frequently used. Physical and occupational therapy are the mainstay of treatment and function by decreasing the pain and improving function of the affected limb [23, 24]. Desensitization of the affected limb through sensory overload using various types of stimuli, contrast baths and massage are among the techniques and modalities that can help the patient overcome the pain [23]. At the same time, a concerted effort should be made to restore as much range of motion and motor strength as possible to prevent limb dysfunction. Physical and occupational therapy are valuable adjuncts in the treatment and are generally safe. However, therapy does require effort and commitment on the part of the patient to participate but, sometimes, access or transportation to see a therapist can be a barrier to treatment.

The use of tissue plasminogen activator (tPA) for selected stroke patients significantly curtails the morbidity and mortality associated with acute ischemic stroke [28]. By salvaging the ischemic penumbra, tPA may also prevent damage to the spinothalamocortical tract, and thus reduce the subsequent risk of post stroke pain [29, 30].

It is important to note that patient with post stroke pain condition is likely to experience not only pain and sensory abnormalities, but also considerable emotional distress. Behavioral therapies, massage, physical therapy and acupuncture are therefore recommended for alleviation of the anxiety, depression and sleep disorders that often accompany chronic pain syndromes such as post stroke pain [30].

Spinocerebellar Ataxia

Spinocerebellar ataxias (SCAs) comprise an extensive and heterogeneous group of neurodegenerative diseases with autosomal dominant inheritance [31]. Despite their inherent heterogeneity, the SCAs present certain consistent characteristics, such as the obvious core features of an ataxic syndrome and its phenomenological correlates, and the pathological substrate of a degenerative process involving the cerebellum and/or its connections.

Machado–Joseph disease is the most common spinocerebellar ataxia, also known as spinocerebellar ataxia type 3 [32] and is a neurodegenerative disease that include ataxia with extracerebellar neurological manifestations, such as dementia, epilepsy, visual disturbances, peripheral neuropathy, supranuclear ophthalmoplegia, pyramidal tract signs, and movement disorders such as parkinsonism, myoclonus, chorea and dystonia [33–35]. Although classically described as affecting the cerebellum, it affects several other brain regions including brainstem, basal ganglia, thalamus, posterior columns, and cerebral cortex. In a small study, nearly 50% of patients reported chronic pain including muscle cramps. This prevalence was similar to that of amyotrophic lateral sclerosis and much higher than in cases of peripheral axonal neuropathy. The study focused into the underlying pathological changes demonstrating axonal excitability significantly greater in SCA3 patients than in normal subjects, probably reflecting axonal regeneration or collateral sprouting [36]. Muscle excitability abnormalities occur in >80% of these patients and peripheral nerve damage correlates with the extent of muscle fasciculations. In addition, widespread neurodegeneration is observed in somatosensory (although pain is not specifically delineated) as well as primary sensory systems with alterations in dopaminergic and cholinergic systems [32]. Sensory symptoms including pain are observed across subtypes of spinocerebellar ataxia, with 48% of subjects complaining of pain or discomfort.

One emerging concept is that the cerebellum may play a role in chronic pain, based on its complex role in cognitive and affective processing. Current data suggest that the cerebellum is an integrator of multiple effector systems including affective processing, pain modulation, as well as sensorimotor processing.

As compared with other neurodegenerative disorders such as Parkinson's disease, quantitative and validated assessment tools are less developed [37]. The patients generally experience problems with mobility, usual activities, pain/discomfort, depression/anxiety, and self-care. Different population surveys have shown that 19% to 64% of patients report pain as a problem in selected SCA conditions [38]. In the same study, multivariate analysis revealed three independent predictors of subjective health status: ataxia severity, extent of noncerebellar involvement, and the presence of depressive syndrome. Although pain is not a primary invalidating factor in such patients, it may influence the quality of life as part of depression-related symptoms cohort and noncerebellar features.

In a recent systematic review reporting data from 1062 publications and 12,141 patients with different neuromuscular disorders, pain was found to be reported in 1 among 30 SCA sufferers [39]. However, pain may often be underestimated though it can be severe when related to dystonia. In SCA conditions, pain can be misdiagnosed and mistreated but successfully ameliorated by, for example, botulinum toxin therapy [40].

There are currently no cures for SCA and treatments (pharmacological therapy and physical therapy) target the symptoms such as pain, spasticity, tremor, stiffness, postural balance, gait disabilities, sleep problems, and depression. However, there are some very preliminary and nonvalidated data suggesting the use of umbilical cord mesenchymal stem cells in SCA [41].

Amyotrophic Lateral Sclerosis

Amyotrophic lateral sclerosis (ALS) is a progressive neurodegenerative disorder characterized by degeneration of upper and lower motor neurons in the cerebral cortex, brainstem, and spinal cord. This results in a characteristic phenotype of muscle weakness, dysphagia, dysarthria, respiratory failure, and eventual death usually within 2–4 years from symptom onset. ALS has traditionally been viewed as a purely motor disease. Because of this misconception, pain has been a largely neglected symptom in ALS patients until recently. Studies have shown that up to 85% of patients with ALS experience pain at some point during the course of their disease. If left untreated, pain has been correlated with a significant decline in quality of life [42].

The three most common sources of pain in ALS patients include musculoskeletal pain, muscle cramps, and spasticity [42]. Although electrodiagnostic studies and skin biopsies show evidence of somatosensory dysfunction, patients with ALS do not commonly endorse neuropathic pain features.

Musculoskeletal pain (or nociceptive pain) originates from injury to non-neural structures, such as bones, ligaments, tendons, or muscle tissue. Muscle atrophy, muscle weakness, and reduced mobility may result in injury to musculoskeletal structures. Peripheral nociceptors in these structures transmit pain signals to the central nervous system, leading to the development of nociceptive pain [43]. Patients may present with articular pain, pain from pressure injuries, and neck or low back pain [44]. In the late stages of ALS, pain may become chronic and patients may complain of diffuse pain that is hard to localize. In these stages, central sensitization is hypothesized to play a role in the maintenance of pain, although this has never been directly studied [44]. Patients with ALS who have been started on mechanical ventilation may develop novel sources of pain, such as pain from suctioning and pain from skin lesions caused by facial pressure from non-invasive ventilation masks [44].

Muscle cramps are another source of pain for ALS patients. Cramps likely originate from neuronal hyperexcitability of unstable motor units. They occur universally in ALS patients, affecting approximately 95% of patients at some point during the disease course and are a major source of pain in a quarter of these patients [45]. Cramps are frequently present during the early stages of the illness and there is a trend towards fewer cramps as the disease progresses [46]. Patients display a wide variability in the frequency and severity cramps from 1 month to the next. If patients do not experience cramps at the time of diagnosis, they tend to never develop frequent cramps as the disease progresses. Those older than 60 years of age and those with limb-onset disease experience more cramps than younger patients and those with bulbar-onset disease [46]. Cramps most commonly occur in the thighs and calves, followed by the hands and feet [46]. They may be worsened by cold temperatures and decreased circulation caused by maintaining muscles in static positions for prolonged periods of time [47].

Lastly, ALS patients may endorse pain from spasticity. Although spasticity itself does not cause pain, it can result in muscle fatigue and painful cramps [48]. If severe, spasticity may immobilize joints and lead to muscle contractures resulting in pressure injuries. Furthermore, spasticity can result in distorted biomechanics causing abnormal postures and gait, thus leading to new pain generators [48].

Treatment

After identifying the cause of pain, the appropriate non-pharmacological and pharmacological interventions should be implemented to appropriately manage pain. There are currently no treatment guidelines available to aid clinicians in managing pain in patients with ALS. Therefore, pain in these patients is managed based on expert opinion largely backed by case series and a small number of randomized controlled trials rather than published guidelines. Two sources of published recommendations are provided by the European Guidelines on the Clinical Management of ALS [46] and the Practice Parameters of the American Academy of Neurology [48].

For patients with musculoskeletal pain, non-steroidal anti-inflammatory drugs (NSAIDs) and acetaminophen are used as first-line treatment options, while opioids are used as second-line options when pain was difficult to control, particularly in advanced disease stages [44]. In these patients, opioids are also used to manage symptoms of respiratory insufficiency, such as poor sleep and dyspnea. Cannabinoids may be an effective option to improve pain in some patients. If used, side effects may include confusion, tachycardia, and amotivational syndrome. For patients with reduced mobility, it is important to initiate a daily exercise regimen consisting of stretching, assistive range of motion (ROM) exercises. Modalities such as ultrasound and laser therapy can be used as adjunct treatment options.

For ALS patients with muscle cramps, levetiracetam has been shown to reduce the severity and frequency of cramps in this population. Common side effects include fatigue, somnolence, and headache. Second-line treatment options include quinine sulfate and mexiletine. Quinine sulfate is commonly used in the off-label treatment and prevention of nocturnal leg cramps of any cause. It carries a black box warning cautioning against serious hematologic reactions and clinicians should monitor complete blood counts when prescribing. Mexiletine carries an off-label indication to manage painful muscle spasms in ALS patients. It is safe and well tolerated at doses of 300 mg per day with dose-dependent adverse effects including cardiac arrhythmias occurring at 900 mg per day. Once prescribed, medications should be weaned once cramps are adequately controlled since the frequency of cramps decreases as the disease progresses. Non-pharmacologic options that may be of benefit include stretching, massage, physical therapy, and hydrotherapy.

The mainstay of treating spasticity in ALS patients is physical therapy consisting of daily stretching, assistive ROM exercises, and moderate physical activity. Neutral-position splints can provide static stretching to the distal extremities. Although not formally studied in this population, baclofen, tizanidine, dantrolene, and benzodiazepines have been used with success as has botulinum toxin A. In ALS patients with intractable spasticity despite oral medications, intrathecal baclofen remains an option.

Clinicians should vigilantly assess ALS patients for pain as this symptom may develop early or late in the disease course and can contribute a significant decline in the patients' quality of life.

Patients with ALS may experience pain from a variety of causes. However, the three most common sources of pain include musculoskeletal pain, muscle cramps, and spasticity. When addressing these sources of pain, it is important to utilize both pharmacologic and non-pharmacologic treatment options. In addition to assessing for pain, clinicians should address factors that could aggravate pain, such as sleep disturbances and depression.

Huntington Disease

Huntington disease (HD) is a fatal neurodegenerative disorder inherited as an autosomal dominant manner and characterized by motor, cognitive, and behavioral changes. It results from a mutation in the huntingtin gene causing abnormal repetition of the CAG DNA sequence eventually resulting in a misfolded gene product. This protein causes degeneration of medium spiny neurons, which are mainly concentrated in the striatum [49]. The striatum primarily regulates the affective and cognitive dimensions of pain and thus plays a role in processing feelings related to pain unpleasantness and the emotional response to pain. The striatum also plays a role in analgesia and contains a high concentration of endogenous opiates and receptors. It is believed that patients with HD experience disturbed pain processing due to the degeneration of medium spiny neurons in the striatum. Additionally, patients with HD often do not report pain even after experiencing significant trauma. This is believed to be related to "unawareness" caused by impaired frontal-striatal networks [50]. A recent systematic review and meta-analysis reported the prevalence of pain to be approximately 41% in this population [51].

Studies evaluating pain in patients with HD are scarce and therefore, there are currently no treatment guidelines available to aid clinicians in managing pain in this population. Common causes of pain in HD include dystonia, chorea, contractures, musculoskeletal injuries including occult fractures, pressure injuries, constipation, and urinary retention [52]. Treatment mainly focuses on managing the underlying disorder. Due to cognitive dysfunction, patients with HD may not endorse pain when questioned or may have significant communication deficiencies that prevent the accurate assessment of pain. Clinicians should monitor for atypical manifestation of pain in this population such as increased confusion, agitation, and depression [53].

Alzheimer's Disease

Alzheimer's disease (AD) is a neurodegenerative disorder and a common form of dementia characterized by cognitive and behavioral impairments. AD is often comorbid with chronic pain with an estimated prevalence of 45.8% [54]; however, this may be underestimated given that some patients with Alzheimer's disease are unable to effectively communicate their pain compared to cognitively intact individuals [55]. Other studies have showed that pain is observed with a higher prevalence in patients with severe dementia [54, 56], and that pain intensity is positively correlated with dementia severity, neuropsychiatric symptoms, depression, agitation, and quality of life [57].

The neuropathophysiology involved in AD affects both pain processing and pain perception. To understand this, a distinction must be made between the medial and lateral pain systems. The medial pain system primarily involves the spinothalamic tract which projects directly to the intralaminar thalamic nuclei, the spinoreticular tract which projects to the reticular formation, and the spinomesencephalic tract which projects to the mesencephalon. The medial pain system is involved in the motivational-affective and cognitive-evaluative features of pain, which involves the memory for pain and the autonomic-neuroendocrine responses evoked by pain. The lateral pain system involves the spinothalamic tract neurons that project to the somatic sensory cortical areas, and it is involved in the sensory-discriminative features of pain, or the intensity, location, quality, and duration of pain [58].

The pathophysiological changes that occur with AD selectively affect most of the medial pain system while leaving the lateral pain system relatively well preserved. This clinically manifests as the perception of unaltered acute pain while there is an overall decrease in chronic pain in AD patients. Pickering et al. found that analgesic consumption in acute pain was not significantly different for AD patients and cognitively intact patients, whereas chronic pain analgesic consumption was significantly lower for AD patients. This is further evidence for the dissociation between the sensory-discriminative of the lateral pain system, and the motivational-affective of the medial pain system aspects of pain in AD patients [59]. Other studies have found that AD patients have fewer of the affective components of pain than non-demented elderly people. Several studies have shown that the pain threshold in response to an electrical stimulus is not changed in AD patients compared to cognitively intact patients, suggesting that the sensory-discriminative component of the lateral pain system is preserved in AD [58].

AD has been associated with neuronal loss in the locus ceruleus of the medial pain system [60]. Conversely, Song et al. proposed a mechanism of how chronic pain can accelerate AD pathogenesis. Chronic pain induces dysfunction in the locus ceruleus noradrenergic system, leading to neuroinflammation and enhanced norepinephrine transmission. This results in increased excitability in specific areas of the brain like the prefrontal cortex and hippocampus, which is suggested to induce microglial proinflammatory activation that promotes further AD pathogenesis [61].

Cognitive impairments in AD include memory deficits and impaired reasoning, which can affect the patient's ability to describe their pain. Furthermore, pain is often ignored, underestimated, or underreported in the elderly with dementia, and thus improperly treated. Pain in this cohort can manifest in various ways, including sleep disorders, decreased mobility, falls, malnutrition, depression, agitation, aggression, delirium, and reduced social participation. This can have serious consequences on health, the ability to perform activities of daily living, and overall quality of life. Prior to treatment, an assessment of pain should be made. While self-assessment scales are considered the gold standard, the presence of cognitive decreases their reliability and utility. The American Geriatrics Society published guidelines in 2002 for assessing behavioral indicators of pain, which includes evaluating for any persistent pain that impacts physical function, psychosocial function, or other aspects of quality of life. This may be supplemented by a physical exam, routine lab work, and evaluating patients' social support systems.

The goal in treating pain may not be to completely eliminate the pain entirely, but to decrease and reduce its intensity, duration, and frequency of the episodes in order to maximize independence in activities of daily living while minimizing adverse effects of the treatments. Treatment of chronic pain includes pharmacologic and non-pharmacologic approaches. Nonpharmacologic approaches include a wide variety of options including therapy, modalities, osteopathic manipulative medicine, acupuncture, and psychological therapy. Multimodal cognitive behavioral therapy has shown to significantly decrease pain. Gagliese et al. proposed that pain in older patients with dementia is the result of an intricate network of interactions between biopsychosocial phenomena, and that treatment of depression in older people with osteoarthritis can have a significant impact on function and pain [62].

When utilizing the pharmacologic approach, polypharmacy in the elderly must be taken into account, as well as age-related differences in pharmacokinetics and pharmacodynamic properties of drugs. Furthermore, a study by Benedetti found that the placebo mechanism was reduced in AD patients, who may require higher dosages of pain medications to obtain the analgesic effect that is normally reached in cognitively healthy individuals [63].

Non-opioid analgesics are recommended first, with gradual increases in dosages in order to monitor for adverse effects and build tolerance to the medication. Acetaminophen is an effective first-line approach for pain in patients with dementia. Other medications include nonsteroidal anti-inflammatory drugs (NSAIDs) , such as ibuprofen or naproxen. NSAIDs have shown to exhibit a "ceiling effect" where further increases in the dose does not correspond with more pain relief; however, these higher doses are associated with an increased risk for adverse effects such as gastrointestinal or cardiovascular disorders which can be life-threatening. The use of opioids in the long-term treatment of pain in the elderly with cognitive deficits lacks evidence. Drugs for neuropathic pain including gabapentinoids should be used cautiously and be monitored for side effects. Tricyclic antidepressants are not recommended because of the anticholinergic side effects as well as other side effects including urinary incontinence, hypotension, sedation, glaucoma, and cardiac arrhythmia. Serotonin and norepinephrine reuptake inhibitors are a good alternative to NSAIDs and opioids due to their ability to raise the pain threshold with a lower side effect profile; for example, duloxetine can be effective and is generally well tolerated. There is insufficient data on the use of antiepileptics for the treatment of pain in patients with dementia [55].

Spinal Muscular Atrophy

Spinal muscular atrophy (SMA) is an autosomal recessive disease characterized by the degeneration of alpha motor neurons in the spinal cord, leading to progressive muscle weakness and paralysis. It is caused by a deletion or mutation in the SMN1 gene. SMN1 is responsible for producing a protein called survival motor neuron protein (SMN) in all somatic cells. Although the exact pathogenesis is not known, it is thought to disrupt cellular functions that are unique to motor neurons leading to the selective degeneration of alpha motor neurons in the spinal cord, which results in progressive muscle weakness and paralysis.

SMA is divided into four types based on age of onset and motor function. SMA type 1 (Werdnig-Hoffman disease) is the most severe and most common type, accounting for about 60% of patients with SMA. It manifests during the first 6 months of age with onset of clinical signs including ataxia, hypotonia, symmetrical flaccid paralysis greater in the lower than upper extremities, and the inability to sit unsupported. Most infants with SMA type 1 die before age two due to bulbar dysfunctions and pulmonary complications. SMA type 2 is usually diagnosed between 6 months of age and 2 years. There is often a delay or failure in meeting motor milestones and are unable to walk independently, but patients achieve the ability to sit unsupported. SMA type 3 (Kugelberg-Welander disease) is typically diagnosed after 18 months of age and before 3 years, although it can be diagnosed much later in teenage years. Patients with SMA type 3 usually meet all major motor milestones, including walking independently; however, some may develop proximal muscle weakness and require wheelchair assistance later in life. They may also have scoliosis and joint contractures, and their disease course is usually slowly progressive. SMA type 4 is very rare, and usually is diagnosed in adulthood. It is characterized by mild motor impairments [64].

SMA patients have muscle weakness that can lead to multifactorial causes of pain, including contracture formation, spinal deformity, limited functional mobility, fractures, osteoporosis, and increased risk of pain. The exact pathogenesis of chronic pain in SMA patients has not been widely explored. Qu et al. studied SMA mice models, and found that there was a pronounced increase in response to both noxious and innocuous stimuli correlated with the hyperexcitability of nociceptive neurons in the dorsal root ganglion. They also found significantly elevated levels of norepinephrine which suggested that there may additionally be a peripheral process that induces pain hypersensitivity. Further exploring the pathophysiological mechanisms can guide future therapeutic approaches to treat chronic pain [65].

A study by Lager et al. showed that pain is a frequent problem in adolescents with SMA, affecting up to 71% adolescents with SMA. Pain was most frequently reported in the neck, back, and legs. This was attributed to a number of causes, including history of spinal surgery with continued pain, vertebral compression fractures due to immobility-induced osteoporosis and corticosteroid treatment. Furthermore, profound muscle weakness may contribute to pain as it can increase the total load on the musculoskeletal system; pain was commonly reported to be worse with sitting and relieved with change in position [66]. Another study by Abresch et al. showed that SMA adult patients did not experience pain to the same degree as other slowly progressive neuromuscular disorders despite significant muscle atrophy and deconditioning, and also that there was no increase in pain sensitivity compared to the general population [53].

Supportive care can help reduce disease impact and burden in SMA patients. Since pain can be exacerbated by muscle overuse and weakness, conservative treatment can include finding ways to conserve energy and achieving a balance between activity and rest. Patients may also benefit from electrical wheelchairs that can recline and tilt. Furthermore, therapy to prevent progression of contractures including stretching and orthotics can be beneficial. Orthoses can also help achieve assisted ambulation. Spinal bracing can be helpful for early prevention of scoliosis, while spinal surgery may be required for others [67].

Multiple Sclerosis

Multiple sclerosis [MS] is the most common immune-mediated inflammatory disease of the central nervous system. It affects women more than men (at a rate of more than 2:1) and this gap is increasing for unknown reasons. For the majority of these patients, the average age at onset is between 28–31 years old and is usually a few years earlier in women than men although it varies based on subtype (earlier in relapsing-remitting [25–28, 68] and later in primary progressive [38–40]) [69].

While no single presenting sign or symptom is pathognomonic for MS some are highly characteristic. These signs and symptoms include optic neuritis, headaches, sensory loss, paresthesias, motor dysfunction, ataxia, Lhermitte's sign, bowel and bladder dysfunction, weakness and *pain*. Pain in MS is not very well understood but certain pain syndromes appear more frequently in MS than the general population and warrant further investigation.

The prevalence of pain over the lifetime of a PwMS has been shown to be above 50% and the comorbidity of pain with depression is around 30% suggesting that chronic pain can leave one feeling helpless and depressed. A study of 157 patients showed that more than two-thirds felt they had insufficient pain care by their physicians suggesting that it is also a frequently undertreated condition in PwMS [69].

When treating pain experienced in MS it is important to distinguish a number of factors such as whether the pain is neuropathic or non-neuropathic, sensory or motor and whether the pain is primary or secondary [70]. Keep in mind that it is often not just one or the other, rather a combination of the two especially as the disease progresses over time.

There are 8 main types of pain experienced by PwMS. They are optic neuritis, central neuropathic pain, dysesthetic extremity pain, trigeminal neuralgia, Lhermitte's sign, painful tonic spasms, back and musculoskeletal pain and headaches. Current treatment of pain associated with MS is largely guided by a few RCTs conducted in patients with other central neuropathic pain conditions (post-stroke, SCI). General first line agents are medications such as gabapentin, pregabalin, lamotrigine and TCAs. As a second line, there is evidence for tramadol, opioid analgesics and SNRIs in the treatment of peripheral neuropathic pain [71, 72].

Starting with optic neuritis; MS is the most common cause of inflammation of the optic nerve and occurs in about 50% of individuals at some point during the course of their illness [72]. Most cases of ON occur in women, typically between 20-40 yrs. old, it is usually monocular and develops over hours to days. Treatment for ON is effective and well established with IV methylprednisolone, typically for 3 days followed by PO prednisone taper over 10 days [73].

Central neuropathic pain defined by Osterberg et al. as "if the distribution of pain was consistent with a CNS lesion and a thorough evaluation for nociceptive and peripheral neuropathic pain was negative, including a detailed history and physical exam, focused blood tests, and electrophysiology" [74]. Their study looked at a sample of 364 MS patients, 27.5% had what was considered definite central neuropathic pain, including 18 with trigeminal neuralgia. Of these, 91% had pain at the time of evaluation, most had constant daily pain and it disproportionately affected the lower extremities. Nearly all patients had abnormal sensory exams, with the most common abnormality being decreased cold sensation, which the authors interpreted as support for the hypothesis that central neuropathic pain in MS patients often results from lesions in spinothalamocortical pathways [74].

Dysesthetic extremity pain (sometimes referred to as central neuropathic extremity pain), is usually a chronic form of pain described as a "burning", typically bilateral, affecting the legs and feet, usually worse at night and can be exacerbated by physical activity [75, 76]. It is thought to be caused by lesions in spinal cord nociceptive pathways affecting the inhibitory function of GABA interneurons, the differentiating factor from central neuropathic pain.

For treating neuropathic pains, the focus is on three targets; reducing CNS activity, enhancing reuptake of serotonin and noradrenaline, and influencing adrenoreceptors. This can be achieved through the action of anticonvulsants, benzodiazepines, baclofen, SSRI's, SNRI's, TCAs and clonidine. Overall evidence is lacking but what does exist, suggests starting with TCAs, then gabapentin/pregabalin and lastly lamotrigine. Should all of those fail to provide relief, the last line is generally opioids.

Trigeminal neuralgia [TN] occurs at roughly 20x the prevalence of the general population and is the presenting symptom of MS in around 14% of cases. Of those with MS who have TN, up to one third are bilateral, they tend to be younger, are less likely to have an ophthalmic nerve distribution and more commonly experience autonomic symptoms including lacrimation, conjunctival injection and rhinorrhea. Treatment of TN is well studied in the general population and carbamazepine or oxcarbazepine are the first line treatment. If initial therapy does not provide adequate relief, alternative medications such as gabapentin, lamotrigine and baclofen have been shown to provide some relief. Surgical interventions following failed medical therapy are available although there is some evidence that surgery may be less effective in PwMS than those without MS [77, 78].

Lhermitte's sign, or more accurately Lhermitte's symptom, is defined as "a transient short-lasting sensation related to neck movement felt in the back of the neck, lower back or other parts of the body". It is associated with MRI lesions in the posterior columns of the cervical spinal cord and is thought to be caused by hypersensitivity of demyelinated cervical sensory axons to stretching [79]. Lhermitte's symptom is generally self-limiting over weeks to months but if it is medically managed, it can be treated in a similar fashion to TN with anticonvulsants as first line agents [80].

Painful tonic spasms [PTS] are referring to a specific type of painful spasm often found in PwMS. Studies have shown that in patients with PTS, they usually occur several times per day, last a couple of minutes, can be triggered by touch, movement, hyperventilation or emotions and can even be preceded by what is described as a "somesthetic aura". MRI lesions associated with PTS have been demonstrated throughout the brainstem and spinal cord, and symptoms are thought to be the result of ephaptic spread of spontaneous discharges generated by demyelinated axons [81].

PTS are treated the same as any other condition involving spasticity, usually starting with physical modalities including stretching, ROM exercises, splinting and casting. From here, there are multiple ways to approach medical management of spasticity. Oral agents include baclofen (GABA B agonist), dantrolene (hydantoin derivative), tizanidine (alpha 2 receptor agonist), gabapentin (voltage gated calcium channel inhibitor), benzodiazepines (GABA A agonist). For more focal spasticity (individual muscle group or joint) chemodenervation may be more effective using Botox or phenol. More generalized spasticity may require intrathecal agents such as baclofen (much more effective for lower extremity spasticity than upper extremity spasticity), clonidine or gabapentin.

Headaches are consistently shown in studies to be more common in PwMS. In one cohort of MS patients, 41% of headaches were migraines (accounting for 22% of the MS patients in the cohort) and the remainder were classified as "muscle contraction headaches". Watkins and Espir found migraine in 27% of MS patients, compared to just 12% of other age and sex matched patients [82]. Keys for migraine management include being mindful of triggers, practicing good sleep habits, losing excess weight, regular aerobic exercise and trying to treat the migraine early (NSAIDs, acetaminophen, triptans, antiemetics). If these fail to achieve an adequate response, it may warrant preventative treatment with beta-blockers, TCAs, anticonvulsants or Botox.

Back and other musculoskeletal pains are under-diagnosed in PwMS. Often in this patient population, back pain is musculoskeletal in nature and a result of prolonged standing or sitting. Musculoskeletal pain is treated similar to how you would manage a patient without MS (PT/OT, physical modalities, exercise, analgesics, lifestyle changes etc.) with a few important caveats. Demyelination makes nerves more vulnerable to heat-related changes so thermoregulation in PwMS becomes more difficult and can lead to Uhthoff's phenomenon (transient worsening of neurologic signs and symptoms in MS, can be physical and cognitive). For this reason, patients should avoid modalities such as hot packs, saunas, hot tubs etc.

This often leads to the question, is it okay for patients with MS to exercise? Yes. Exercise is helpful for PwMS with no evidence for deleterious effects as long as the intensity, duration and frequency are matched with the patient's symptoms, heat tolerance, strength and endurance.

Evidence for MS specific pain management is lacking and much of how we treat it is based on patients with similar pain without MS. What we do know, is that PwMS experience specific pain syndromes at higher rates than the general population. Work with them to find out what they're experiencing, what treatments are providing relief and what are not. Pain can be a huge barrier to quality of life and effective management can breathe new life into an often discouraging disease.

Neurofibromatosis

Neurofibromatosis [NF] is an autosomal dominant disease of the nervous system. There are three distinct types of neurofibromatosis that present differently both clinically and genetically: NF1, NF2 and schwannomatosis. Of the three, NF1 is the most common and is often recognized by its two hallmark features, café-au-lait spots and neurofibromas. This section will be discussing pain specific to NF1.

Pain location and acuity plays a large role in surveillance of current tumors, new tumors and malignant transformation of known tumors. Because of this, guidelines incorporate changes in pain to their recommendations for new imaging when assessing tumors [83].

Current focus on managing pain in NF1 is on management of symptomatic tumors and is primarily treated with surgery. In a study by Buono et al., all of the 255 patients who participated reported having had at least 1 surgery to remove an NF1 tumor. This is often problematic given the tumors are of nerves themselves, in close proximity to vascular structures, and tumor regrowth is common. Nearly half of the 255 patients experienced complications following surgery including permanent weakness affecting their activities of daily living [84].

The large prevalence of this population utilizing surgery for management of tumor related pain illustrates that it is as or more heavily relied on for relief than medications alone. Neuropathic pain is inevitable and the frequently utilized agents include gabapentin, pregabalin and TCA's. From here the addition of SNRI's and certain anticonvulsants can be trialed. Opioids can be appropriate when disease has progressed beyond the confines of the nervous system, treatment is limited by comorbidities or other options have been exhausted.

While it has been shown by Meldrum that chronic pain symptoms, specifically tumor-related, do not respond well to opioids, medical management with opioids is common in this patient population [85]. One study demonstrated that 17% of patients actively take opioids to manage their pain [86]. When this subgroup was looked at more closely, they reported higher levels of pain and interference with daily life suggesting that opioid induced hyperalgesia may be contributing to the experienced pain.

Some alternative therapies have shown promise when combined with surgical and medical management. Particularly yoga, massage therapy and physical therapy have shown efficacy with improving pain thresholds [87]. Multiple studies looking at populations with similar pain prevalence and symptoms have shown that complementary therapies can be effective in reducing both chronic and acute pain [88]. Psychology plays an often understated role in the experience of pain and should always be incorporated into the treatment plan. Helping manage expectations, anxiety and future potentials is vital to helping guide patients through their disease.

References

1. Antonini A, Tinazzi M, Abbruzzese G, Berardelli A, Chaudhuri KR, Defazio G, et al. Pain in Parkinson's disease: facts and uncertainties. Eur J Neurol. 2018;25(7):917–e69.
2. Rana AQ, Kabir A, Jesudasan M, Siddiqui I, Khondker S. Pain in Parkinson's disease: analysis and literature review. Clin Neurol Neurosurg. 2013;115(11):2313–7.
3. Qureshi AR, Rana AQ, Malik SH, Rizvi SFH, Akhter S, Vannabouathong C, et al. Comprehensive examination of therapies for pain in Parkinson's disease: a systematic review and meta-analysis. Neuroepidemiology. 2018;51(3–4):190–206.

4. Ford B. Pain in Parkinson's disease. Clin Neurosci (New York, NY). 1998;5(2):63–72.
5. Rukavina K, Leta V, Sportelli C, Buhidma Y, Duty S, Malcangio M, Chaudhuri KR. Pain in Parkinson's disease: new concepts in pathogenesis and treatment. Curr Opin Neurol. 2019;32(4):579–88.
6. Quittenbaum BH, Grahn B. Quality of life and pain in Parkinson's disease: a controlled cross-sectional study. Parkinsonism Relat Disord. 2004;10(3):129–36.
7. Todor DR, Mu HT, Milhorat TH. Pain and syringomyelia: a review. Neurosurg Focus. 2000;8(3):1–6.
8. Hatem SM, Attal N, Ducreux D, Gautron M, Parker F, Plaghki L, Bouhassira D. Clinical, functional and structural determinants of central pain in syringomyelia. Brain. 2010;133(11):3409–22.
9. Milhorat TH, Kotzen RM, Mu HT, Capocelli AL Jr, Milhorat RH. Dysesthetic pain in patients with syringomyelia. Neurosurgery. 1996;38(5):940–7.
10. Zorowitz RD, Smout RJ, Gassaway JA, Horn SD. Usage of pain medications during stroke rehabilitation: the post-stroke rehabilitation outcomes project (PSROP). Top Stroke Rehabil Fall. 2005;12(4):37–49.
11. Bowsher D, Leijon G, Thuomas KA. Central poststroke pain: correlation of MRI with clinical pain characteristics and sensory abnormalities. Neurology. 1998;51:1352–8.
12. Garcia-Larrea L, Perchet C, Creac'h C, Convers P, Peyron R, Laurent B, et al. Operculo-insular pain (parasylvian pain): a distinct central pain syndrome. Brain. 2010;133:2528–39.
13. Berthier M, Starkstein S, Leiguarda R. Asymbolia for pain: a sensory-limbic disconnection syndrome. Ann Neurol. 1988;24:41.
14. Hong JH, Bai DS, Jeong JY, Choi BY, Chang CH, Kim SH, et al. Injury of the spino-thalamo-cortical pathway is necessary for central post-stroke pain. Eur Neurol. 2010;64:163–8.
15. Lumer ED, Edelman GM, Tononi G. Neural dynamics in a model of the thalamocortical system. I. Layers, loops and the emergence of fast synchronous rhythms. Cereb Cortex. 1997;7:207–27.
16. Borsook D, Becerra L, Hargreaves R. Biomarkers for chronic pain and analgesia part 1: the need, reality, challenges, and solutions. Discovery Med. 2011a;11:197–207.
17. Seghier ML, Lazeyras F, Vuilleumier P, Schnider A, Carota A. Functional magnetic resonance imaging and diffusion tensor imaging in a case of central poststroke pain. J Pain. 2005;6:208–12.
18. Henry J, Lalloo C, Yashpal K. Central poststroke pain: an abstruse outcome. Pain Res Manag. 2008;13(1):41–9.
19. Yang S, Grabois M, Brian B. Postroke-pain. Pract Pain Manag. 2011;9:5.
20. Koyama S, Katayama Y, Maejima S, Hirayama T, Fujii M, Tsubokawa T. Thalamic neuronal hyperactivity following transection of the spinothalamic tract in the cat: involvement of N-methyl-D-aspartate receptor. Brain Res. 1993;612:345–50.
21. Hansson P. Post-stroke pain case study: clinical characteristics, therapeutic options and long-term follow-up. Eur J Neurol. 2004;11(Suppl 1):22–30.
22. Leijon G, Boivie J. Central post-stroke pain – a controlled trial of amitriptyline and carbamazepine. Pain. 1989;36:27–36.
23. Lampl C, Yazdi K, Röper C. Amitriptyline in the prophylaxis of central poststroke pain. Preliminary results of 39 patients in a placebo-controlled, long-term study. Stroke. 2002;33:3030–2.
24. McQuay HJ, Tramèr M, Nye BA, Carroll D, Wiffen PJ, Moore RA. A systematic review of antidepressants in neuropathic pain. Pain. 1996;68:217–27.
25. Attal N, Guirimand F, Brasseur L, Gaude V, Chauvin M, Bouhassira D. Effects of IV morphine in central pain: a randomized placebo-controlled study. Neurology. 2000;58:554–63.
26. Rowbotham MC, Twilling L, Davies PS, Reisner L, Taylor K, Mohr D. Oral opioid therapy for chronic peripheral and central neuropathic pain. N Engl J Med. 2003;348:1223–32.
27. Vick PG, Lamer TJ. Treatment of central post-stroke pain with oral ketamine. Pain. 2001;92:311–3.

28. The National Institute of Neurological Disorders and Stroke rt-PA Stroke Study Group. Tissue plasminogen activator for acute ischemic stroke. N Engl J Med. 1995;333:1581–7.
29. Gordon A. Best practice guidelines for treatment of central pain after stroke. In: Henry JL, Panju A, Yashpal K, editors. Central neuropathic pain: focus on poststroke pain. Seattle: IASP Press; 2007.
30. Backonja MM, Serra J. Pharmacologic management part 2: lesser-studied neuropathic pain diseases. Pain Med. 2004;5(Suppl 1):S49–59.
31. Klockgether T, Lüdtke R, Kramer B, Abele M, Bürk K, Schöls L, et al. The natural history of degenerative ataxia: a retrospective study in 466 patients. Brain. 1998;121:589–00.
32. Rub U, Brunt ER, Deller T. New insights into the pathoanatomy of spinocerebellar ataxia type 3 (Machado-Joseph disease). Curr Opin Neurol. 2008;21:111–6.
33. Teive HAG. Spinocerebellar degenerations in Japan. New insights from an epidemiological study. Neuroepidemiology. 2009;32:184–5.
34. Harding AE. The hereditary ataxias and related disorders. Edinburgh: Churchill Livingstone; 1984. p. 129–65.
35. Durr A. Autosomal dominant cerebellar ataxias: polyglutamine expansions and beyond. Lancet Neurol. 2010;9:885–94.
36. França MC Jr, D'AbreuA NA, Lopes-Cendes I. Mucle excitability abnormalities in Machado-Joseph disease. Arch Neurol. 2008;65(4):525–9.
37. Johansson J, Forsgren L, Sandgren O, Brice A, Holmgren G, Holmberg M. Expanded CAG repeats in Swedish spinocerebellar ataxia type 7 (SCA7) patients: effect of CAG repeat length on the clinical manifestation. Hum Mol Genet. 1998;7(2):171–6. https://doi.org/10.1093/hmg/7.2.171.
38. Szende A, Williams A, editors. Measuring self-reported population health: an international perspective based on EQ-5D. Budapest: SpringMed Publishing: Euro-Qol Group; 2004.
39. Rossi M, Perez-Lloret S, Doldan L, et al. Autosomal dominant cerebellar ataxias: a systematic review of clinical features. Eur J Neurol. 2014;21(4):607–15. https://doi.org/10.1111/ene.12350.
40. Whaley N, Uitti R. Clumsy gait and leg pain. In: Reich S, editor. Movement disorders: 100 instructive cases. Boca Raton: Taylor & Francis Group; 2008. p. 239–44.
41. Miao X, Wu X, Shi W. Umbilical cord mesenchymal stem cells in neurological disorders: a clinical study. Indian J Biochem Biophys. 2015;52(2):140–6.
42. Chiò A, et al. Pain in amyotrophic lateral sclerosis. The Lancet. Neurology. 2017;16(2):144–57. https://doi.org/10.1016/S1474-4422(16)30358-1.
43. de Tommaso M, Arendt-Nielsen L, Defrin R, Kunz M, Pickering G, Valeriani M. Pain in neurodegenerative disease: current knowledge and future perspectives. Behav Neurol. 2016;2016:7576292.
44. Chiò A, Canosa A, Gallo S, Moglia C, Ilardi A, Cammarosano S, Papurello D, Calvo A. Pain in amyotrophic lateral sclerosis: a population-based controlled study. Eur J Neurol. 2012;19(4):551–5.
45. Caress JB, Ciarlone SL, Sullivan EA, Griffin LP, Cartwright MS. Natural history of muscle cramps in amyotrophic lateral sclerosis. Muscle Nerve. 2016;53(4):513–7.
46. EFNS Task Force on Diagnosis and Management of Amyotrophic Lateral Sclerosis, et al. EFNS guidelines on the clinical management of amyotrophic lateral sclerosis (MALS)--revised report of an EFNS task force. Eur J Neurol. 2012;19(3):360–75. https://doi.org/10.1111/j.1468-1331.2011.03501.x.
47. Handy CR, et al. Pain in amyotrophic lateral sclerosis: a neglected aspect of disease. Neurol Res Int. 2011;2011:403808. https://doi.org/10.1155/2011/403808.
48. Miller RG, et al. Practice parameter update: the care of the patient with amyotrophic lateral sclerosis: multidisciplinary care, symptom management, and cognitive/behavioral impairment (an evidence-based review): report of the quality standards subcommittee of the American Academy of Neurology. Neurology. 2009;73(15):1227–33. https://doi.org/10.1212/WNL.0b013e3181bc01a4.

49. Jimenez-Sanchez M, et al. Huntington's disease: mechanisms of pathogenesis and therapeutic strategies. Cold Spring Harbor perspectives in medicine. 2017;7(7):a024240.
50. Wheelock V. The motor disorder. In: Nance M, Paulsen JS, Rosenblatt A, Wheelock V, editors. A Physician's Guide to the Management of Huntington's Disease. 3rd ed. Huntington's Disease Society of America; 2011. p. 39.
51. Sprenger GP, et al. The prevalence and the burden of pain in patients with Huntington disease: a systematic review and meta-analysis. Pain. 2019;160(4):773–83.
52. Suchowersky O. Huntington disease: management. In: Post TW, Hurtig HI, Eichler AF, editors. UptoDate; 2021.
53. Abresch RT, Carter GT. Assessment of pain and health-related quality of life in slowly progressive neuromuscular disease. Am J Hospice Palliative Care. 2002;19(1):39–48.
54. van Kooten J, Smalbrugge M. Prevalence of pain in nursing home residents: the role of dementia stage and dementia subtypes. J Am Med Dir Assoc. 2017;18(6):522–7.
55. Cravello L, Di Santo S. Chronic pain in the elderly with cognitive decline: a narrative review. Pain Ther. 2019;8(1):53–65.
56. van Kooten J, Binnekade TT. A review of pain prevalence in Alzheimer's, vascular, frontotemporal and lewy body dementias. Dement Geriatr Cogn Disord. 2016;41:220–32.
57. Rajkumar AP, Ballard C. Epidemiology of pain in people with dementia living in care homes: longitudinal course, prevalence, and treatment implications. J Am Med Dir Assoc. 2017;18(5):453.e1–6.
58. Scherder EJA, Sergeant JA. Pain processing in dementia and its relation to neuropathology. The Lancet Neurology. 2003;2(11):677–86.
59. Pickering G, Jourdan D. Acute versus chronic pain treatment in Alzheimer's disease. Eur J Pain. 2006;10:379–84.
60. Zarow C, Lyness SA. Neuronal loss is greater in the locus coeruleus than nucleus basalis and substantia nigra in Alzheimer and Parkinson diseases. Arch Neurol. 2003;60:337–41.
61. Song Cao DW. The link between chronic pain and Alzheimer's disease. J Neuroinflammation. 2019;16(204):1–11.
62. Gagliese L, Gauthier LR. Pain, aging, and dementia: towards a biopsychosocial model. Prog Neuro-Psychopharmacol Biol Psychiatry. 2018;87:207–15.
63. Benedetti F, Arduino C. Loss of expectation-related mechanisms in Alzheimer's disease makes analgesic therapies less effective. Pain. 2006;121(1–2):133–44.
64. D'Amico A, M. E. Spinal muscular atrophy. Orphanet J Rare Dis. 2011;6(71):1–10.
65. Qu R, Yao F. SMN deficiency causes pain hypersensitivity in a mild SMA mouse model through enhancing excitability of nociceptive dorsal root ganglion neurons. Nat Sci Rep. 2019;9(6493):1–15.
66. Lager C, Kroksmark AK. Pain in adolescents with spinal muscular atrophy and Duchenne and Becker muscular dystrophy. Eur J Paediatr Neurol. 2015;19:537–46.
67. Dubowitz V. Muscle disorders in childhood. Philadelphia, PA: W.B Saunders; 1978.
68. Gladstone D, Black S. Overview of current and emerging therapies for acute stroke. In: Henry JL, Panju A, Yashpal K, editors. Central neuropathic pain: focus on Poststroke pain. Seattle: IASP Press; 2007. p. 13–25.
69. Pöllmann W, Feneberg W, Erasmus L-P. Pain in multiple sclerosis--a still underestimated problem. The 1 year prevalence of pain syndromes, significance and quality of care of multiple sclerosis inpatients. The Neurologist. 2004;75:135–40.
70. O'Connor AB, Schwid SR, Herrmann DN, Markman JD, Dworkin RH. Pain associated with multiple sclerosis: systematic review and proposed classification. Pain. 2008;137(1):96–111.
71. Dworkin RH, Backonja M, Rowbotham MC, Allen RR, Argoff CR, Bennett GJ, et al. Advances in neuropathic pain: diagnosis, mechanisms, and treatment recommendations. Archiv Neurol. 2003;60:1524–34.
72. Finnerup NB, Otto M, Jensen TS, Sindrup SH. Algorithm for neuropathic pain treatment: an evidence based proposal. Pain. 2005;118:289–305.

73. Beck RW, Cleary PA, Anderson MM Jr, Keltner JL, Shults WT, Kaufman DI, Buckley EG, Corbett JJ, Kupersmith MJ, Miller NR, et al. A randomized, controlled trial of corticosteroids in the treatment of acute optic neuritis. New England J Med. 1992;326(9):581–8.
74. Osterberg A, Boivie J, Thuomas KA. Central pain in multiple sclerosis: prevalence and clinical characteristics. Eur J Pain. 2005;9:531–42.
75. Solaro C, Brichetto G, Amato MP, Cocco E, Colombo B, D'Aleo A, et al. The prevalence of pain in multiple sclerosis: a multicenter cross-sectional study. Neurology. 2004;63:919–21.
76. Indaco A, Iachetta C, Nappi C, Socci L, Carrieri PB. Chronic and acute pain syndromes in patients with multiple sclerosis. Acta Sci Neurol (Napoli). 1994;16:97–102.
77. Broggi G, Ferroli P, Franzini A, Pluderi M, La Mantia L, Milanese C. Role of microvascular decompression in trigeminal neuralgia and multiple sclerosis. Lancet. 1999;354:1878–9.
78. Sandell T, Eide PK. The effect of microvascular decompression in patients with multiple sclerosis and trigeminal neuralgia. Neurosurgery. 2010;67:749–53.
79. Kanchandani R, Howe JG. Lhermitte's sign in multiple sclerosis: a clinical survey and review of the literature. J Neurol Neurosurg Psychiat. 1982;45:308–12.
80. Al-Araji AH, Oger J. Reappraisal of Lhermitte's sign in multiple sclerosis. Multiple Sclerosis J. 2005;11:398–402.
81. Spissu A, Cannas A, Ferrigno P, Pelaghi AE, Spissu M. Anatomic correlates of painful tonic spasms in multiple sclerosis. Movement Disord. 1999;14:331–5.
82. Watkins SM, Espir MLE. Migraine and multiple sclerosis. J Neurol Neurosurg Psychiatry. 1969;32:35–7.
83. Stewart DR, Korf BR, Nathanson KL, Stevenson DA, Yohay K, American College of Medical Genetics. Care of adults with neurofibromatosis type 1: a clinical practice resource of the American College of Medical Genetics and Genomics (ACMG). Genet Med. 2018;20:671–82.
84. Buono FD, Grau LE, Sprong ME, Morford KL, Johnson KJ, Gutmann DH. Pain symptomology, functional impact, and treatment of people with Neurofibromatosis type 1. J Pain Res. 2019;12:2555.
85. Meldrum ML, American Medical Association. A capsule history of pain management. J Am Med Assoc. 2003;290:2470–5.
86. Daubresse M, et al. Ambulatory diagnosis and treatment of nonmalignant pain in the United States, 2000–2010. Medical Care. 2013;51(10):870–88.
87. Thomas D-A, Maslin B, Legler A, Springer E, Asgerally A, Vadivelu N. Role of Alternative Therapies for Chronic Pain Syndromes. Curr Pain Headache Rep. May 2016;20(5):1–7.
88. Krebs EE, Bair MJ, Damush TM, Tu W, Wu J, Kroenke K. Comparative responsiveness of pain outcome measures among primary care patients with musculoskeletal pain. Medical Care. 2010;48(11):1007.

Chapter 9
Complex Regional Pain Syndrome and Interventions

Helen Gharaei

Introduction

Complex Regional Pain Syndrome (CRPS) is outlined as a painful and disabling condition accompanied by physical changes within the affected extremity, characterized by allodynia, edema, baldness, and sudomotor and dilatation dysfunction. The CRPS is a life-altering condition that generally affects the extremities after a trauma or nerve injury. The physiologic changes that follow as a result of the inciting injury are complex. In CRPS type I (reflex sympathetic dystrophy), small injuries or fractures initiate the onset of symptoms without evidence of nerve damage in the affected limb while CRPS type II (causalgia) develops once an injury to a large supplemental nerve happened with evidence of nerve damage in the affected limb. CRPS type 1 accounts for about 90% of CRPS [1]. However, some research has identified evidence of nerve damage in CRPS-I which puts into question as to whether the disorder is always divided into two types. Nevertheless, the treatment is similar [2].

Unfortunately, pain and disability related to CRPS frequently result in co-morbidities that produce a vicious cycle of pain and depression. It is distinct from other pain syndromes due to the presence of autonomic dysfunction, inflammatory changes, and a scarcity of dermatomal distribution. This condition is ambiguous in nature. It has been historically challenging to diagnose, laborious to treat, and the pathophysiology behind it has not been fully defined.

H. Gharaei (✉)
ASA Pain Clinic, Tehran, Iran

© The Author(s), under exclusive license to Springer Nature Switzerland AG 2022
J. de Castro, Y. El Miedany (eds.), *Advances in Chronic and Neuropathic Pain*, Contemporary Rheumatology, https://doi.org/10.1007/978-3-031-10687-3_9

History

Ambroise Paré (1510–1590), the father of modern surgery, was the first to describe a disorder that could be related to the current concept of CRPS. He successfully treated a severe and persistent pain syndrome that occurred to King Charles IX of France after a phlebotomy [3]. The first written description of CRPS was made by Denmark who published a case report of a soldier wounded by a bullet that passed over his arm during the siege of Badajuz (1812) [4].

In 1864, Silas Weir Mitchell, in collaboration with George Morehouse and William Keen, published a monograph entitled "Bullet Wounds and Other Injuries," which soon became the benchmark for diagnosing and treating nerve damage until World War I. A syndrome characterized by a typical chronic burning pain that is located at the end of the peripheral nerve injury site and is associated with skin disorders was described by the author and was highly suggestive of this disease and now became the hallmarks of what we now call CRPS. This clinical condition was later named "causalgia" in "Nerve Injuries and Their Consequences", which is the second book published by Mitchell in 1872. It was later coined by Ruble Danglison in the first edition of the Medical Dictionary in 1874 [5, 6].

Another milestone in the history of the CRPS is made by Paul Sudek. In 1900, at the 29th Congress of the German Surgical Association, Sudeck presented an article entitled "Acute Inflammatory Bone Atrophy" which describes the results of his experiments on patients undergoing X-ray examinations which he was called "Sudeck atrophy" and is still a common term to define algodystrophy [7].

Another turning point in the history of CRPS was the hypothesis that the sympathetic nervous system plays a major role in the signs and symptoms of the disease. This hypothesis was accepted by Rene Leriche (1917) who described a patient with chronic hand pain and numbness after a bullet wound to the right arm. He performed the first sympathectomy on the patient and noted complete resolution of the pain syndrome within 2 weeks [8]. James E. Evans, then emphasized the term "sympathetic reflex dystrophy" (RSD) [9]. Philip S. Foisie, also described a persistent but low-grade arterial spasm after a soft tissue injury, which can lead to severe pain syndrome characterized by allodynia, edema, muscle atrophy, osteoporosis, joint stiffness, and decreased mobility. He argued that RSD might be better defined as a "traumatic arterial vasospasm" [10].

In the 1950s, Algology, a new field of medicine, was born as a branch of anesthesia. John Bonica (1953) was the first to propose the stages for RSD with three types of clinical imaginations [11] and these stages were used as the basis for the next diagnostic criteria (Table 9.1).

John Bonica also found the first scientific association dedicated to the study of pain in 1973: The International Association for the Study of Pain (IASP). One of the several goals of the society was to standardize the classification of chronic pain. The first IASP conference was held in 1988 and the second one was in 1993 where they formulated and described the distinct characteristics of CRPS type I and CRPS type II [12]. Other diagnostic criteria for CRPS have been proposed by Peter Veldmann

Table 9.1 Bonica three stages of the RSD

Stage 1 (acute) from the moment of the trauma to 3 months after	• Erythema • Calor • Edema • Marked hyperhidrosis a distribution of the pain not related to root nor nerve involvement • Limited range of motion and reduced muscle strength	Negative X-ray examination, but a positive scintigraphy showing hyperaccumulation
Stage 2 (dystrophic)	• Severe pain • Edematous skin • Decreased hair growth • Discoloration with cyanotic areas • Persistent hyperhidrosis • Muscle weakness and limited range of motion of the affected joint or joints	
Stage 3 (atrophic) from 6 weeks onwards	• Decreased but still disabling pain that improves with rest and worsens with passive movements • The skin could be atrophic, thin, dry, sometimes ulcerated, cold, mottled or cyanotic • There could be loss of joint range of motion and muscle strength with tendon atrophy, contractures, tremors and dystonia determining a significant motor impairment of the affected limb	Radiographic examination shows inhomogeneous regional osteoporosis (Sudeck's atrophy)

(1993) who criticized the subset in the steps suggested by IASP experts, and identified less common cold forms, and the more common hot forms [13]. Norman Harden and Stephen Bruehlc conducted two papers in 1999 in a multicenter study to test the internal validity and external validity of IASP criteria [14, 15]. A new classification system was proposed during the Consensus Conference in Budapest in 2003. This study supports the validity of the Budapest diagnostic criteria for CRPS and demonstrates their superiority over current IASP criteria. The results of this study support suggestions for accepting the Budapest criteria as a standard for diagnosing clinical CRPS [16].

Epidemiology

Many epidemiological studies have been performed, and there appears to be regional variations in terms of presentation. The diversity in these studies highlights the challenges of diagnosing CRPS. Because this is a clinical diagnosis, physicians will often have different results using different criteria.

An epidemiological study in USA by Sandroni et al. (2003) showed an incidence rate of 5.46 per 100,000 and a prevalence of 20.57 per 100,000. The female to male ratio was 4:1 with a mean age of 46 years and the upper/lower limb ratio was 2:1. All cases reported an inciting event and fracture was the most common stimulus (46%). An excellent correlation was observed between signs and symptoms, with vasomotor symptoms being the most common. Three-phase bone scan and autonomic testing diagnosed the disease in more than 80% of cases. Seventy-four percent of patients treated spontaneously recovered. These results suggest that invasive treatment of CRPS may not be necessary in most cases [17].

Another study in Netherlands by De Mos et al. (2007) estimated the overall incidence of CRPS at 26.2 per 100,000. Women were affected at least three times more often than men. The highest incidence occurred in women between 61 to 70 years old. The upper limb was more affected than the lower limb and fracture was the most common cause (44%). Menopausal women appear to be at the highest risk for CRPS [18].

The German epidemiological study by Ott and Maihofner (2018) reported an incidence of 71% and 29% between men and women, respectively. They also showed that the upper limb was more prone to CRPS (70% of patients), with CRPS I occuring more frequently than CRPS II (88% and 12%, respectively) [19].

Korean epidemiological study by Kim et al. (2018) showed that the difference between men and women was much narrower and the age with the highest incidence was much higher than the previous report. They also found that the pelvis, thighs, and lower limbs were more likely to be affected than the upper limbs in their patient population [20].

Denmark epidemiological study by Petersen et al. (2018), risk factors for CRPS were determined and the following ratios were found: women: men was 4:1, initial diagnosis of upper extremity: lower extremity was 2.5:, and surgical treatment: non-surgical was 3:1. The mean age was 47.5 ± 13.7 years and no gender differences were observed. Antebrachial fractures (23%) and CTS (9%) were the most common initial conditions [21].

According to UK study, CRPS is not a common disease. It has an incidence rate of 6.28 per 100,000 people per year for both types 1 and 2. According to the National Institute of Neurological Disorders and Stroke, the disease can occur at any age, is rare in the elderly and children under 10, and peaks at the age of 40 [22].

Pathophysiology

It is unlikely that a unique linear mechanism will be discovered behind the development of CRPS. According to the most common pathology model, CRPS is a detailed combination of various factors.

For example, peripheral mechanisms explain how hypoxia due to vasoconstriction and endothelial dysfunction leads to a decrease in nitric oxide levels and an increase in endothelin-1 levels in the affected limb. There is a sterile inflammation caused by an elevated levels of proinflammatory cytokines such as interleukin-6 and tumor necrosis factor-alpha. A neurogenic inflammation by the excretion of neuropeptides from C-fibers and a high level of substance P, bradykinin, and calcitonin gene peptide were also observed. Neurosensitivity is caused by the peripheral degeneration of small fiber neurons in the skin of damaged limbs, leading to improper nerve firing [23–25] and catecholamine sensitivity after injury [26]. The researchers reported significant degeneration of large motor Aα nerve fibers, while Aδ nerve fibers survived. They hypothesized that neural signaling imbalance may occur peripherally, increasing Aδ activity and increasing pain. Nevertheless, long-term changes in the peripheral nervous system appear to play an important role [27]. There is also an increase in the expression of α1-adrenoceptors in CRPS-affected organs [28]. Changes in circulating catecholamines can explain clinical development of warm-to-cold limb. In the acute phase, studies show a decrease in circulating norepinephrine, which potentially leads to vasodilation, edema, and warmness. It is believed that over time, this leads to an increase in peripheral catecholamine sensitivity, which in turn leads to excessive vasoconstriction and hyperhidrosis, leading to cooling limb in the chronic phase of the disease [22]. Clinically, an increase in the number of alpha-1 receptors in the affected limb, increased sensitivity of peripheral alpha adrenergic receptors, and chemical coupling between sympathetic neurons and CRPS-induced limb pain caused sympathetic dysfunction and lead to variable vasoconstriction, hypoxia, and sweating abnormalities and involuntary movements characterized by dystonia, and decreased range of motion [29].

Continuous activation of the peripheral nerve after injury has been shown to increase the firing effect of synaptic pain in the dorsal horn and lead to central sensitization [30]. Central mechanisms, such as (super) spinal sensitization via *N*-methyl-D-aspartate and neurokinin-1 receptors have also been described [31]. CRPS patients due to damaged limbs experience a smaller view of the sensorimotor cortex than the normal limbs [32]. There is cortical reorganization characterized by the significant contraction of the extension of the cortical view of the hand at the injured side, shifting of the hand to the cortical area of the lip, and the reorganization of the opposite side of the S1 cortex. These reorganization are associated with CRPS pain, mechanical hyperalgesia, and neuropathic pain [33]. Recent study showed that S1 representation of the CRPS hand is comparable between affected and unaffected hand map [34].

There is also an evidence of autoimmune-mediated reaction in the development of CRPS. Autoantibodies are believed to be produced against the structures of the autonomic nervous system causing exacerbation of inflammation and symptoms [35]. The mast cells were shown to decrease around atrophied cutaneous nerve fibers in the affected limbs. The researchers hypothesized that abnormal nerve-mast cell interaction occurs, leading to long-term inflammation and delayed tissue repair in CRPS [36]. Research studies have shown that up to 70% of these patients have anti-autonomic antibodies to immunoglobulin G in their serum [37].

The genetic impact on the development of CRPS is currently under investigation and showed that family relationships were associated with early-onset and increased incidence of multi-member involvement [38]. Discovering specific microRNA signatures (miRNAs) is another interesting way to study genetics. These small noncoding fragments of RNA have been shown to directly alter gene expression [37, 39] However, the genetic link is not definitive. A paradoxical study in 2016 examined more than 200,000 single nucleotide polymorphisms between CRPS patients and control groups and found no significant difference in expression between the two [40].

There is evidence that certain mental states can predispose a patient to illness. Patients with post-traumatic stress disorder (PTSD) significantly showed increased CRPS compared with controls [41]. In many of these patients, PTSD precedes the onset of CRPS as indicated by their medical history. In fact, psychological stress seems to affect the progression of the disease. Patients with higher levels of anxiety, disability perception, and fear of pain have been shown to worsen the course of the disease [42].

Clinical Presentation

CRPS describes an array of painful conditions that are characterized by a continuing (spontaneous and/or evoked) pain that is seemingly disproportionate to a given trauma or any inciting event. To wit, an unexpected prolongation of recovery of an uncomplicated fracture characterized this disease. Pain may vacillate between allodynia, signs of autonomic instability, and sensory dysfunction of the skin which include hyperalgesia and mechanical allodynia and hypoalgesia and mechanical hypoesthesia. There are also motor dysfunction which include a reduction in the "range of motion" of affected joints and/or weakness, tremor, involuntary movements, bradykinesia, and dystonia along with an abnormality of cerebral motor processing which are unusually associated with a peripheral process and deep tendon reflex findings. A fracture, or crushing injury or a forceful trauma to the arm is the most common initial event when it occurs in the upper extremity. It usually starts in the limb as an extreme pain, swelling, limited range of motion, and trophic changes in the skin and bones with nearly all patients showing sweating abnormalities (hypohydrosis or hyperhydrosis). It may initially affects one limb (asymmetrical distal extremity pain) and then spreads throughout the body with sensory abnormalities affecting the most distal part of the extremities ("stocking-glove" pattern). Furthermore, the affected area usually manifest symptoms beyond the site of the original injury with varying degrees of pain over time such that pain and other symptoms are often exacerbated with exertion of the affected extremity [43].

To quantify the severity of the disease, Harden et al. (2010) developed the CRPS Severity Score (CSS) . Higher scores were not only positively associated with increased pain and functional limitations, but were also used as a measure to detect the disease and to monitor response to a given treatment (Table 9.2) [16, 44].

Table 9.2 CRPS severity score

Symptoms that were self-reported	Symptoms observed at the time of examination
Allodynia	Hyperpathia to pinprick
Temperature asymmetry	Allodynia
Skin color asymmetry	Temperature asymmetry to palpation
Sweating asymmetry	Skin color asymmetry
Trophic changes	Sweating asymmetry
Motor changes	Asymmetric edema
Decreased range of motion	Trophic changes
Asymmetric edema	Motor changes
	Decreased active range of motion

The clinical progression of the disease can usually be divided into three stages:

1. An acute early stage, with inflammatory symptoms
2. Dystrophic stage characterized by a gradual decrease in edema
3. An atrophic stage can then be seen in which atrophy and skin contractions become common

The first symptoms usually appear within a few weeks after the injury and the affected limb is very painful, erythematous, swollen, and warm. Allodynia, hyperalgesia, trophic changes in the skin and nail growth, and muscle weakness may be present. The affected area is limited and does not have a specific nerve distribution. As the disorder progresses, the pain exacerbates and spreads. Voluntary motor control decreases, negative sensory symptoms (hypostasis, hypoalgesia, and hypothermia) develop, and the limbs become cold, dark, and sweaty. Myoclonus, tremor and dystonia may also occur. Over time, the clinical symptoms can spread to other parts of the body even affecting the contralateral or bilateral sides. A subset of patients with CRPS becomes chronic, and after a long period of illness (>5 years) develop other features such as urological symptoms, syncope, and even mild cognitive impairments. The acute phase and dystrophy are reversible, while the form of atrophy is irreversible [45].

Three distinct vascular regulation patterns related to the duration of the disorder were also identified:

1. In the "warm" (acute) pattern, the affected limb was warmer and the amount of perfusion was greater in CRPS limb.
2. In the "moderate" pattern, the limbs were either warmer or colder.
3. In the "cold" (chronic) pattern, skin temperature and perfusion were lower.

It is suggested that in CRPS I, unilateral inhibition of sympathetic vasoconstrictor neurons leads to warmer limb in the acute phase. Secondary changes in neurovascular transmission may lead to vascular contraction and cold skin in chronic CRPS I, while sympathetic activity is still depressed [46].

Three possible subtypes of CRPS is also described that is useful clinically:

1. Relatively limited syndrome with predominant vasomotor symptoms,
2. Relatively limited syndrome with predominant neuropathic pain/sensory abnormalities,
3. Florid CRPS syndrome, described as "classic RSD"

Subgroup 3 showed the highest levels of motor/trophic symptoms and possible changes due to osteopenia in bone scans, despite the shortest duration of pain in the three groups. The EMG/NCV test indicates that subgroup 2 may reflect CRPS-Type 2 [2].

Diagnosis

The diagnosis and treatment of CRPS has been a challenge to health care providers. Diagnosis is based upon criteria obtained from the medical history and physical examination. Due to the great clinical diversity and heterogeneity of the cause, the diagnosis is not easy. There are many non-standard diagnostic benchmark systems. The new diagnostic criteria were developed by the International Association for the Study of Pain (IASP) based on classification in the consensus workshop in 1994. Subsequent validation research using these criteria have encountered problems differentiating the disease with the possibility of over-diagnosis. In the fall of 2003, diagnostic criteria were reviewed in Budapest which were adopted in 2012 as a new international standard for the diagnosis of CRPS by the IASP and could reduce the CRPS diagnosis by about 50%. The most commonly used criteria are the main IASP criteria and the modified Harden and Bruehl's diagnostic criteria. The criteria described by Veldman are often used in the Netherlands (Table 9.3). All criteria are essentially empirically determined and have overlapping parameters to some extent. However, the IASP criteria is the most sensitive, while the modified criteria according to Harden and Bruehl is the most specific [16, 42, 47].

No diagnostic test is considered definitive for CRPS, there are no laboratory tests to diagnose or eliminate it completely. However, other methods can help with the diagnosis. Thermography may be the most common and the most basic diagnostic method used wherein changes of 1 °C or more are considered diagnostic [48].

Standard radiographs can be normal in the early stages (bone mineral depletion occurred within 3–6 weeks of the onset of symptoms, and this change may continue for up to 2 years after the symptoms have resolved). In the absence of clinical signs (autonomic changes and dystrophy) and radiographic examination findings, further tests such as MRI and scintigraphy are done for accurate evaluation. MRI imaging scans show low signal intensity in T1-w images and high signal intensity in STIR or T2-w fat suppression images. These changes indicate an increase in the intracellular and extracellular fluid of the bone marrow, which results from the formation and repair of bone (differential diagnosis on MRI should be made for infection, osteonecrosis, and post-traumatic brain edema). A three-stage bone scan may be

Table 9.3 Different diagnostic criteria for CRPS

Dutch criteria (Veldman 1993)	IASP criteria (Merskey 1994)	Budapest clinical diagnostic criteria for CRPS (2003)	Modified diagnostic criteria (Harden 2007)
1. 4 or 5 of the following symptoms:	1. Develops after tissue damage (CRPS type—1) or nerve damage (CRPS type—2)	1. Continuing pain, which is disproportionate to any inciting event	1. Continuous pain, disproportionate to the inciting event.
(a) Inexplicable diffuse pain	2. Continuous pain, allodynia or hyperalgesia disproportional to the inciting event.	2. Must report at least one symptom in three of the four following categories:	2. Patients should have at least 1 symptom in each of the following categories and 1 sign in 2 or more categories.
(b) Difference in skin color between affected and contralateral extremity	3. Evidence at some time of edema, abnormal skin blood flow and sudomotor abnormalities in the region of pain.	(a) Sensory: reports of hyperesthesia and/or allodynia	Categories:
(c) Diffuse edema	4. Other causes of pain or dysfunction are excluded.	(b) Vasomotor: reports of temperature asymmetry and/or skin color changes and/or skin color asymmetry	1. Sensory (allodynia, hyperalgesia, hypoesthesia)
(d) Difference in skin temperature between affected and contralateral extremity	Criteria 2, 3, and 4 must be fulfilled	(c) Sudomotor/edema: reports of edema and/or sweating changes and/or sweating asymmetry	2. Vasomotor (temperature or skin color abnormalities)
(e) Limited "active range of motion"		(d) Motor/trophic: reports of decreased range of motion and/or motor dysfunction (weakness, tremor, dystonia) and/or trophic changes (hair, nail, skin)	3. Sudomotor (edema or sweating abnormalities)
2. The occurrence or increase of above—mentioned symptoms with use of the involved extremity.		3. Must display at least one sign at time of evaluation in two or more of the following categories:	4. Motor/trophic (muscle weakness, tremor, hair, nail, skin abnormalities)

(continued)

Table 9.3 (continued)

Dutch criteria (Veldman 1993)	IASP criteria (Merskey 1994)	Budapest clinical diagnostic criteria for CRPS (2003)	Modified diagnostic criteria (Harden 2007)
3. Above—mentioned symptoms are present in an area that is greater than the area of original trauma or surgery and distal to this area.		(a) Sensory: evidence of hyperalgesia (to pinprick) and/or allodynia (to light touch and/or deep somatic pressure and/or joint movement)	
		(b) Vasomotor: evidence of temperature asymmetry and/or skin color changes and/or asymmetry	
		(c) Sudomotor/edema: evidence of edema and/or sweating changes and/or sweating asymmetry	
		(d) Motor/trophic: evidence of decreased range of motion and/or motor dysfunction (weakness, tremor, dystonia) and/or trophic changes (hair, nail, skin)	
		There is no other diagnosis that better explains the signs and symptoms	

positive a few days after the onset of symptoms. Tc99m-MDP increases uptake, indicating a focal increase in capillary permeability, hyperemia, and osteoblastic activity [49]. Three-phase bone scan may show increased absorption of technetium Tc99m bisphosphonate due to increased bone metabolism, although it has no benefit in the management of CRPS and should not be used as a confirmatory measure [50, 51].

Electromyography has shown some validity in some specific patients. Myoclonus, which occurs in CRPS patients, is thought to be distinct from other types of myoclonus and may be detected by electromyography. However, only 11–36% of patients showed myoclonus, greatly limiting its sensitivity as a diagnostic tool [52].

Musculoskeletal ultrasound can also be used to describe physical differences in muscle tissue in CRPS patients, CRPS-affected muscles have significant myoglobular deviation, whereas muscles affected by chronic neuropathic pain have a normal structure [53].

Painful hypersensitivity in persistent CRPS is maintained by autoantibodies, which act by sensitizing pain receptors A and C. Twenty-seven (33%) of the 82 CRPS patients whose serum was available tested positive for ANA, indicating that autoantibodies may be associated with the pathophysiology of CRPS, at least in a subset of patients [54, 55].

Treatment

CRPS treatment guidelines recommend a multidisciplinary approach including physiotherapy, occupational therapy, and psychotherapy (with coping mechanisms for pain, relaxation training, thermal biofeedback, and graded exposure therapy) to improve movement, mobility, quality of life, and the patient ability to manage pain [56]. The graded motor imagery and mirror therapy have the best available data that could improve pain and function in CRPS I patients [57].

Intense exercise therapy is critical to the effective treatment of CRPS and the reduction in the reported high incidence of recurrence in patients treated with physiotherapy alone and cognitive-behavioral therapy. Electrical nerve stimulation (TENS) reduces CRPS 2 pain and when delivered contralateral to a nerve injury best reduces allodynia in a combination of high- and low-frequency [58]. Many CRPS 1 patients receiving neurofeedback training report a significant short-term reduction in their pain experience as well as improvement of symptoms [59].

Pharmacologic Therapy

Based on overlapping pathophysiologic mechanisms of CRPS different pharmacological treatment is recommended. Commonly used drugs are nonsteroidal anti-inflammatory drugs (NSAIDs) such as naproxen or ibuprofen, tramadol, antidepressants such as amitriptyline, doxepin or trazodone; anticonvulsants (e.g. gabapentin), clonidine, clonazepam, baclofen, topical capsaicin cream, lidocaine 5 patch [60].

The effect of NSAIDs in reducing pain in some neuropathic conditions have not been well demonstrated. However, inflammation is involved in CRPS, especially in the early months of the syndrome and may respond effectively to NSAID. Systemic corticosteroids have been studied in various trials and have generally had positive results [61, 62]. A short course of steroids may be indicated in early CRPS with prominent inflammation, but contraindicated for a long course [56].

Neuropathic pain medications for CRPS have not been extensively studied. The use of neuropathic pain medications to treat CRPS is based on their usefulness in the treatment of other neuropathic diseases. Evidence of their use in CRPS is limited; some of these medications include amitriptyline, doxepin, nortriptyline, desipramine, imipramine, and trazodone, serotonin-norepinephrine reuptake inhibitors

(SNRIs) duloxetine and venlafaxine. The use of other neuropathic pain medications by pain physicians to treat CRPS is experimental and is based on the preference and experience of each provider [63, 64]. Gabapentin and amitriptyline were effective in reducing pain intensity and improving sleep [65]. Carbamazepine, another anticonvulsant also showed pain relief [66].

Bisphosphonates (e.g., pamidronate, clodronate, alendronate) are one of the most widely used drugs for the treatment of osteoporosis, but as a treatment for CRPS the mechanism of pain relief is unclear. Some theories include the ability of bisphosphonates to modulate inflammation, inhibit the growth and migration of bone marrow cells, and reduce bone marrow acidity [67, 68]. In patients with acute CRPS-1, Neridronate was associated with clinical benefits compared with placebo control group [69].

Anesthetic doses of ketamine, an NMDA receptor antagonist, were used in patients with severe refractory CRPS that was spreading [70]. Intranasal calcitonin showed improvement in pain intensity, but not in all studies [71].

One possible mechanism of CRPS is that it is triggered by an exaggerated inflammatory response to tissue damage caused by the overproduction of oxygen-mediated radicals, so free-radical scavengers (alpha lipoic acid, dimethyl sulfoxide [DMSO], *N*-acetylcysteine [NAC], and vitamin C) have been studied with some success for the treatment of CRPS [72, 73]. There is also the possibility that vitamin C may be effective in preventing CRPS but due to the varied results and the overall quality of evidence, it is unclear whether vitamin C is generally effective in reducing the prevalence of CRPS after fractures and limb surgeries [74, 75].

Alpha-adrenoceptor antagonists (such as phentolamine, phenoxybenzamine, clonidine, and reserpine) have been used clinically to treat CRPS without good results from prospective randomized trials. Patients who have symptoms of vasomotor hyperactivity leading to cold (intermittent) CRPS may respond to alpha-1 adrenergic blockers such as phenoxybenzamine and trazosine or calcium channel blockers such as nifedipine [43]. Oral clonidine has not been shown to be significantly effective in neuropathic pain and its use is challenging due to its characteristic side effects. It is mostly used as an intrathecal agent [76–78]. The transdermal clonidine patch in four CRPS patients with sympathetic pain has shown some benefits. It is also suggested that oral terazosin may be effective in treating sympathetically maintained pain in patients with CRPS. Oral nifedipine or oral phenoxybenzamine was useful for controlling severe vasoconstriction in two uncontrolled cases of patients with CRPS. Intravenous phentolamine has been used to assess pain maintained by the sympathetic, and is not commonly used clinically, however, it may be used to make a diagnosis [77–83].

Transdermal clonidine and the fentanyl patch, lidocaine patch 5%, eutectic mixture of local anesthetics (EMLA) cream, dimethyl sulfoxide (DMSO), and capsaicin introduced based on their effect on neuropathic pain, but none of which has been directly studied in CRPS. Intravenous lidocaine is used both therapeutically and diagnostically to assess the responsiveness to a subsequent oral sodium channel blocker (e.g., mexiletine, oxcarbazepine, and carbamazepine) [60, 64, 84–86]. Bier block with methylprednisolone and lidocaine in CRPS type I does not provide long-term benefit in CRPS. While its short-term benefit is not superior to placebo [87].

There is considerable controversy about the use of opiates to treat chronic noncancerous pain, and this is especially true in CRPS. Opioids are generally thought to be less effective in chronic neuropathic pain conditions than in acute and subacute pain conditions. However, there is good evidence that opiates can reduce pain and improve quality of life in patients with neuropathic pain. However, there are no controlled studies showing long-term improvement in opioid-treated neuropathic pain [88–90].

The auto-antigenicity of KRT16 in a murine CRPS model and CRPS patients further reinforce the idea of autoimmune involvement in CRPS, suggesting that new diagnostic tests and treatment strategies may be developed to follow these findings [90]. The use of new immunomodulatory and anti-inflammatory drugs such as thalidomide and lenalidomide (an alpha tumor necrosis factor inhibitor) may offer a new approach to treating CRPS [91]. Low dose naltrexone has unique properties to specifically help the disease cascade of CRPS including attenuation of microglial cells involved in pain transmission, decreased proinflammatory cytokines and toll-like receptor antagonism 4 (TLR4), and stimulation of endorphin secretion. Naltrexone is currently approved for the management of alcohol and opioid disorders. Previous reports have shown that about one-tenth of the dose used for these approved indications may be beneficial for patients with CRPS. A company is developing a new low-dose naltrexone formulation which is due for evaluation [92, 93]. Treatment with low-dose intravenous immunoglobulin (IVIG) may significantly reduce pain in refractory CRPS [94]. Although a trial in 2016 showed that it was "not effective in relieving pain in patients with moderate to severe CRPS between 1 and 5 years of age" [95]. Plasma replacement therapy is also effective in a subset of patients with severe and long-term CRPS [96].

Interventional Therapy

Botulinum toxin type A (BTA) prevents release of acetylcholine from cholinergic nerve terminals, and therefore, intradermal injection of BTX-A has direct analgesic effects in patients with focal chronic neuropathic pain associated with allodynia [97]. BTA-enhanced sympathetic blocks for the treatment of CRPS [98].

CRPS is a very painful condition where patients are unable to move the affected limb much. Because ligaments are very sensitive to immobility, also called stress deprivation, they never heal, although other injuries, such as bone fractures, heal. This unhealed ligament injury continues to activate the sympathetic nervous system, and the patient continues with chronic symptoms, including severe burning pain from CRPS. Ligament relaxation often activates the sympathetic nervous system, and prolotherapy not only relieves pain by stimulating ligament regeneration, but also relieves sympathetic hyperactivity and CRPS-related symptoms [99]. Nerve stimulation which occur through repetitive muscle contractions and a sudden change in the direction of the sensory nerves move between the muscular and facial layers. Cutaneous nerve trauma may cause nerve edema in the proximal and distal regions of the lesion. With perineural prolotherapy, dextrose binds to presynaptic calcium channels and prevents the release of nerve-damaging peptides, thereby reducing nerve inflammation, restoring the normal flow of nerve growth factors, and facilitating nerve repair and produces an almost immediate analgesic effect from hours to days [100]. Stem cell therapy is a new type of regeneration therapy and really an advanced type of prolotherapy. It also has the ability to increase blood flow to damaged tissue and help heal the injured area at the same time. It is a good alternative to RSD treatment and its effect could be monitored by neuro-musculoskeletal thermology [101].

Part of the pathophysiology of CRPS is thought to be related to an autoimmune disorder in the affected limb with an exaggerated response to catecholamines which subsequently causes pain. Sympathetic blocks may facilitate the ratio of sympathetic pain at that point and be of therapeutic benefit, but they cannot exclude or rule out the diagnosis of CRPS. Stellate ganglion blocks and thoracic sympathetic block (T2–T3) are useful in the treatment of sympathetic block of upper extremity pain and lumbar sympathetic block for the lower extremity. Also, a catheter with a stationary sympathetic chain provides continuous pain relief, while it has no motor or sensory dysfunction and may be very effective in allowing the PT to continue working. Single-shot sympathetic blocks must be coordinated with PT sessions, so the patient is painless in all sessions. The successful block is usually controlled by increasing the temperature of the lower part [102–104] (Figs. 9.1 and 9.2).

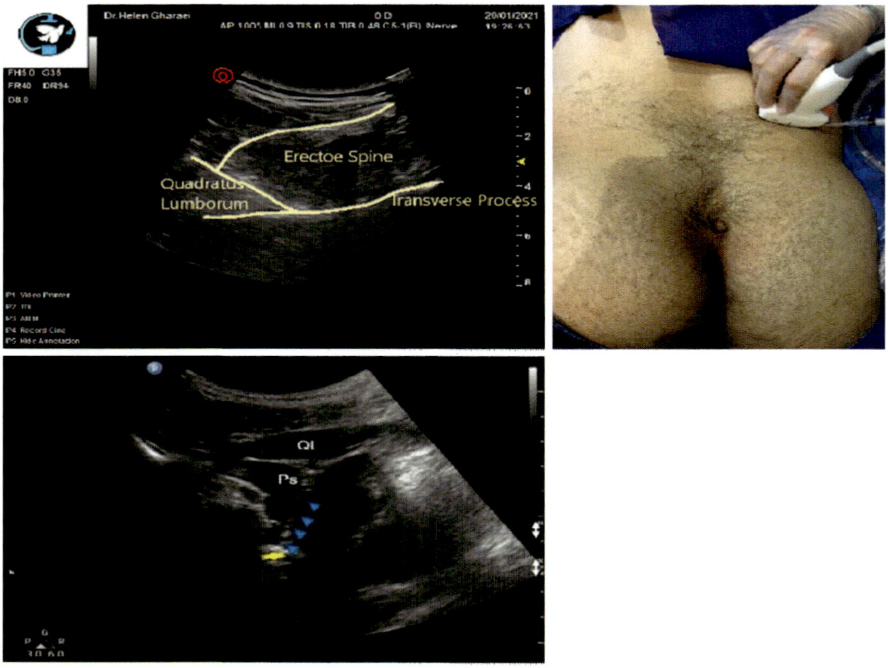

Fig. 9.1 Ultrasound-guided lumbar sympathetic block at L3 inter-transverse space. After visualization of the transverse process by turning the medial side of the probe clock-wise in order to see the anterior border of the vertebral body and psoas muscle. Arrow heads point to a needle shaft and a yellow star shows the anterior fascia of the psoas major muscle. *Ps* psoas major muscle, *QL* quadratus lumborum muscle

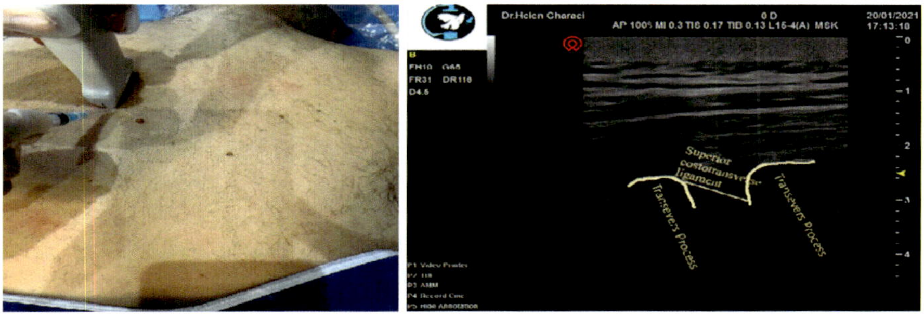

Fig. 9.2 Ultrasound-guided thoracic paravertebral (between the T2 and T3). After passing the ligament, inject drug

Brachial plexus block is used to treat the somatic part of the CRPS-affected upper limb pain. Different approaches to the current block exist including the supraclavicular block, interscalene block, axillary block and the infraclavicular block with the latter being the most common. Continuous popliteal blocks, sciatic peripheral nerve block and saphenous peripheral nerve blockade are of use in treating the somatic part of CRPS lower extremity pain. Continuous epidural analgesia allows a similar level of pain management for PT. Continuous peripheral nerve catheters reduce pain and facilitate intensive physiotherapy and practical rehabilitation, they resulted in resolution of physical changes associated with CRPS and a decrease need for pharmacological drugs, including opioids. Peripheral nerve blockade treats the symptoms. However, it cannot suppress activity at the dorsal root ganglion and it does not address the chronic sensitization within the disease process. Peripheral nerve catheters have the advantage of continuous epidural infusion and can be used in upper extremity disease, provide unilateral analgesia, provide limited and localized sympathetic blockade, and have no effect on bladder or bowel function. However, continuous peripheral nerve block should be more comfortable at home than continuous epidural analgesia. The use of disposable pumps reduces hospitalization such that this treatment can be continued at home. Stationary epidural catheters, although usually effective in relieving pain, cause additional motor block and/or sensation that the patient cannot participate in PT effectively. This may be harmful because any limb immobilization appears to worsen CRPS [105–109].

For patients with upper extremity CRPS type 1 who experience incurable neuropathic pain that is largely limited to the distribution of a peripheral nerve may benefit from implantation of a percutaneous PNS when other options have failed and thus provide pain relief. Peripheral nerve stimulation to the left ulnar nerve may be used for the treatment of patients with complex type 1 pain syndrome following injury to the left fifth finger [110]. Peripheral nerve stimulation is a useful way to improve function and reduce long-term pain in patients who suffer from CRPS types I and II [111]. Wireless peripheral nerve stimulation (WPNS) has unique properties due to its minimally invasive technique. This system does not involve implanting a battery or its connections. In the case of CRPS I, which affects the upper extremities, a WPNS with radial and median nerve coverage provides good pain relief [112]. The plexus stimulation, such as brachial plexus stimulation, has long been used in the treatment of complex regional pain syndrome of the upper extremities [113]. In refractory cases, neuromodulatory option such as SCS stimulation or DRG stimulation may be considered, in very elite cases. Sympathectomy is also useful for this condition [105, 108] (Figs. 9.3, 9.4, and 9.5).

Neuropathic pain is defined as "pain from a lesion or disease of the somatosensory system." Deep brain stimulation (DBS) has been the central implantable nerve stimulation of choice for chronic pain. Some neurosurgeons advocate DBS and its newer target, the anterior cingulate cortex (ACC), while stimulating the motor cortex as "the hall's last chance" [114]. There are good evidences for interventional therapy of CRPS (Table 9.4) [43, 115].

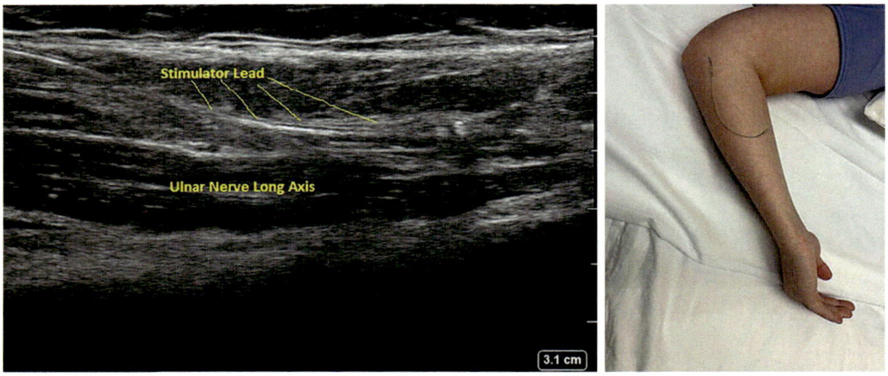

Fig. 9.3 Administration of percutaneous peripheral nerve stimulation in CRPS Type 1 following a crush injury to the fifth digit

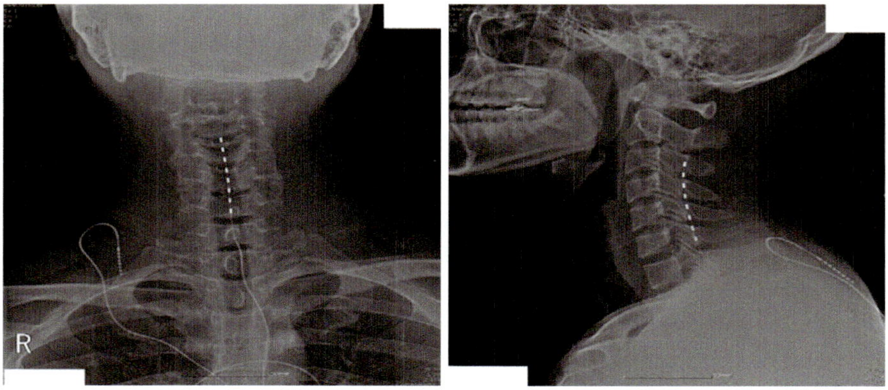

Fig. 9.4 SCS lead position; the catheter enter from T6 and 7 interspaces with final position at the right side of the C3 body in a refractory case of right arm CRPS

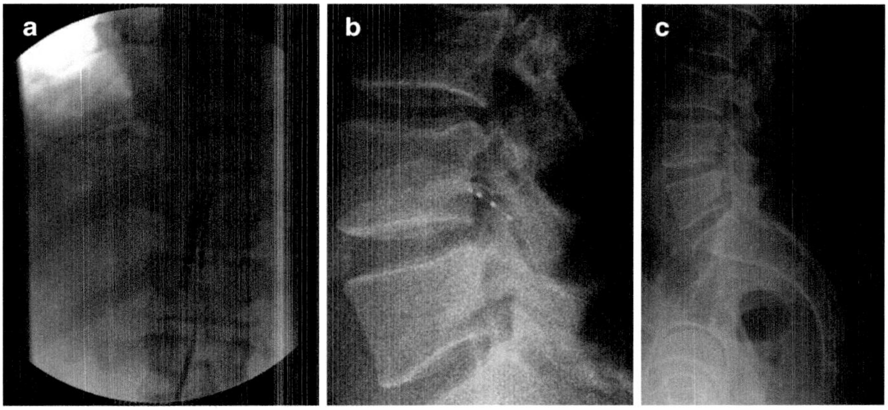

Fig. 9.5 CRPS recurrence 2 years after midtibial amputation, L4 dorsal root ganglion stimulation achieved substantial pain relief after a failed trial of SCS

Table 9.4 Evidence based medicine for interventional pain management in CRPS

Treatment	Recommendations in 2010	Grade level of evidence in 2015	Recommendations in 2018
• Sympathetic blocks with local anesthetics (sympathetic blocks of the ganglion stellatum for CRPS in the arm)	2B+	Moderate	Moderate against
• Thoracic block (T2–T3) with ropivacaine and triamcinolone	2A−	Low	Weak
• IV regional blocks with guanethidine	2B+	Moderate	Moderate against
• Spinal cord stimulation	2C+	Moderate	Moderate
• DRG stimulation (for lower extremity CRPS)		Moderate	Moderate
• Peripheral nerve stimulation		Very low	Very weak
• Low-dose IV ketamine		Moderate	Weak

Algorithmic Approach to CRPS Pain Management

The primary treatment of CRPS consists of early active mobilization by physical therapy combined with pharmacological pain treatment. An early diagnosis is mandatory for therapeutic success and functional outcome. The therapeutic approach with more possibilities of success in the early stages is primarily pharmacological. When conservative treatment with physical and medical treatment fail, multidisciplinary evaluation should be considered. Physical therapy with active mobilization and graded motor imagery treatment, together with a symptom oriented pharmacological treatment, is the best initial approach of CRPS. When there is no

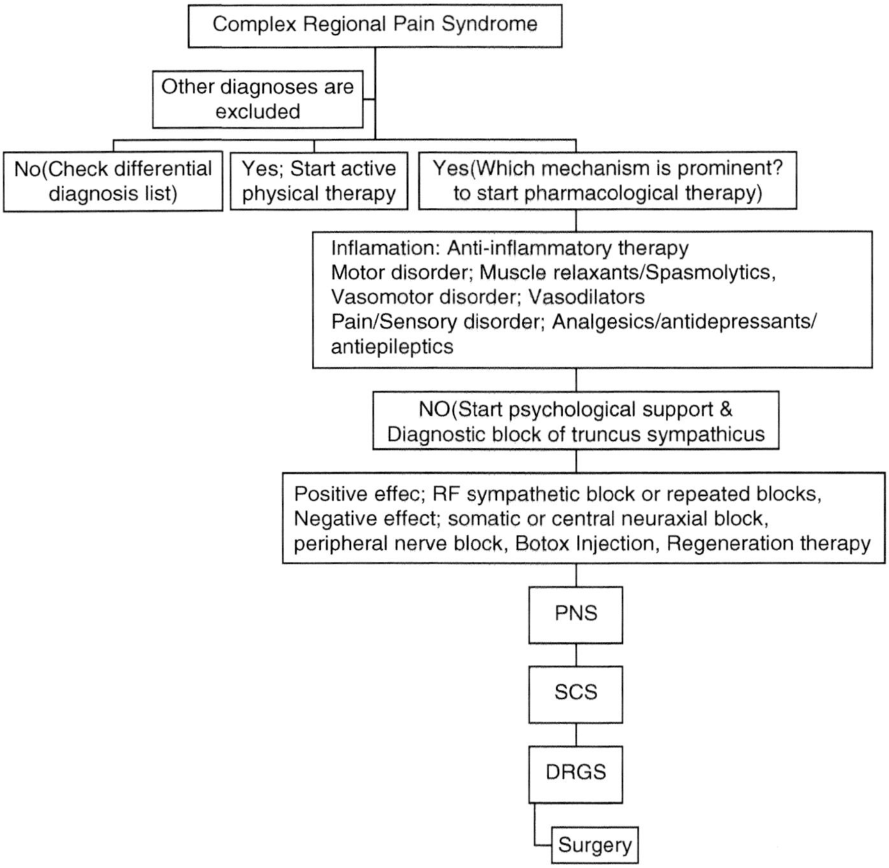

Fig. 9.6 Algorithmic approach to CRPS pain management

improvement in pain and dysfunction, interventional pain management including sympathetic blockade may be performed. If this block is effective, it may be followed by repeated injections or RF treatment. If symptoms persist, a continuous epidural infusion, intermittent or continuous plexus brachialis block in combination with exercise therapy may be useful. And in refractory cases, SCS after a successful trial stimulation period may yield positive results [43] (Fig. 9.6).

Conclusion

Currently, there are no drugs approved by FDA specifically for the treatment of CRPS. Early diagnosis is still the key in the success of therapeutic intervention. Interventional pain management in CRPS is a great chance given to us to resolve these difficult cases in the early stages while patients with CRPS have negative bone scans. Chronic CRPS, or a predominantly cold illness are less likely to respond to any treatment modalities [67, 68]. I recommend to start with less invasive and less expensive intervention especially in low income country and a judicious use of any intervention regardless of the country of origin as soon as possible without leaving these cases unsolved.

References

1. National Institute of Neurological Disorders and Stroke. Complex regional pain syndrome. https://www.ninds.nih.gov/Disorders/Patient-Caregiver-Education/Fact-Sheets/Complex-Regional-Pain-Syndrome-FactSheet#:~:text=Complex%20regional%20pain%20syndrome%20(CRPS,peripheral%20and%20central%20nervous%20systems. Accessed 14 Dec 2020.
2. Bruehl S, Harden RN, Galer BS, Saltz S, Backonja M, Stanton-Hicks M. Complex regional pain syndrome: are there distinct subtypes and sequential stages of the syndrome? Pain. 2002;95:119–24.
3. Paré A. Of the cure of wounds of the nervous system. The collected works of Ambroise Pare. New York: Milford House; 1634.
4. Denmark A. An example of symptoms resembling tic Douleureux, produced by a wound in the radial nerve. Med Chir Trans. 1813;4:48–52.
5. Mitchell SW. Injuries of nerves and their consequences. Philadelphia: JB Lippincott; 1872.
6. Dunglison R. A dictionary of medical science. Philadelphia: Blanchard & Lea; 1874.
7. Sudeck P. Über die akute entzündliche Knochenatrophie. Arch Klin Chir. 1900;62:147–56.
8. De la Leriche R. causalgie envisagee comme une nevrite due sympathique et de son traitment par la denudation et l'excision des plexus nerveux peri-arteriels. Presse Med. 1916;24:178–80.
9. Evans JA. Reflex sympathetic dystrophy. Surg Clin N Am. 1946;26:780–90.
10. Foisie PS. Traumatic arterial vasospasm. N Engl J Med. 1947;237:295–302.
11. Bonica JJ. The management of pain. Philadelphia: Lea & Febiger; 1953.
12. Merskey H, Bogduk N. International Association for the Study of Pain Task Force on Taxonomy: classification of chronic pain: descriptions of chronic pain syndromes and definitions of pain terms. 2nd ed. Seattle, WA: IASP Press; 1994.
13. Veldman PH, Reynen HM, Arntz IE, Goris RJ. Signs and symptoms of reflex sympathetic dystrophy: prospective study of 829 patients. Lancet. 1993;342(8878):1012–6.
14. Harden RN, Bruehl S, Galer BS, Saltz S, Bertram M, Backonja M, Gayles R, Rudin N, Bhugra MK, Stanton-Hicks M. Complex regional pain syndrome: are the IASP diagnostic criteria valid and sufficiently comprehensive? Pain. 1999;83(2):211–9.
15. Bruehl S, Harden RN, Galer BS, Saltz S, Bertram M, Backonja M, Gayles R, Rudin N, Bhugra MK, Stanton-Hicks M. External validation of IASP diagnostic criteria for complex regional pain syndrome and proposed research diagnostic criteria. International Association for the Study of Pain. Pain. 1999;81(1–2):147–54.
16. Harden RN, Bruehl S, Perez RS, Birklein F, Marinus J, Maihofner C, Lubenow T, Buvanendran A, Mackey S, Graciosa J, Mogilevski M, Ramsden C, Chont M, Vatine JJ. Validation of proposed diagnostic criteria (the "Budapest criteria") for complex regional pain syndrome. Pain. 2010;150(2):268–74.
17. Sandroni P, Benrud-Larson LM, RL MC, Low PA. Complex regional pain syndrome type I: incidence and prevalence in Olmsted county, a population-based study. Pain. 2003;103:199–207.
18. de Mos M, de Bruijn AG, Huygen FJ, Dieleman JP, Stricker BH, Sturkenboom MC. The incidence of complex regional pain syndrome: a population-based study. Pain. 2007;129:12–20.

19. Ott S, Maihofner C. Signs and symptoms in 1,043 patients with complex regional pain syndrome. J Pain. 2018;19:599–611.
20. Kim H, Lee CH, Kim SH, Kim YD. Epidemiology of complex regional pain syndrome in Korea: an electronic population health data study. PLoS One. 2018;13:e0198147.
21. Petersen PB, Mikkelsen KL, Lauritzen JB, Krogsgaard MR. Risk factors for post-treatment complex regional pain syndrome (CRPS): an analysis of 647 cases of CRPS from the Danish Patient Compensation Association. Pain Pract. 2018;18:341–9.
22. Goh EL, Chidambaram S, Ma D. Complex regional pain syndrome: a recent update. Burns Trauma. 2017;5:2.
23. Groeneweg JG, Huygen FJ, Heijmans-Antonissen C, Niehof S, Zijlstra FJ. Increased endothelin-1 and diminished nitric oxide levels in blister fluids of patients with intermediate cold type complex regional pain syndrome type 1. BMC Musculoskelet Disord. 2006;7:91.
24. Birklein F, Schmelz M. Neuropeptides, neurogenic inflammation and complex regional pain syndrome (CRPS). Neurosci Lett. 2008;437:199–202.
25. Oaklander AL, Fields HL. Is reflex sympathetic dystrophy/complex regional pain syndrome type Ia small-fiber neuropathy? Ann Neurol. 2009;65:629–38.
26. Janig W, Baron R. Complex regional pain syndrome: mystery explained? Lancet Neurol. 2003;2:687–97.
27. Yvon A, Faroni A, Reid AJ, Lees VC. Selective fiber degeneration in the peripheral nerve of a patient with severe complex regional pain syndrome. Front Neurosci. 2018;12:207.
28. Finch PM, Drummond ES, Dawson LF, Phillips JK, Drummond PD. Up-regulation of cutaneous alpha1-adrenoceptors in complex regional pain syndrome type I. Pain Med. 2014;15:1945–56.
29. Gibbs GF, Drummond PD, Finch PM, Phillips JK. Unravelling the pathophysiology of complex regional pain syndrome: focus on sympathetically. Clin Exp Pharmacol Physiol. 2008;35(7):717–24.
30. Woolf CJ. Central sensitization: implications for the diagnosis and treatment of pain. Pain. 2011;152:S2–S15.
31. de Mos M, Sturkenboom MC, Huygen FJ. Current understandings on complex regional pain syndrome. Pain Pract. 2009;9:86–99.
32. Di Pietro F, McAuley JH, Parkitny L. Primary somatosensory cortex function in complex regional pain syndrome: a systematic review and meta-analysis. J Pain. 2013;14:1001–18.
33. Maihöfner C, Handwerker HO, Neundörfer B, Birklein F. Patterns of cortical reorganization in complex regional pain syndrome. Neurology. 2003;61(12):1707–15.
34. Mancini F, Wang AP, Schira MM, Isherwood ZJ, McAuley JH, Iannetti GD, Sereno MI, Moseley GL, Rae CD. Fine-grained mapping of cortical somatotopies in chronic complex regional pain syndrome. J Neurosci. 2019;39(46):9185–96.
35. Blaes F, Schmitz K, Tschernatsch M. Autoimmune etiology of complex regional pain syndrome (M. Sudeck). Neurology. 2004;63:1734–6.
36. Morellini N, Finch PM, Goebel A, Drummond PD. Dermal nerve fibre and mast cell density, and proximity of mast cells to nerve fibres in the skin of patients with complex regional pain syndrome. Pain. 2018;159:2021–9.
37. Birklein F, Ajit SK, Goebel A, Perez R, Sommer C. Complex regional pain syndrome - phenotypic characteristics and potential biomarkers. Nat Rev Neurol. 2018;14:272–84.
38. de Rooij AM, de Mos M, Sturkenboom MC, Marinus J, van den Maagdenberg AM, van Hilten JJ. Familial occurrence of complex regional pain syndrome. Eur J Pain. 2009;13:171–7.
39. Orlova IA, Alexander GM, Qureshi RA. MicroRNA modulation in complex regional pain syndrome. J Transl Med. 2011;9:195.
40. Janicki PK, Alexander GM, Eckert J, Postula M, Schwartzman RJ. Analysis of common single nucleotide polymorphisms in complex regional pain syndrome: genome wide association study approach and pooled DNA strategy. Pain Med. 2016;17:2344–52.
41. Speck V, Schlereth T, Birklein F, Maihofner C. Increased prevalence of posttraumatic stress disorder in CRPS. Eur J Pain. 2017;21:466–73.

42. Urits I, Shen AH, Jones MR, Viswanath O, Kaye AD. Complex regional pain syndrome, current concepts and treatment options. Curr Pain Headache Rep. 2018;22:10.
43. van Eijs F, Stanton-Hicks M, Van Zundert J, Faber CG, Lubenow TR, Mekhail N, van Kleef M, Huygen F. Evidence-based interventional pain medicine according to clinical diagnoses. 16. Complex regional pain syndrome. Pain Pract. 2011;11(1):70–87.
44. Harden RN, Bruehl S, Perez RS. Development of a severity score for CRPS. Pain. 2010;151:870–6.
45. Giannotti S, Bottai V, Dell'Osso G, Bugelli G, Celli F, Cazzella N, Guido G. Algodystrophy: complex regional pain syndrome and incomplete forms. Clin Cases Miner Bone Metab. 2016;13(1):11–4.
46. Wasner G, Schattschneider J, Heckmann K, Maier C, Baron R. Vascular abnormalities in reflex sympathetic dystrophy (CRPS I): mechanisms and diagnostic value. Brain. 2001;124(Pt 3):587–99.
47. Harden RN, Maihofner C, Abousaad E. A prospective, multisite, international validation of the complex regional pain syndrome severity score. Pain. 2017;158:1430–6.
48. Jeon SG, Choi EJ, Lee PB. Do severity score and skin temperature asymmetry correlate with the subjective pain score in the patients with complex regional pain syndrome? Korean J Pain. 2014;27:339–44.
49. Korompilias AV, Karantanas AH, Lykissas MG, Beris AE. Bone marrow edema syndrome. Skelet Radiol. 2009;38(5):425–36.
50. Wertli MM, Brunner F, Steurer J, Held U. Usefulness of bone scintigraphy for the diagnosis of complex regional pain syndrome 1: a systematic review and Bayesian meta-analysis. PLoS One. 2017;12(3):e0173688.
51. Ringer R, Wertli M, Bachmann LM, Buck FM, Brunner F. Concordance of qualitative bone scintigraphy results with presence of clinical complex regional pain syndrome 1: meta-analysis of test accuracy studies. Eur J Pain. 2012;16:1347–56.
52. Munts AG, Van Rootselaar AF, Van Der Meer JN, Koelman JH, Van Hilten JJ, Tijssen MA. Clinical and neurophysiological characterization of myoclonus in complex regional pain syndrome. Mov Disord. 2008;23:581–7.
53. Vas L, Pai R. Musculoskeletal ultrasonography to distinguish muscle changes in complex regional pain syndrome type 1 from those of neuropathic pain: an observational study. Pain Pract. 2016;16:E1–3.
54. Cuhadar U, Gentry C, Vastani N, Sensi S, Bevan S, Goebel A, Andersson DA. Autoantibodies produce pain in complex regional pain syndrome by sensitizing nociceptors. Pain. 2019;160(12):2855–65.
55. Dirckx M, Schreurs MWJ, de Mos M, Stronks DL, Huygen FJPM. The prevalence of autoantibodies in complex regional pain syndrome type I. Mediat Inflamm. 2015;2015:718201.
56. Harden RN, Oaklander AL, Burton AW. Complex regional pain syndrome: practical diagnostic and treatment guidelines, 4th edition. Pain Med. 2013;14:180–229.
57. Smart KM, Wand BM, O'Connell NE. Physiotherapy for pain and disability in adults with complex regional pain syndrome (CRPS) types I and II. Cochrane Database Syst Rev. 2016;2:CD010853.
58. Somers DL, Clemente FR. Transcutaneous electrical nerve stimulation for the management of neuropathic pain: the effects of frequency and electrode position on prevention of allodynia in a rat model of complex regional pain syndrome type II. Phys Ther. 2006;86(5):698–709.
59. Jensen MP, Caroline Grierson RN, Tracy-Smitm V, Bacigalupi SC, Othmer S. Neurofeedback treatment for pain associated with complex regional pain syndrome type I. J Neurother. 2008;8:45–53.
60. Clinical practice guidelines–third edition. International Research Foundation for RSD/CRPS. www.rsdfoundation.org/en/en_ clinical_practice_guidelines.html. Accessed 1 Apr 2009.
61. Breuer AJ, Mainka T, Hansel N, Maier C, Krumova EK. Short-term treatment with parecoxib for complex regional pain syndrome: a randomized, placebo-controlled double-blind trial. Pain Physician. 2014;17:127–37.

62. Eckmann MS, Ramamurthy S, Griffin JG. Intravenous regional ketorolac and lidocaine in the treatment of complex regional pain syndrome of the lower extremity: a randomized, double-blinded, crossover study. Clin J Pain. 2011;27:203–6.
63. Collins SL, Moore RA, McQuay H, et al. Antidepressants and anticonvulsants for diabetic neuropathy and postherpetic neuralgia: a quantitative systematic review. J Pain Symptom Manag. 2000;20:449–58.
64. Dworkin RH, O'Connor AB, Backonja M, et al. Pharmacologic management of neuropathic pain: evidence-based recommendations. Pain. 2007;132:237–51.
65. Brown S, Johnston B, Amaria K. A randomized controlled trial of amitriptyline versus gabapentin for complex regional pain syndrome type I and neuropathic pain in children. Scand J Pain. 2016;13:156–63.
66. Harke H, Gretenkort P, Ladleif HU, Rahman S, Harke O. The response of neuropathic pain and pain in complex regional pain syndrome I to carbamazepine and sustained-release morphine in patients pretreated with spinal cord stimulation: a double-blinded randomized study. Anesth Analg. 2001;92:488–95.
67. Varenna M, Adami S, Sinigaglia L. Bisphosphonates in complex regional pain syndrome type I: how do they work? Clin Exp Rheumatol. 2014;32:451–4.
68. Chevreau M, Romand X, Gaudin P, Juvin R, Baillet A. Bisphosphonates for treatment of complex regional pain syndrome type 1: a systematic literature review and meta-analysis of randomized controlled trials versus placebo. Joint Bone Spine. 2017;84:393–9.
69. Varenna M, Braga V, Gatti D, et al. Intramuscular neridronate for the treatment of complex regional pain syndrome type 1: a randomized, double-blind, placebo-controlled study. Ther Adv Musculoskelet Dis. 2021;13:1759720X211014020.
70. Kiefer RT, Rohr P, Ploppa A, et al. Efficacy of ketamine in anesthetic dosage for the treatment of refractory complex regional pain syndrome: an open-label phase II study. Pain Med. 2008;9:1173–201.
71. Perez R, Kwakkel G, Zuurmond W, et al. Treatment of reflex sympathetic dystrophy (CPRS type I): a research synthesis of 21 randomized clinical trials. J Pain Symptom Manage. 2001;21:511–26.
72. Zuurmond WW, Langendijk PN, Bezemer PD, et al. Treatment of acute reflex sympathetic dystrophy with DMSO 50% in a fatty cream. Acta Anaesthesiol Scand. 1996;40:364–7.
73. Zollinger PE, Tuinebreijer WE, Kreis RW, Breederveld RS. Effect of vitamin C on frequency of reflex sympathetic dystrophy in wrist fractures: a randomised trial. Lancet. 1999;354:2025–8.
74. Besse JL, Gadeyne S, Galand-Desme S, Lerat JL, Moyen B. Effect of vitamin C on prevention of complex regional pain syndrome type I in foot and ankle surgery. Foot Ankle Surg. 2009;15:179–82.
75. Lichtman DM, Bindra RR, Boyer MI. American Academy of Orthopaedic Surgeons clinical practice guideline on: the treatment of distal radius fractures. J Bone Jt Surg Am. 2011;93:775–8.
76. Te AE. A modern rationale for the use of phenoxybenzamine in urinary tract disorders and other conditions. Clin Ther. 2002;24:851–61.
77. Muizelaar JP, Kleyer M, Hertogs IA, DeLange DC. Complex regional pain syndrome (reflex sympathetic dystrophy and causalgia): management with the calcium channel blocker nifedipine and/or the alpha-sympathetic blocker phenoxybenzamine in 59 patients. Clin Neurol Neurosurg. 1997;99:26–30.
78. Raja SN, Turnquist JL, Meleka S, Campbell JN. Monitoring adequacy of alpha-adrenoceptor blockade following systemic phentolamine administration. Pain. 1996;64:197–204.
79. Davis KD, Treede RD, Raja SN, et al. Topical application of clonidine relieves hyperalgesia in patients with sympathetically maintained pain. Pain. 1991;47:309–17.
80. Stevens DS, Robins VF, Price HM. Treatment of sympathetically maintained pain with terazosin. Reg Anesth. 1993;18:318–21.

81. Prough DS, McLeskey CH, Poehling GG, et al. Efficacy of oral nifedipine in the treatment of reflex sympathetic dystrophy. Anesthesiology. 1985;62:796–9.
82. Inchiosa MA, Kizelshteyn G. Treatment of complex regional pain syndrome type 1 with oral phenoxybenzamine: rationale and case reports. Pain Pract. 2008;8:125–32.
83. Raja SN, Treede RD, Davis KD, et al. Systemic alpha-adrenergic blockage with phentolamine: a diagnostic test for sympathetically maintained pain. Anesthesiology. 1991;74:691–8.
84. Mackey S, Feinberg S. Pharmacologic therapies for complex regional pain syndrome. Curr Pain Headache Rep. 2007;11(1):38–43.
85. Mao J, Chen LL. Systemic lidocaine for neuropathic pain relief. Pain. 2000;87:7–17.
86. Attal N, Brasseur L, Chauvin M, et al. Effects of single and repeated applications of a eutectic mixture of local anaesthetics (EMLA) cream on spontaneous and evoked pain in postherpetic neuralgia. Pain. 1999;81:203–9.
87. Taskaynatan MA, Ozgul A, Tan AK, Dincer K, Kalyon TA. Bier block with methylprednisolone and lidocaine in CRPS type I: a randomized, double-blinded, placebo-controlled study. Reg Anesth Pain Med. 2004;29(5):408–12.
88. Dellemijn P. Are opioids effective in relieving neuropathic pain? Pain. 1999;80:453–62.
89. Watson CP, Babul N. Efficacy of oxycodone in neuropathic pain: a randomized trial in postherpetic neuralgia. Neurology. 1998;50:1837–41.
90. Tajerian M, Hung V, Khan H, et al. Identification of KRT16 as a target of an autoantibody response in complex regional pain syndrome. Exp Neurol. 2017;287:14–20.
91. Asher C, Furnish T. Lenalidomide and thalidomide in the treatment of chronic pain. Expert Opin Drug Saf. 2013;12(3):367–74.
92. FDA grants Orphan Drug status to Soin Therapeutics for low dose naltrexone (LDN) to treat complex regional pain syndrome (CRPS). News release. September 9, 2021.
93. Taylor SS, Noor N, Urits I, et al. Complex regional pain syndrome: a comprehensive review. Pain Ther. Published online June 24, 2021.
94. Goebel A, Baranowski A, Maurer K, Ambler G. Intravenous immunoglobulin treatment of the complex regional pain syndrome: a randomized trial. Ann Intern Med. 2010;3:152–8.
95. Hopes dwindle for new CRPS treatment. BLB Chronic Pain Solicitors Dec 21st, 2016. https://www.blbchronicpain.co.uk/news/hopes-dwindle-for-new-crps-treatment/.
96. Aradillas E, Schwartzman RJ, Grothusen JR, Goebel A, Alexander GM. Plasma exchange therapy in patients with complex regional pain syndrome. Pain Physician. 2015;18:383–94.
97. Ranoux D, Attal N, Morain F, Bouhassira D. Botulinum toxin type a induces direct analgesic effects in chronic neuropathic pain. Ann Neurol. 2008;64:274–83.
98. Ian Carroll J, Clark D, Mackey S. Sympathetic block with botulinum toxin to treat complex regional pain syndrome. Ann Neurol. 2009;65(3):348–51.
99. Hauser RA, Debra K, Brinker RN. The theoretical basis for and treatment of complex regional pain syndrome with prolotherapy. J Prolother. 2010;2(2):356–70.
100. Thor JA, Hanapi NHM, Halil H, Suhaimi A. Perineural injection therapy in the management of complex regional pain syndrome: a sweet solution to pain. Pain Med. 2017;18(10):2041–5.
101. Schwartz RG. Stem cells for the treatment of complex regional pain syndrome (CRPS)/reflex sympathetic dystrophy (RSD): a case study. Pan Am J Med Thermol. 2014;1(2):89–92.
102. O'Connell NE, Wand BM, Gibson W, Carr DB, Birklein F, Stanton TR. Local anaesthetic sympathetic blockade for complex regional pain syndrome. Cochrane Database Syst Rev. 2016;7(7):CD004598.
103. Moon JY, Choi JK, Shin JY, Chon SW, Dev S. A brief report on a technical description of ultrasound-guided lumbar sympathetic block. Korean J Pain. 2017;30(1):66–70.
104. Kim J, Lee HJ, Lee YJ, Lee CS, Yoo Y, Moon JY. Ultrasound-guided thoracic paravertebral block as a sympathetic blockade for upper extremity neuropathic pain: a prospective pilot study. J Pain Res. 2020;13:3395–403.
105. Martin DP, Bhalla T, Rehman S, Tobias JD. Successive multisite peripheral nerve catheters for treatment of complex regional pain syndrome type I. Pediatrics. 2013;131(1):e323–6.

106. Margic K, Pirc J. The treatment of complex regional pain syndrome (CRPS) involving upper extremity with continuous sensory analgesia. Eur J Pain. 2003;7(1):43–7.
107. Dadure C, Motais F, Ricard C, Raux O, Troncin R, Capdevila X. Continuous peripheral nerve blocks at home for treatment of recurrent complex regional pain syndrome I in children. Anesthesiology. 2005;102(2):387–91.
108. Goebel A, Lewis S, Phillip R, Sharma M. Dorsal root ganglion stimulation for complex regional pain syndrome (CRPS) recurrence after amputation for CRPS, and failure of conventional spinal cord stimulation. Pain Pract. 2018;18(1):104–8.
109. Gharaei H. Continuous peripheral nerve catheters in pediatric complex regional pain syndrome. Anesth Pain Med. 2015;5(1):e23414.
110. Fritz AV, Ferreira-Dos-Santos G, Hurdle M, et al. Ultrasound-guided percutaneous peripheral nerve stimulation for the treatment of complex regional pain syndrome type 1 following a crush injury to the fifth digit: a rare case report. Cureus. 2019;11(12):e6506.
111. Chmiela MA, Hendrickson M, Hale J, Liang C, Telefus P, Sagir A, Stanton-Hicks M. Direct peripheral nerve stimulation for the treatment of complex regional pain syndrome: a 30-year review. Neuromodulation. 2021;24(6):971–82.
112. Herschkowitz D, Kubias J. Wireless peripheral nerve stimulation for complex regional pain syndrome type I of the upper extremity: a case illustration introducing a novel technology. Scand J Pain. 2018;18(3):555–60.
113. Frederico TN, Freitas TS. Peripheral nerve stimulation of the brachial plexus for chronic refractory CRPS pain of the upper limb: description of a new technique and case series. Pain Med. 2020;21(1):S18–26.
114. Farrell SM, Green A, Aziz T. The current state of deep brain stimulation for chronic pain and its context in other forms of neuromodulation. Brain Sci. 2018;8(8):158.
115. Huygen F, Kallewaard JW, Tulder MV, Boxem KV, Vissers K, van Kleef M, Van Zundert J. "Evidence-based interventional pain medicine according to clinical diagnoses": update 2019. Pain Pract. 2019;19(6):664–75.

Chapter 10
Introduction to Central Pain Syndromes and Painful Peripheral Neuropathy

Daniel Wang and George C. Chang Chien

Introduction

The International Association for the Study of Pain (IASP) describes neuropathic pain as pain caused by a lesion or disease of the somatosensory system. The types of neuropathic pain can be further segmented into pathways arising from the peripheral nervous system as well as those arising from the central nervous system depending on the location of interest. Neuropathic pain originating from the peripheral nervous system is more common. They can be further broken down into painful neuropathies originating from autoimmune/infectious diseases, systemic diseases, genetic conditions, or injury/acquired conditions [1]. Patients with peripheral neuropathy present with a wide range of issues and do not necessarily experience pain [1]. They may report with hyperalgesia (normally painful stimuli causing exaggerated pain), allodynia (normally non-painful stimuli causing pain), hyperpathia (repetitive stimulation causing prolonged persistent pain), paresthesia (atypical non painful sensations that is not unpleasant) and dysesthesia (atypical painful sensation that is unpleasant) [1].

D. Wang
Kansas City University, Kansas City, MO, USA

G. C. C. Chien (✉)
Pain Management, Ventura County Medical Center, Ventura, CA, USA

Physical Medicine and Rehabilitation, Pain Medicine, Ventura County Medical Center, Ventura, CA, USA

GCC Institute Regenerative Medicine, Newport Beach, CA, USA

© The Author(s), under exclusive license to Springer Nature Switzerland AG 2022

J. de Castro, Y. El Miedany (eds.), *Advances in Chronic and Neuropathic Pain*, Contemporary Rheumatology, https://doi.org/10.1007/978-3-031-10687-3_10

Painful neuropathies originating from the central nervous system (CNS) develop from diseases affecting the spinal cord, brainstem, or brain. These are deemed as Central Pain Syndromes (CPS) or Central Neuropathic Pain (CNP). There is a wide range of Central Pain-associated injuries that result from infectious, vascular, demyelinating, traumatic, or neoplastic etiologies. Some of the most common issues originate from stroke, and spinal cord injury (SCI) [1]. This chapter will first focus on neuropathic pain as a result of issues to the central nervous system and then later to the peripheral nervous system.

Central Pain Syndromes

History and Definitions

In the early nineteenth century, German neurologist Dr. Edinger first proposed the theory of a central pain in public literature [2]. Until that point, there had only been case reports detailing pain originating from the spinal cord or brain. This led to further case studies mentioning pain due to specific locations in the CNS (brainstem, thalamus, internal capsule, cortex, etc.). In the early twentieth century, Roussy and Dejerine found that thalamic lesions caused pain with other associated symptoms. This was later termed as "thalamic syndrome." [3]. Sometime later, Holmes and Head published literature further detailed the relationship between thalamic issues and central pain (CP) [4]. Holmes further found comparable pains that were associated with spinal cord injuries in WWI soldiers. Though it was becoming more known that CPs could arise from pain outside of the thalamus, the exact origin remained unknown. In the 1960s, however, Pagni and Cassinari published a monumental review that detailed the relationship between CP occurring as a result of a spinothalamic tract lesion [5].

Even with these findings, the terms "central pain syndrome" and "thalamic syndrome" remain synonymous. The increase in functional neurophysiologic testing and neuroimaging technology (MRI and CT scans) have led to increased evidence and literature supporting that lesions along anywhere in the CNS could lead to CP [2]. This has finally led to the term "Central Pain Syndrome" being increasingly adopted to indicate this change in thought.

Clinical Characteristics

CP can sometimes present similarly to neuropathies. Common presenting symptoms include tingling, burning, pins and needles, electrical, stabbing, itching, and many more feelings that can happen as an isolated instance or in various combinations.

The severity of pain is variable among patients, ranging from some mild discomfort to severe pain. The literature has pointed to several factors including psychological mood comorbidities, pain components, and scale of neurological deficits that possibly impact pain severity [2]. Specifically for neurological sensory deficits, literature indicates the thermal and pinprick sensations correlate with areas of greatest pain severity, and two-point discrimination, tactile sensation, and vibration were unaffected in areas of pain [2].

Furthermore, CP can present with varying traits in different combinations in the same person [3]. These traits can be broken down into continuous, intermittent, or evoked symptoms [6, 7]. Intermittent pain is often more severe and spontaneous when compared to continuous pain. Evoked pain is induced and often leads to hyperalgesia (normally painful stimuli causing increased pain), allodynia (normally non-painful stimuli causing pain), and hyperesthesia (normal stimuli causing increased sensitivity). Patients commonly present with a variation of severe intermittent pain and a dull continuous pain [8]. Generally, the more variations of pain present, the more severe the perceived pain. Patients with incomplete sensory deficits compared to those with complete sensory deficits will typically have an increased pain severity because they show extreme evoked pain in the impaired areas of sensory loss [3].

Aside from the intensity and descriptive characteristics, pain can negatively affect quality of life and function [9]. Pain and functional limitations often correlate with sleeping complications and depression 1 year after stroke [10]. Thus, it is vital to evaluate sleep and psychological mood impairments when diagnosing, evaluating, or treating CP. Challenges in either may alter the severity of pain perception.

Diagnosis

Diagnosing and classifying CP has been a continuous conversation between clinicians and researchers. Because CP is a type of neuropathic pain, the existence of typical neuropathy will often lead to further analysis.

Currently, there are several official neuropathic pain scales including the Neuropathic Pain Questionnaire [16], Douleur Neuropathique 4 (DN4) [17], and Leeds Assessment of Neuropathic Symptoms and Signs (LANSS) pain scale [11]. These were created to assist in indicating the presence of neuropathic pain. These scales, however, are limited in defining CP. The Neuropathic pain System Inventory (NPSI) does break down neuropathic pain into further components which slightly helps classify CP [12]. However, it is limited in specificity and sensitivity [2]. As such, these scales are not intended to be used as a gold standard diagnostic tool, but rather in combination with a thorough history, physical examination, and other forms of additional testing [2].

The neuropathic pain grading system is used to determine, to a certain degree, the presence of neuropathic pain. It was created based on the definition detailed by the IASP mentioning that "neuropathic pain caused by a lesion or disease of the somatosensory nervous system." For neuropathic pain to occur, history and distribution of pain, sensory deficits on physical examination, and lesion location confirmed on imaging must coincide [13].

Several limitations must be considered when diagnosing CP. The existence of neuropathic pain does not indicate whether it is a central nervous system (CNS) or peripheral nervous system (PNS) problem (i.e. burning sensations can be indicated in central poststroke pain [CPSP] and diabetic neuropathy). Further, CP can coexist with other pain manifestations, which can make the diagnosis inaccurate (i.e. patients with CPSP can exhibit coexistent pain affecting the same extremity). Lastly, patients with CP clinically present with a high degree of variability.

CP is a multifactorial issue because it shares many coinciding criteria with other pain conditions [2]. This further complicates the diagnosis, evaluation, and management. A common clinical scenario to see includes neurologically limited patients that have decreased mobility; thus, they are at an increased risk of musculoskeletal injuries. One study examined the relationship between stroke patients diagnosed with CP syndrome and the existence of myofascial pain (MP) [14]. It was concluded that for stroke patients, the existence of MP cannot be eliminated and can possibly be a comorbidity. As exemplified in the aforementioned example, other diagnoses of pain must be considered; otherwise, ineffective treatment plans could happen.

Because of the difficulties in diagnosing CP, the American Pain Society Pain Taxonomy published a multifactorial framework associated with multiple sclerosis, SCI, and stroke [15]. These suggestions include five factors: "(1) core diagnostic criteria, (2) common features, (3) common medical and psychiatric comorbidities, (4) neurobiological, psychosocial, and functional consequences, and (5) putative neurobiological and psychosocial mechanisms, risk factors, and protective factors."

Central Post Stroke Pain

Definition and Prevalence

Stroke often induces many complications such as chronic pain. Every year, approximately 795,000 strokes happen in the United States, and an incidence of 3.73 per 1000 person-years [2]. Literature shows that one-fifth to half of stroke patients experience some pain. Pain is further segmented into stroke-related and non-stroke-related. In the former, there are sub-conditions that typically happen as a result of stroke. These conditions include headaches, CP, complex regional pain syndrome, myofascial pain, and spasticity [16]. In the latter it tends to be explained by pre-comorbidities such as polyneuropathy.

Central post stroke pain (CPSP) syndrome is a sensory irregularity or pain that is localized to the area of cerebrovascular impact following a stroke [2]. As an example, an infarct in the right hemisphere of the brain can cause left-sided hemiplegia may result in pain in those left-sided extremities. When considering all stroke types, the prevalence of CPSP is significantly variable; the incidence is typically 2–8% [9]. The variability can stem from variability in study design and definitions [7, 17]. Further, CPSP can often go undiagnosed by physicians as a result of the lack of a specific CP scale and as a result of patients not mentioning it; this often leads to differences in studies [18]. Studies suggest that risk factors for CPSP include tobacco use, depression comorbidities, and motor/sensory deficits [19, 20]. Some studies also suggest young age to be a risk factor, although this is highly variable [9]. Further, the progression is significantly correlated with depression and severity of stroke impairments, and other pain issues [17]. Specifically, in one of the biggest studies in thalamic CPSP, right-sided infarctions were more associated with CPSP than left-sided infarctions. This finding is significant because the right hemisphere is vital for pain control [9]. Screening and recognizing CPSP should include cognitive and functional deficits as well as emotional health.

Onset

Typically, CPSP onset is approximately 3–6 months. Although, there has been huge variability of up to 18 months [2]. This pain felt at a later onset, which can be both instant or gradual, is thought to be correlated with the sensory and motor improvements as time progresses [21]. Additionally, it can precede neurological improvements. As stated previously in the chapter, pain can be intermittent, continuous, or evoked. Continuous pain is most common and is typically dull, while evoked and intermittent pain are typically severe [3, 18].

The significant variability of CPSP symptoms presents challenges in diagnosing CPSP for clinicians. As such, there has been increased research to determine standard patterns and traits that clearly point to CP instead of other pain conditions [22]. Despite pain sensations such as shooting, tingling, and burning are not specific enough to CP, a vital trait is examining where the area of pain distribution is. For example, if there is pain that correlates with the area of a lesion in the CNS, these symptoms can be traced back to the CNS.

Diagnostic Standards

Diagnosis for CPSP includes a framework created by AAPT that is based on neuropathic pain [15]. Firstly, there should be a diagnostic test that confirms the stroke. Secondly, continuous or recurring pain after stroke after the onset for up to 1 year. Thirdly, pain that has a duration for a minimum of 3 months. Fourthly, pain will be distributed in the area affected by the stroke as mentioned earlier. Fifthly, sensory changes in the distribution of the insult, which can be either a positive or negative sign. Lastly, all other diagnoses must be ruled out that cannot explain the pain [15].

Location

Typically, stroke location is more critical to the risk for CPSP than stroke etiology. Thalamic and lateral medullary lesions have the highest incidence of CPSP [2]. The "thalamic pain syndrome" as coined by Dejerine and Roussy, is a common example of CPSP. With that said, further studies have indicated most patients with CPSP have non-thalamic strokes [2]. Studies suggest that insults in the cerebral cortex, medullary tract, and spinothalamic tract (which all regulate pain) are correlated with the etiology of CPSP.

Infarcts within the cerebral cortex are typically not associated with CPSP. Despite that, lesions in the cerebral structures involved in pain regulation, including the medial operculum posterior insular cortex, are partly responsible for the development of CP [23]. These specific brain areas are a receiving area for the spinothalamic tract and tightly intertwined with the sensory and limbic cortices, both of which are involved in pain processing [23]. The medullary tract includes the trigeminothalamic pathway, where one of its functions is to regulate pain within the face. Lesions involving this can lead to strokes such as the Lateral Medullary stroke or "Wallenberg" Syndrome. These patients have atypical pain and temperature sensations on the ipsilateral face and contralateral portion of the body [9]. Lastly, the spinothalamic tract is further responsible for both pain and temperature sensations.

Mechanism

The specific CPSP pathophysiology is still being studied today. There are several proposed working theories that include central disinhibition and sensitization.

In the early 1900s, insults to the lateral thalamus were proposed to affect CPSP. Specifically, the pain was suggested to be a result of insult to the GABAergic inhibitory pathway, which thus disinhibits the pathway from controlling pain. This theory was later confirmed by SPECT studies; now, it is the widely approved mechanism of CPSP [7, 34]. It was later found that spinothalamic pathway (which regulates pain and temperature) insults can lead to disinhibition and thus increased thalamic activity and pain sensations [2]. This is further supported by several studies that show decreased temperature and pinprick pain sensations in the progression of CP [7, 24].

Central sensitization is an abnormal condition resulting from chronic pain. It is not to be confused with central neuropathic pain. Central sensitization is where a loss of inhibition or increased neuron activity leads to allodynia and/or hyperalgesia [25]. In contrast, CP is more general and simply refers to pain that results from CNS injury. Central sensitization is one of the main driving factors for chronic pain. This is seen in several studies for post-stroke subjects, where an atypical thalamic burst firing caused further neuronal hyperexcitability and central sensitization [26]. Central sensitization can be tracked clinically by examining hypersensitive areas and measuring activity when applying stimuli.

Neuronal hyperexcitability is best examined through firing patterns in the thalamus. One study proposes two different neuronal firing patterns that are both controlled by neurotransmitters: (1) single-spike depolarization and (2) bursts during hyperpolarization [27]. Modulation of firing patterns is controlled by cholinergic, noradrenergic, and serotonergic variables and impact pain patterns [28]. For example, noradrenaline and serotonin increased GABAnergic transmission. This in turn explains why treating CPSP with antidepressants is a viable treatment. Studies involving pathways using opioid receptors suggest that decreased opioid receptor binding is correlated with CPSP [29]. Having said that, opioid use is often contraindicated in post stroke patients [30].

Spinal Cord Injury Central Pain

Definition and Prevalence

Patients with SCI can experience CP as well. In this patient population, this refers to neuropathic pain as a sequela of damage to the CNS, specifically the spinal cord. The International Spinal Cord Injury Pain Classification indicates that below-level neuropathic pain and some cases of at-level neuropathic pain can indicate central neuropathic pain. One important distinction in at-level neuropathic pain is that it can represent both peripheral (nerve root) and/or central (dorsal horn) pain depending on its specific location. The official prevalence of CP in SCI patients is highly variable. It was complicated by the lack of categorization by earlier literature and a latency in presentation in some post-SCI pain types such as below-level neuropathic pain [31, 32]. Despite that, studies indicate approximately 31% of patients with SCI had at-level lesions and 31% had below-level neuropathic pain 12 months after injury [33]. This CP significantly impacts function and quality of life in patients with SCI.

Localization

As stated before, SCI consists of both at-level lesions and below-level lesions. At-level CP is neuropathic pain that specifically involves the dorsal horn. It involves a segmental manifestation within the dermatome or up to three dermatomes below the lesion level [33]. As such, this is commonly mentioned as "transitional zone" or "segmental" pain. To reemphasize, this is not to be confused with at-level neuropathic pain that involves nerve roots ultimately leading to peripheral neuropathic pain [34]. This pain is either evoked or spontaneous. Evoked pain presents with common characteristics involving hyperalgesia, allodynia, wind-up pain, and after-sensations [33]. The pain can typically be traced with the dermatome of the lesion and can be unilateral or bilateral.

Below-level SCI neuropathic pain represents solely CP. It has previously been called "deafferentation central pain" [31]. In contrast to at-level CP in SCI patients, below-level CP involves pain manifestation more than three dermatomes below the lesion level [33]. Clinically, below-level CP presents similarly to at-level CP. However, below-level is commonly described as patch, asymmetric, and not typically dermatome. It can sometimes come from a specific body part.

Mechanism

The pathophysiology of at-level and below-level CP in SCI patients is not well defined. It is typically correlated with excitotoxic and neurochemical changes. Literature points to amino acids (glutamate) and post-inflammatory cytokines temporarily released at the site of the SCI lesion [35, 36]. This partly gives rise to many pathological alterations in the spinal cord. It involves "increased sensitivity due to loss of normal neuronal input, removal of inhibitory influences, increased efficacy of alternative synapses and deafferentation, hyperexcitability of spinal and/or thalamic neurons, and further alterations in cellular activity of neurochemical and excitatory amino acids due to changes in ion channels and transport activity" [36].

Recent literature also indicates that the neuroimmune system can contribute to chronic pain, specifically in the microglia. Microglia are known to be phagocytes that are activated after pathological causes such as infection, injury, disease, and seizures. The theory is that in SCI patients that have lesions in the spinothalamic tract, there is microglial activation that directly fires the surviving spinothalamic tract neurons [36]. When mobilized, microglial cells create nitric acid, proinflammatory cytokines, and excitatory amino acids which all regulate pain following neural injury create neuronal hyperexcitability in the dorsal horn [36]. Further, microglial insults are correlated with neuropathic and psychological pain-related behaviors (hyperalgesia, allodynia) and are theorized to contribute to the progression of chronic CP [36].

Lastly, there are structural changes in the gray/white matter at the lesion level. These anatomical changes modify the equilibrium the spinothalamic tract has with other tracts such as the dorsal column and spinoreticulothalamic tract; this can ultimately play a part in the progression of CP [34].

Treatment

Pharmacotherapy

The treatment options for CP are still being studied and are highly variable and challenging. There have been several studies that indicate effective treatments for CP. However, there are only a few and go against the general acknowledgement that pain resolution is unlikely. Certain pharmacological drugs have been proven to be effective solutions such as antidepressants, and anticonvulsants, and cannabinoids, opioids, and steroids. The pharmacotherapy treatment is summarized in Table 1.1 in Appendix.

Table 1.1 Pharmacotherapy information for central pain syndrome

Drug class	Agent	Mechanism	Effective dosage (mg QD)	Side effects/common notable adverse events and *precautions
Anticonvulsant	Gabapentin	Regulates Ca+ voltage-gated channels in neural synapses	1800 minimum	Sedation, confusion, edema, dizziness, tremor
	Pregabalin	Voltage-gated Ca+ channel (VGCC) antagonist	410–460	Sedation, confusion, edema, dizziness, tremor, euphoria
	Lamotrigine	Stabilizes Na+ channel blockade through neuronal membrane	200–400	Rash (Stevens-Johnson syndrome), abdominal pain, diarrhea, headache, dizziness
	Carbamazepine	Na+ membrane stabilizer and channel blocker	500–760	Stevens-Johnson syndrome, hematologic suppression, aplastic anemia, hepatic dysfunction, hyponatremia, nausea, dizziness, drowsiness
				*Monitor CBC and LFTs
Antidepressants	Amitriptyline	Inhibiting the reuptake of serotonin and norepinephrine (SNRI)	75 minimum	Sedation, blurred vision, dry mouth, orthostatic hypotension, confusion, weight gain, constipation, urinary retention
				*Risk of suicidal tendencies
				*Risk of serotonin syndrome
				*Risk of cardiac arrhythmias
	Duloxetine	SNRI and adrenergic agonist	60	Sedation, fatigue, nausea, dizziness, hyperhidrosis
				*Risk of suicidal tendencies
				*Risk of serotonin syndrome
				*Risk of cardiac arrhythmias
				*Risk of increased bleeding
				*Risk of withdrawal symptoms with abrupt discontinuation

(continued)

Table 1.1 (continued)

Drug class	Agent	Mechanism	Effective dosage (mg QD)	Side effects/common notable adverse events and *precautions
NMDA antagonist	Ketamine	Blocks the NMDA excitatory receptor	Highly variable in RCTs	Hypertension, respiratory depressions, hallucinations *Risk of cardiac issues
Opioid	Tramadol	Inhibition of the pre- and postsynaptic CNS and PNS neurons		Sedation, dizziness, nausea, confusion, respiratory depression, constipation, urinary retention
	Morphine			
	Oxycodone			
Steroid	Methylprednisolone	Not officially established		Confusion, nausea, restlessness, abdominal pain, weight gain, hyperglycemia
Cannabinoids	Tetrahydrocannabinol			Hypotension, palpitations, dry mouth, hallucinations, paranoia
	Cannabinol			

QD once a day, *CBC* complete blood cell count, *LFT* liver function test, *RCT* randomized control trial

Neuropathic Pain Meds

Randomized control trial data supports the use of anticonvulsants and antidepressants as first-line therapy for CP [37]. Anticonvulsants such as gabapentin and pregabalin have been well supported as the treatment for neuropathic pain due to the tolerability and price [34, 35]. Pregabalin has been tested more in CP disorders such as CPSP and SCI pain. For example, Gabapentin was effective for SCI-related central pain [38] and two trials showed pregabalin was effective for SCI central pain [39, 40]. Several studies have also pointed to show that pregabalin improves anxiety and sleep in patients with post-stroke CP.

Antidepressants such as amitriptyline and duloxetine are also used as first-line therapy for treating CP. The mechanism occurs through blocking reuptake of norepinephrine and serotonin reuptake inhibitors. In one study, amitriptyline (goal of minimum 75 mg/day) was effective for CPSP [41]. For SCI, studies show mixed results for amitriptyline [42]. Duloxetine (60 mg/day) was shown to be clinically effective for Multiple Sclerosis-related neuropathic pain. However, these antidepressant agents are shown to have side effects such as serotonin syndrome and emerging suicidality [9].

Some studies support the use of other neuropathic agents as second-line therapy. These agents can often include lamotrigine and carbamazepine. Studies on carbamazepine for CP are mixed. One study shows positive results; however, the study design was poorly powered and thus the conclusions were limited [34, 35, 43].

Given in certain doses (200-400 mg/day), Lamotrigine is effective for CPSP and for incomplete lesions of SCI for below-level and at-level CP [9]. However, both of these agents are used after first-line therapy because of a higher rate of adverse events and side effects [41, 44].

Nonneuropathic Pain Medications

Ketamine , an *N*-methyl-D-aspartate (NDMA) antagonist, is thought to have an antinociceptive effect in many disorders including CP. The proposed mechanism is that it "resets the CNS" because it blocks the excitation of the NMDA receptor [45]. Additionally, ketamine is thought to have an effect on the Hyperpolarization Activated Cyclic Nucleotide Gated Potassium Channel 1 (HCN1) on neurons involved in nociception as well as microglia, which are both involved in pain [46]. Intravenous (IV) fusion of ketamine has also been studied in patients with SCI-related CP and has been shown to temporarily reduce pain according to the Visual Analogue Scale (VAS) scores [45, 47].

Methylprednisolone was also proposed as a possible treatment option for CPSP. In one study, a group of stroke patients with CPSP were treated with methylprednisolone and showed a large decrease in pain, specifically numerical rating scale score, and a minor decrease in as-needed pain medications [52]. The treatment involved a taper scheduling starting from a 6-day taper at 24 mg, and eventual decrease of dosing by 4 mg on each subsequent and consecutive day.

Opioids are proposed as a therapeutic option for patients with unmanageable and uncompromising CP. In one study, a group of patients were treated with oxycodone, morphine, and tramadol, eventually leading to better management of the CP. Nonetheless, the potential for adverse events and side effects are widely known, specifically drug abuse. This can limit long-term use. It is worth noting that clinicians should follow proper clinical practice guidelines and appropriate recommendations to protect patients from the negative effects of opioids [56, 57].

Non-pharmacotherapy

Medical cannabinoids and cannabis have gained extreme popularity as alternative or adjunct therapy to conventional pharmacologic therapy. There have been mixed outcomes in the use of cannabinoids in neuropathic pain, specifically central spinal cord pain [35]. However, there have been positive results as well [48]. Because of the nature of how new this treatment is, current research is limited, and thus more is needed to develop a larger sample size and determine efficacy. Of note, cannabis is still classified as a Schedule 1 medication. Patients with CNS impairments have a critically increased risk of adverse effects secondary to neural impairments such as impaired judgement and motor coordination [48].

Central Pain can take a large mental toll on patients. It is a complex stressor, specifically in patients with neurological impairments. Thus, there are several studies that indicate that behavioral and psychological therapy and treatments are effective in the management of pain disorders, especially CP [35, 49]. Other treatments not from the aforementioned studies include biofeedback, cognitive behavioral techniques, and hypnosis. These methods focus on other aspects of pain such as emotional and occupational functions. They can be utilized in combination with pharmacologic medical treatment.

Some alternative medical therapies such as acupuncture and transcutaneous electrical stimulation (TENS) are utilized to treat CP. In several studies, acupuncture has been shown to treat neuropathic pain and CP in patients with SCI [50]. However, it should be noted that there are a limited number of consistent studies on acupuncture for CP. The design and methods of each study vary widely. TENS is a treatment modality where electrical impulses are sent through electrodes placed where pain is located at or trigger points. One theory for how TENS works is that it activates large afferent nerve fibers, which then activates descending inhibitory fibers within the CNS [51]. This ultimately modifies the perception of pain through blocking the transmission of pain signals. Another theory is that the nerve stimulation increases the number of endorphins, which is the body's natural chemical that is used to decrease and block the perception of pain [51]. However, just like acupuncture therapy, it is worth noting that research on TENS therapy is limited. Of the studies that are available, TENS may be beneficial in the treatment of CP.

There are various current studies that are utilizing interventions for the management of CP. Some of these include botulinum toxin injections for central neuropathic pain and caloric vestibular stimulation for CPSP. Recently, studies on botulinum toxin (BTX) and its effects sensory nerves and on central neuropathic pain have been conducted. Several studies have shown that the effects of BTX on neuropathic pain after SCI, MS, and stroke show that it can be considered as a treatment option for CP [9]. One study had two patients with spinal cord lesions who had at-level CP and oral medications were not effective [52, 53]. The patients were given BTX-A treatment and there was a significant decrease in pain perception. There are many other studies with at-level CP in patients with SCI that corroborate this. Additionally, caloric vestibular stimulation has been shown to have beneficial effects for the treatment of CP. In several cases, it significantly reduced pain with a benefit of at least 7 weeks [54]. Additionally, another study showed improved motor skills and reduced pain and somatosensory delusions in a CPSP female patient [55]. The author postulated that the reflex activates the posterior insula which in turn inhibits the sensation of pain arising from the anterior cingulate, which was backed by behavioral and imaging evidence. However, like the previously mentioned studies, more research is needed to increase sample size and determine efficacy of the treatments.

Interventional/Surgical

Given the refractory nature of CP states, various interventional procedures and forms of surgery have been proposed to either impair afferent nociceptive signaling or regulate the signaling (neuromodulation) to ultimately treat patients with refractory CP [2]. Lesioning, which is surgically creating a destructive lesion, is often most commonly applied to the spinal cord and includes various methods. Given a successful procedure, lesioning is most effective for treating allodynia and paroxysmal shooting pain [9]. However, pain usually returns after a number of years. Combined with the surgical risks, lesioning is now done infrequently [56].

Neuromodulation has also been studied for the treatment of CP states and includes repetitive transcranial magnetic stimulation (rTMS), spinal cord stimulation, motor cortex stipulation (MCS), and deep brain stimulation (DBS). The former is a method is a noninvasive procedure that utilizes magnetic fields that delivers impulses to stimulate nerve cells in the brain to improve symptoms of depression. One study treated patients with CPSP and trigeminal neuralgia with rTMS for 5 days. Fifteen days later at a follow-up visit, the patients expressed long-lasting pain improvement [2].

Spinal cord stimulation (or also called dorsal column stimulation) involves placing several stimulating electrical contacts in the epidural space in the spine near the region that supplies the nerves to the painful areas, specifically parallel to the posterior sensory columns of the spinal cord [9]. However, there is minimal literature on this approach to treat pain in patients with both SCI-related CP. Further, the neuromodulation signal needs to impair the afferent nociceptive signaling or activate descending inhibitory pathways above the central lesion. Thus, spinal cord stimulation is ineffective for CPSP and is more effective for thoracic spinal lesions where it can be applied to the early thoracic or cervical spine [9]. However, incomplete SCI injuries are more likely to be treatable because there is incomplete or no Wallerian degeneration of ascending sensory pathways, unlike complete SCI [9]. Additionally, patients with SCI often undergo surgical fixation. The resulting surgical hardware often impairs the patient's original anatomy and renders the patient unable to have spinal cord stimulation. Having said this, there is minimal backing of interventional approaches to treat CP permanently; the efficacy of the procedure for CP states tends to decrease as time progresses [9].

Motor cortex stimulation involves placing electrodes on the surface of the brain to regulate pain signals. Imaging has shown that epidural MCS can possibly activate structures involved in the evaluation of pain rather than the regulation of pain intensity [9]. The theory is that by activating fourth-order neurons in the precentral gyrus (motor function), nociceptive inputs from the cortex were blocked, ultimately decreasing pain. Further, evidence shows that pain decrease is associated with an increase in blood flow in the cingulate gyrus. This may indicate that motor cortex stimulation may also have a mechanism through decreasing the emotional aspect of pain (suffering) [57]. This treatment modality is most appropriate for arm- and face-predominant CP-related disorders. This aligns with the fact that the superficial portions of the homunculus are the hand and face. Almost two-thirds of patients with CPSP have clinically significant improvement with MCS [58]. In some studies, this treatment also shows promise in atypical facial CP [58].

Lastly, deep brain stimulation is where a surgically implanted device with electrodes is implanted in deep structures of the brain involving the supratentorial nuclei, often near the thalamus, periaqueductal gray matter, and globus pallidus [9].

It regulates sensory inputs and outputs through unclear mechanisms of action. Classically, the periventricular and periaqueductal gray matter have been the targets to ultimately release endogenous opioids [57]. The nucleus accumbens and ventral thalamus also are promising targets for the treatment of CP through activating inhibitory pathways [57]. The efficacy also varies widely based on the CP type, but positive results have been achieved. As mentioned before, DBS is generally less effective for patients with SCI-related CP [59]. However, for patients with CPSP, several studies show that DBS can be anywhere from 50 to 80% effective in pain relief [58]. One study further showed that slightly over half of the patients were able to taper down their pain medications [60, 61].

A multifactorial treatment approach involving the conventional pharmacotherapy treatment as first-line, as well as non-pharmacotherapy approaches and interventions should be employed simultaneously. The ultimate goal is to provide the appropriate medical treatment while achieving an optimal function and quality of life for the patient.

Conclusion

Chronic pain syndrome is a clinical state that is still very challenging to treat even with the many efforts to understand this condition. Some of these difficulties include diagnosis difficulty due to the various presentations in diagnosis and many mechanisms of action and pathophysiology as well as the wide spectrum of treatment outcomes. It is often difficult to recognize due to the delay (up to years) in onset and sensory inabilities from the CNS lesion. Theoretically, CP should be seriously considered when the pain is associated with spinothalamic tract sensory loss and is localized to the region of neurological impairment.

However, one thing is certain: early screening and recognition of CP syndrome is critical and is a vital component in the treatment of patients. It is most common in patients with functional deterioration from CNS conditions. The ideal treatment approach is a multifactorial pain plan that includes pharmacotherapy and non-pharmacotherapy medications, and interventional/surgical modalities if needed. Specifically, DBS has shown to be effective in several studies.

Incomplete management of pain, especially as it relates to CP syndrome, can ultimately lead to significant decrease in function and quality of life. Further direction could include creating a proactive approach or method of identifying patients who are at "high-risk" for developing CP. This would theoretically lead to better clinical outcomes. Additionally, more research into the mechanisms of action and pathophysiology may aid in the overall treatment of CP. Current treatments need to be looked at more deeply to understand pathophysiology as well. Specifically, patients may benefit from looking more into advanced neuromodulation techniques.

Painful Neuropathies (PNS)

Definitions and Prevalence

As mentioned before in the introduction to CP, according to the IASP, neuropathic pain is defined as pain caused by a lesion or disease involving the somatosensory nervous system. Neuropathic pain can be further segmented into peripheral vs. central neuropathies depending on the lesion location. The rest of this chapter will be focused on neuropathic pain as a result of issues to the peripheral nervous system.

Unlike patients with central neuropathy pain, patients with peripheral neuropathic pain have a lesser chance of experiencing pain [62]. In one study with patients with diabetic neuropathy, the prevalence of peripheral pain was approximately one-fifth of the cohort. These types of neuropathies can affect multiple nerves (peripheral neuropathy) or only one nerve or nerve group (mononeuropathy) at a time. Specifically, mononeuropathy is typically the result of damage to a single nerve or nerve group by inflammation, local compression, prolonged pressure, or trauma [63]. Most patients, however, suffer from polyneuropathy. Both types of insults cause similar changes in sensations of pain. This pain can be induced and often leads to hyperalgesia (normally painful stimuli causing exaggerated pain), allodynia (normally non-painful stimuli causing pain), hyperpathia (repetitive stimulation causing prolonged persistent pain), paresthesia (atypical non painful sensations that is not unpleasant) and dysesthesia (atypical painful sensation that is unpleasant) [62]. There is also a type of neuropathy called neuritis, where a nerve can undergo inflammation. Neuritis is typically caused by a bacterial or viral infection. One typical example is acute inflammatory demyelinating polyneuropathy (AIDP). This is an autoimmune process that is characterized by progressive areflexic weakness and mild sensory changes [62].

Describing the incidence and prevalence of neuropathic pain is particularly difficult to estimate given the diversity of related clinical entities and lack of validated diagnostic tools. However, there has been recent development of basic screening-tools based on symptoms and validation of a number of assessment tools. These have facilitated an estimation of the prevalence of neuropathic pain to range from 7% to 10% in the general population [64]. Further, some quality-of-life studies show that it can be associated with sleep conditions, depression, and physical function impairments. It is also more commonly seen in females and in patients older than 50 years of age [65].

Mechanisms/Pathophysiology

Various mechanisms of pain due to peripheral nerve injury have been proposed and have been under investigation. Acquiring a fundamental understanding of the mechanisms of neuropathic pain can lead to finding optimal therapeutic options. Several small sensory fibers, which include myelinated Aβ, and Aδ fibers and unmyelinated C fibers, are involved with neuropathic pain. Once nerve insults occur, voltage-gated sodium channels build up around the impaired site and along the axon. This leads to hyperexcitability and action potential activation [66]. Specific membrane stabilizers and sodium channel blockers act on this mechanism to treat patients with neuropathic pain [67]. Additionally, transient receptor potential vanilloid type 1 (TRPV1) channels are a factor in neuropathic pain. Nerve insults cause a decrease in TRPV1 receptor activation on that nerve and an increase in C fibers. The valladolid firing rate increases with heat. This results in overactive nerve activity which can present as burning pain and heat hyperalgesia [67]. Capsaicin is a TRPV1 agonist that results in an influx and buildup of intracellular calcium resulting in permanent dysfunctionalities of nociceptive nerve fibers [68].

Atypical ectopic neuronal activity in primary afferent fibers and in the dorsal root ganglion (DRG) can lead to dysregulation of the synthesis and function of sodium channel, specifically the tetrodotoxin-resistance channel [69]. Fiber cross-excitation and ephaptic interactions, sympathetic sensory coupling, and nociceptor sensitization can also be involved [69]. Additionally, Nerve insults can cause sprouting of sympathetic postganglionic fibers in the dorsal root ganglion (DRG) and the peripheral nerves. More specifically, sympathetic innervation of the DRG may impact the development and maintenance of sympathetically maintained neuropathic pain. After nerve insult, the axons upregulate α-adrenoreceptors and increase uptake of many neurotransmitters from postganglionic sympathetic terminals. This can be treated therapeutically with sympathetic blocks or α1-antagonists [69].

Additionally, CNS alterations can happen after a peripheral nerve insult. Changes include fluctuations in the inhibitory regulation in the spinal cord. The disinhibition is regulated through multiple pathways. Research has shown that gamma-aminobutyric acid (GABA) and opioid receptors have been downregulated [66]. Cholecystokinin, an opioid receptor inhibitor, is increased in expression while GABA, an inhibitory neurotransmitter, is decreased in the dorsal horn [66]. Ultimately, these alterations in disinhibition lead to a heightened perception of pain. Thus, pharmacotherapy targeting GABA receptors or simulating descending inhibition such as clonidine can treat patients with neuropathic pain. Overall, further study into the pathophysiology of peripheral nerve injury is needed.

Diagnosis

Patients with peripheral neuropathic pain can present differently from those with nociceptive pain. As mentioned in the beginning of this section, the patient with peripheral pain can experience hyperalgesia, allodynia, hyperpathia, paresthesia and dysesthesia. Questionnaires have been developed as screening tools and first-line treatment to find patients with neuropathic pain and require active participation from patients to describe their symptoms. Some of these screening questionnaires include ID-Pain, Douleur-Neuropathique 4 (DN4), Neuropathic pain Questionnaire

(NPQ), and painDETECT [70]. Although there are multiple screening questionnaires and they are used as first-line, their accuracy and efficacy remain largely undetermined.

As part of the diagnosis of peripheral neuropathic pain, a thorough physical examination should be done. This should include a complete sensory examination involving temperature, pinprick, vibration, light touch, and temporal summation. Temperature can be tested by applying cold and hot stimuli; pinprick sensations can be tested with a sharp tool such as a sharp pin; light touch can be tested by applying a low-density object to skin such as cotton wool; vibration can be tested using a tuning fork; and temporal summation can be tested with repeated and equal-intensity noxious stimuli [71]. If a patient has peripheral neuropathic pain and is undergoing physical exam testing, it is often described in a pattern of a stock glove distribution of changed sensory perception.

Diagnostic testing involving electrodiagnostic testing (EDX) may be useful in patients with peripheral neuropathic pain. This specific testing is one of the most common and involves two components: nerve conduction studies (NCS) and electromyography (EMG). The former, also called a nerve conduction velocity (NCV) test, measures the velocity of an electrical impulse that is applied to the targeted nerve through electrode patches on the skin. The latter identifies electrical activity of muscle tissue as a visual display or audible signal through electrodes attached to the skin. Together, EDX is used to support confirmation of nerve damage and possible neuropathy. Further, it helps to determine whether the pathology is due to axonal or demyelinating and if it is a polyneuropathy or mononeuropathy [62]. However, since EDX tests primary large fibers, EDX can present as clinically normal if the painful peripheral neuropathy only affects small fibers, resulting in a pseudo-false negative outcome [72]. As such, skin biopsy is one way to test for small fibers in patients with peripheral neuropathy. However, its outcomes are minimally accurate at best and there is generally not much support between pain and abnormal atypical skin biopsy findings [73].

Another way to test for both small and large sensory nerve fiber function in peripheral neuropathies is through quantitative sensory testing (QST). This is vital since as mentioned before, conventional sensory EDX only assesses for large fibers. The tool involves patient psychological involvement and lacks the objectivity of EDX, specifically NCS [62]. Thus, the results can change and have high variability due to extraneous factors such as boredom, drowsiness, confusion, and distraction [62]. Because QST has many limitations, it is not meant to be an isolated diagnostic tool, but rather as a supplement to aid in the interpretation of the patient's clinical presentation [74]. Further, the results of QST do not influence or alter the therapeutic plan for patients with neuropathic pain. Laboratory testing can further aid in determining causes of neuropathic pain stemming from bacterial or viral infections, genetic, metabolic, and toxic causes.

Since the IASP redefined neuropathic pain in 2008, the redefinition has been widely accepted. The proposed grading system of possible, probably, and definite neuropathic pain from 2008 was intended to determine the chances of neuropathic pain. "Possible" neuropathic pain involves a history of relevant neurological lesion or disease and pain distribution that is neuroanatomically plausible [13]. "Probably" neuropathic pain has the history mentioned in possible neuropathic pain as well as a physical examination that indicates the pain is associated with sensory signs in the same neuroanatomically plausible distribution. "Definitive" neuropathic pain has both the history and examination findings mentioned in probably neuropathic pain as well as confirmatory tests that verify a lesion or disease of the somatosensory nervous system that explains the pain [13]. Having said that, there have been several reviews that indicate that although the redefinition has widely been accepted, the adoption of the grading system has been used to a lesser extent.

Painful Neuropathies

To reiterate, this latter half of the chapter will hone in on peripheral neuropathies. These peripheral neuropathies that have painful peripheral presentations can be segmented into autoimmune and infectious, resulting from systemic disease, injury/acquired, and genetics. Painful peripheral neuropathies (PPNs) have a wide spectrum of pathophysiology. Because the PPNs origins can be very different, a complete history and physical exam is vital in order to use the appropriate supplemental diagnostic testing (such as EDX) and therapeutic treatments. Reviewing all PPNs in-depth is outside the scope of this introductory chapter to CP and PPN. Thus, the rest of this chapter will highlight some, not all, of the PPNs that present. The painful neuropathies are briefly organized in Table 1.2 in Appendix.

Table 1.2 Brief list of causes of painful peripheral neuropathies

Cause	Type of neuropathy
Infectious and autoimmune	Guillain-Barre syndrome/acute inflammatory demyelinating polyneuropathy (AIDP)
	Chronic inflammatory demyelinating polyneuropathy (CIDP)
Systemic diseases	Diabetic painful polyneuropathy
Injury and acquired	Complex regional pain syndrome
	Nutritional deficiency-induced peripheral neuropathy
	Chemotherapy-induced peripheral neuropathy (CIPN)
Hereditary	Charcot-Marie-tooth disease
	Hereditary sensory autonomic neuropathy
	Painful channelopathies
Drug-induced	Chemotherapeutics
	Antibiotics
	Cardiovascular agents
	NRTIs

Infectious and Autoimmune Painful Peripheral Neuropathies

Guillain-Barre Syndrome (GBS) and Chronic Inflammatory Demyelinating Polyneuropathy (CIPD)

Acute Inflammatory demyelinating polyneuropathy (AIDP), also known as Guillain-Barre Syndrome (GBS), and chronic inflammatory demyelinating polyneuropathy (CIDP) are among the most acquired immune-mediated polyneuropathies. GBS can have PPN such as paresthesia and numbness in their extremities. However, the main hallmark is extensive motor muscle weakness and cramping in an ascending pattern from legs to arms. Difficulty breathing may also occur and call for a neurological emergency in case of respiratory arrest. GBS can have many causes, but one of the most frequent is campylobacter jejuni infections which lead to complement and antibodies against nerve ganglions to attack the nodes of Ranvier [62].

GBS is the leading cause of acute flaccid paralysis in developed countries such as the United States with an annual incidence of 0.6–2.7 per 100,000 persons [75]. Around 33% of patients diagnosed with GBS present with pain, and approximately 89% of patients with GBS are eventually affected with pain [62]. Mechanisms of pain in GBS are inflammation and compression of the nerve roots resulting from segmental demyelination in large and small motor and sensory nerves and spiral roots with secondary axonal degeneration. Other than treating the underlying cause of GBS, pain is typically treated with pharmacotherapy involving anti-epileptics such as carbamazepine and gabapentin, antidepressants, analgesics including opiate drugs. Steroids have also been shown to be effective but come with risks and complications with long-term use [76].

CIDP is a chronic form of GBS and may present with slowly progressive and diffuse sensory and motor symptoms after approximately 8 weeks. The peak incidence of CIDP happens in middle age (40s–60s). There are two patterns that predominate: relapsing-remitting (20–65%) and progressive [77]. The relapsing and remitting form, unlike GBS, occurs more often in young adults in their 20s, whereas older patients may present with more chronic progressive polyneuropathy. Prevalence largely varies because of changing adherence to diagnostic criteria, from 1 to 9 per 100,000 persons [77]. Of those, 13–17% have severe pain [77]. Some diagnostic criteria include the well-known Asbury and Cornblath electrodiagnostic criteria for demyelination and the American Academy of Neurology research criteria for, which is known for its high specificity [75]. The most frequently used diagnostic criteria tool used is published by the European Federation of Neurological Societies, which balances specificity and sensitivity [75]. Some common treatments CIDP involve intravenous immunoglobulins (IVIG), plasma exchange, and corticosteroids. Further, neuropathic pain may also be treated with pharmacotherapy involving anti-epileptics, antidepressants, and analgesics.

Post-herpetic Neuralgia

Post-herpetic neuralgia (PHN) is the most common long-term sequelae of varicella-zoster virus (VZV) reactivation, also known as herpes zoster or shingles . VZV is the viral cause of the formerly common childhood condition, varicella, classically known as chickenpox . Before vaccinations, approximately 90% of American adults tested positive for VZV. Although the number may start to decrease in the future, there is still an annual incidence of one million cases in the United States and manifests itself in approximately 20% of patients with shingles [62].

The hallmark of PHN is a lancinating, burning, and/or electrical pain in a unilateral dermatomal pattern for three or more months. Some widely accepted risk factors include immunosuppression and increasing age [78]. The American Academy of Neurology recommends that the treatment should include neuropathic pharmacotherapy and lidocaine patch 5% (approved by FDA for PHN). However, like most treatments, the most successful are multi-modal. In fact, some physicians will focus more on the prevention in high-risk populations such as elderly and infirm because of the often refractory and crippling nature of PHN in already delicate patient populations. Additionally, the VZV vaccine is recommended for patients over 60 years of age and may help prevent PHN. Interventional procedures can be used as a last line of defense which include nerve blocks to the impacted dermatome and neuromodulation [78].

Painful Peripheral Neuropathies Resulting from Systemic Diseases

Diabetic Painful Polyneuropathy

Diabetic painful polyneuropathy (PPN) is the most common and serious peripheral painful neuropathy with a known cause [79]. Studies have reported a large range of prevalence, with 8–30% of patients that diabetic polyneuropathy reporting pain. The variation may be attributed to varying study designs and definitions of DPN. Although the specific pathophysiology of hyperglycemia-induced PPN is yet to be described, neurovascular and nerve insults are likely causes. Axonal degeneration and atrophy, peripheral sensitization, and changed peripheral neurovascular flow, all lead to diabetic PPN. However, increasing evidence has shown that not only hyperglycemia, but also factors such as type 2 vs. type 1 diabetes, obesity, smoking, female sex, and diabetes duration may be linked to painful DPN. Diabetic PPN affects multiple peripheral sensory and motor nerves that branch out from the spinal cord into the upper and lower extremities in the classic "stocking and glove" distribution. They typically affect the longest nerves, those that extend from the spine to the feet. This can present classically present as paresthesia such as tingling, burning, or stabbing, and electric sensations [79].

Treatment of diabetic PPN, like most PPNs, requires a multifactorial approach. Hyperglycemic regulation is critical in a preventative manner in type 1 diabetes but not as much in type 2 diabetes [79]. Other approaches include pain medications, anti-epileptics such as gabapentin, tricyclic antidepressants (TCAs), topical creams, TENS therapy, hypnosis, relaxation training, biofeedback training, and acupuncture [80].

Injury and Acquired Painful Peripheral Neuropathies

Complex Regional Pain Syndrome

Complex regional pain syndrome (CRPS) is a neuropathic painful condition that is defined by symptoms such as allodynia, trophic changes, hyperalgesia, and motor dysfunction. It typically occurs as a result of varying degrees of trauma, with fracture being the most common occurring in >40% of CRPS cases [81]. Some other common inciting events include surgery, crush injuries, sprains, and contusions.

There are two types of CRPS: type I, formerly known as reflex sympathetic dystrophy and occurs in the absence of nerve trauma, and type II, formerly known as causalgia and occurs in the presence of nerve trauma. They are clinically indistinguishable and follow a regional pattern (hence the name) rather than a nerve distribution or dermatome pattern. It presents initially most commonly the distal extremities and spread proximally or to the contralateral extremity. It is further broken down into sympathetically maintained (SMP) versus sympathetically independent (SIP) and "cold" versus "warm."

Using the IASP diagnostic criteria, the incidence in the United States is 5.46 per 100,000 person-years and 0.82 per 100,000 person-years for CRPS type I and type II, respectively. It is found to have peaks between ages 50 and 70 years, to be three to four times more common in women than in men, and to be found more in the upper limbs.

Currently, CRPS is diagnosed clinically by a set of decision rules for proposed clinical criteria developed by the Budapest consensus pane (sensitivity 85% and specificity 70%) [81]. The criteria, illustrated in Table 1.3 in Appendix, consists of four categories: sensory, vasomotor, sudomotor/edema, and motor/trophic. The first category, sensory, reports hyperalgesia and/or allodynia, which is when a normally non-painful stimulus causes pain. Patients may report wind, shoes, and gloves may cause pain in a distal extremity such as hands and feet. The second category, vasomotor, involves temperature and/or skin color asymmetry and/or changes. The third category, sudomotor/edema, involves edema and/or sweating changes and/or asymmetry. The fourth and final category, motor/trophic, involves decreased range of motion, motor dysfunction (weakness, dystonia, tremor), and/or trophic changes (hair, skin, nails). For this specific criterion, the patient must report at least one symptom in three of the categories and at least two of the categories at the time of evaluation. Lastly, one final criterion is that there should be no other condition that can better explain the signs and symptoms presented by the patient.

Developing a treatment plan in a prudent and aggressive manner is vital to delay an unfavorable outcome such as spread to different limbs peripherally and to the spinal cord and brain centrally. Patients should seek a treatment plan from a pain

Table 1.3 Budapest diagnostic criteria for CRPS

Requirement #	Criteria details
1	Continuing pain, which is disproportionate to any inciting event
2	Must report at least one symptom in three of the four following categories:
	1. *Sensory*: Reports of hyperalgesia and/or allodynia
	2. *Vasomotor*: Reports of temperature asymmetry and/or skin color changes and/or skin color asymmetry
	3. *Sudomotor/edema*: Reports of edema and/or sweating changes and/or sweating asymmetry
	4. *Motor/trophic*: Reports of decreased range of motion and/or motor dysfunction (weakness, tremor, dystonia) and/or trophic changes (hair, skin, nails)
3	Must display at least one sign at the time of evaluation in two or more of the following categories:
	1. *Sensory*: Evidence of hyperalgesia (to pinprick) and/or allodynia (to light touch or deep somatic pressure)
	2. *Vasomotor*: Evidence of temperature asymmetry and/or skin color changes and/or asymmetry
	3. *Sudomotor/edema*: Edema and/or sweating changes and/or sweating asymmetry
	4. *Motor/trophic*: Evidence of decreased range of motion and/or motor dysfunction (weakness, tremor, dystonia) and/or trophic changes (hair, skin, nails)
4	No other diagnosis that better explains the signs and symptoms.

clinician who has experience treating this disorder. Further, comprehensive treatment involves a multimodal strategy with a rehabilitation program driving the treatment. Treatments can involve oral corticosteroids (for warm CRP), anti-epileptics (gabapentin), analgesics (duloxetine), transdermal lidocaine, and opioids. Nonpharmacologic therapy including physical therapy, psychological therapy is also vital. Lastly, more interventional techniques may be used if pain is severe, such as spinal cord stimulation (SCS), DRG stimulation, ketamine infusions, and intrathecal drug pumps [82].

Nutritional Deficiency-Induced Peripheral Neuropathy

Malnutrition can affect all areas of the nervous system and can thus lead to PPNs. Pain is also one of many symptoms that can present for the patient. General risk factors for malnutrition can include eating disorders, alcohol abuse, older age, pregnancy, lower socioeconomic status (SES), and homelessness [83]. Thiamine deficiency can commonly lead to two conditions: beriberi and Wernicke-Korsakoff's syndrome . Beriberi has two subtypes: dry, which does not include heart failure, and wet, which includes heart failure. Additionally, thiamine deficiency due to chronic alcoholism can typically lead to Wernicke-Korsakoff's syndrome. Both of these

Table 1.4 Summary of nutritional-induced neuropathies

System	Sub-system	Nutritional toxicity or deficiency
Cardiovascular	Cardiac	Thiamine deficiency (wet beriberi)
Central nervous system	Cognitive	Lead toxicity, arsenic toxicity, mercury toxicity, disulfiram toxicity, vitamin B12 deficiency (pellagra), thiamine deficiency (Wernicke-Korsakoff syndrome)
	Corticospinal	Vitamin B12 deficiency, copper deficiency
	Cerebellum	Vitamin E deficiency, mercury toxicity
	Posterior column	Vitamin B12 deficiency, copper deficiency
Gastrointestinal	Intestinal	Vitamin E deficiency, thallium toxicity, lead toxicity, arsenic toxicity
	Liver	Vitamin E deficiency, arsenic toxicity
Hematologic	Anemia	Vitamin B12 deficiency, copper deficiency, lead toxicity
	Pancytopenia	Arsenic toxicity
Integument	Skin	Thiamine deficiency (beriberi), lead toxicity, thallium toxicity (alopecia), arsenic toxicity (alopecia)
	Nails	Thallium toxicity (Mees lines), arsenic toxicity (Mees lines)
Musculoskeletal	Muscle	Vitamin E deficiency (myopathy)
Renal	Kidneys	Mercury toxicity

conditions can manifest themselves with PPN that act similarly to Guillain Barre Syndrome which can include burning pain, paresthesia, muscle weakness and fatigue. If left untreated, it can eventually lead to ascending paralysis and weakness in the legs and sensorimotor neuropathy in the hands [83].

Cobalamin deficiency can also lead to PPN. It is absorbed in the terminal ileum. Thus, deficiency can be caused by pernicious anemia, gastrointestinal surgeries, malabsorption, and weight reduction surgery. Additionally, as cobalamin is only found in animals , vegetarians who follow a strict vegan diet must supplement with cobalamin. When cobalamin is deficient, this leads to altered metabolism of homocysteine and lack of tetrafolate and the creation of succinyl coenzyme A. Without these reactions, this can lead to deficient purine and pyrimidine synthesis and myelin sheath formation, respectively [83]. A summary of some nutritional deficiencies and their associated pathologies are listed in Table 1.4 in Appendix.

Chemotherapy-Induced Peripheral Neuropathy (CIPN)

Chemotherapy-induced peripheral neuropathy (CIPN) is a frequent side effect of chemotherapeutic agents with a prevalence from 19% to over 85% [84]. This specific neuropathy is mostly sensory in nature that may also present with a wide spectrum of motor changes. Because of its high occurrence in cancer patients, CIPN presents a major challenge for both current patients, survivors, and their clinicians; there is no clear-cut defined solution to treating CIPN. Traditional antineoplastic agents that cause CIPN include platinum-based chemotherapies, vinca alkaloids, taxanes, epothilones (ixabepilone), proteasome inhibitors (bortezomib,), and immunomodulatory drugs (thalidomide). The most potent are the platinum-based therapeutics, taxanes, ixabepilone, and thalidomide; the relatively less toxic are vinca alkaloids and bortezomib [84].

The platinum-based antineoplastic agents (i.e. cisplatin, oxaliplatin, carboplatin) have many discussed mechanisms. The PPN is most likely initiated by the buildup of platinum adducts in the trigeminal ganglion (TG) and dorsal root ganglion (DRG) neurons [84]. Additionally, some patients experience paradoxical intensification of symptoms despite cessation of the platinum drug. This phenomenon is called "coasting" and presents a particular challenge for clinicians since there are no indications that point to a reduction in the dosage to mitigate the symptoms [84]. Vinca alkaloids (i.e. vincristine, vinblastine, vinorelbine, vindesine) inhibit the assembly of microtubules and induce sensorimotor neuropathy that is dose-dependent, often in a stocking-glove distribution. Taxanes (i.e. paclitaxel, docetaxel, cabazitaxel) typically present as a sensory dominant neuropathy that is proportional to the dose and length. Thus, symptoms tend to improve after stopping the treatment. Epothilones are a relatively new class of antineoplastic agents and thus research on the mechanisms of epothilone-induced CIPN is minimal. However, it is postulated that the mechanism is somewhat similar to that of taxanes due to preventing the disassembly of microtubule. Proteasome inhibitors (bortezomib) are dose-dependent and cause distal and symmetrical sensory PN accompanied by neuropathic pain syndrome after drug termination. Thalidomide-induced PPN is proposed to be dose dependent and may be from its antiangiogenic effect, which is postulated to be responsible for the ischemia and hypoxia of nerve fibers followed by damage of the sensory neurons [84].

Hereditary Painful Peripheral Neuropathies

Charcot-Marie-Tooth Disease

Charcot-Marie-Tooth disease (CMT), also known as hereditary motor and sensory neuropathy (HMSN), is the most common hereditary neuromuscular disease and occurs with a prevalence of 1 in 2500. It is a group of diseases with approximately 4 genes (PMP22, GJB1, MPZ, MFN2) that account for 8–90% of CMT-causing mutations that are detectable [85]. There are two main types: the demyelinating form CMT1, and the axonal type, CMT2. The CMT1 primarily affects Schwann cells and the myelin-forming glial cells in the peripheral nerves [85]. The CMT2 directly affects the axons of peripheral neurons. Autosomal dominant CMT (AD-CMT) is the most common pattern, followed by X-linked CMT. Autosomal recessive forms are rare. Because of these inheritance statistics, people with CMTs will have a 50% chance of transmission to further generations by the affected parent

[85]. In addition to PPN, patients will exhibit slowly progressive distal extremity atrophy and weakness, starting in the feet and legs. Deep tendon reflexes can be decreased or absent and foot deformities (most often pes cavus) can be an early sign.

Hereditary Sensory Autonomic Neuropathy

Hereditary sensory autonomic neuropathy (HSAN) has a much lower prevalence than CMT disease. It primarily causes a loss of large unmyelinated and myelinated sensory fibers. There are several subtypes and classifications. HSAN I (also known as hereditary sensory radicular neuropathy and hereditary sensory neuropathy type I) is the most common form of HSAN [86]. It typically shows progressive degeneration of DRG and motor neurons. This leads to distal sensory loss and eventually distal muscle atrophy and weakness and a certain degree of deafness. Brief sharp leg pain is typically the initial symptom followed by some foot ulcers and reduced sensation in the legs. It is inherited in an autosomal dominant pattern. At least thus far have been found in this disorder (HSANIA-HSANIE). Symptom onset is typically during early adulthood. HSAN II is caused by a loss of touch, pressure, pain, and temperature sensations [86]. Fractures in the digits often occur in early childhood and eventually lead to mutilation of the fingers and toes. It is inherited in an autosomal recessive pattern. HSAN III, also known as Riley-Day Syndrome or familial dysautonomia, is inherited in an autosomal recessive pattern [87]. It is a progressive sensorimotor neuropathy, but sympathetic autonomic dysfunction causes most of the clinical symptoms. HSAN IV, also known as congenital insensitivity to pain with anhidrosis (CIPA), is inherited in an autosomal recessive pattern. It typically presents in infancy and has a profound loss of pain sensitivity and thermoregulation [86]. Lastly, HSAN V has a loss of pain and temperature, but most other sensations are preserved.

Painful Channelopathies

Channelopathies are a group of disorders that involve genetic mutations affecting pain receptors. Voltage-gated sodium channels are responsible for conducting action potentials in the peripheral nociceptive pathway where Nav1.8, Na1.7, and Na1.9 sodium channels (encoded by *SCN9A*, *SCN9B*, *SCN9C*) are expressed [88]. Clinical pathologies that result from mutations in these genes include erythromelalgia, and paroxysmal extreme pain disorder, small-fiber neuropathy (SFN), and dysautonomia, and acromesomelic. The onset is variable and can occur early from birth to later in life in adulthood. There are currently no cures for the conditions. Treatment only consists of symptom regulation. Of note, genetic mutations in the SCN9A and SCN11A genes which affect the Na1.7 and Na1.9 voltage-gated channels, respectively, cause a loss of pain perception [88].

Drug-Induced Painful Neuropathy (DIPN)

In general, drug-induced peripheral neuropathy (DIPN) is most often seen in chemotherapeutic agents, antibiotics, cardiovascular agents, immunosuppressants, and NRTIs. Most of these neuropathies involve damaging the dorsal root ganglia. Some groups follow certain trends more so than others. Chemotherapeutics, for example, often show consistent side effects while others are prescribed more frequently such as statins [89]. Additionally, DIPN occurs more in patients with comorbidities such as diabetes. It is relatively difficult to treat, but drugs such as gabapentin and duloxetine have been used to aid in pain symptoms. Additionally, neuromodulation has been promising and is growing through further randomized control trials and studies [89]. The drug-induced painful neuropathies are summarized in Table 1.5 in Appendix.

Table 1.5 Drug-induced painful peripheral neuropathy

Group	Agents	Incidence	Pathophysiology	Neuropathy
Chemotherapeutics	Vinca alkaloids	All grade: up to 96%; severe (grades 3–4): up to 37%	Microtubule-mediated axonal and cellular transport dysfunction	Sensory; distal lower extremities and ascends proximally
	Platinum	30–40%	Irreversible DNA cross-linking and neuronal apoptosis	Chronic sensory neuropathy
	Bortezomib and thalidomide	Bortezomib: 37–64%, severe up to 33%; thalidomide: 23–70%, severe up to 13%	Mitochondrial calcium release leading to apoptosis cascade activation	Bortezomib: Small fiber sensory neuropathy with burning pain, distal lower extremities; thalidomide: sensory neuropathy, primarily in distal extremities
	Epothilones	15–64%	Microtubule dysfunction	Primarily sensory deficits
	Arsenic trioxides	2–42%	Demyelination and acute axonal damage	Sensory and chronic motor polyneuropathy
	Taxanes	Monotherapy: up to 30?%; combined therapy with platinum: 70%	Interfere with calcium signaling; interfere with tubulin depolymerization in axonal transport	Primarily sensory deficits; motor deficits if severe

Table 1.5 (continued)

Group	Agents	Incidence	Pathophysiology	Neuropathy
Antibiotics	Isoniazid	2–44%	Disruption of vitamin B6 synthesis	Sensory peripheral neuropathy
	Ethambutol	1–18%	Unclear; possibly due to protein inhibition and mitochondrial toxicity	Optic neuritis and neuropathy
	Linezolid	13–20%	Axonal degeneration, binds to neuronal rNA	Sensory peripheral neuropathy and optic neuropathy
Immunosuppressants	Interferon-α inhibitors—adalimumab, etanercept, infliximab	Rare	Immune-mediated myelin degeneration, vessel occlusion leading to nerve ischemia, induction of anti-GM antibodies	Acute axonal polyneuropathy, demyelinating polyneuropathy, chronic inflammatory demyelinating polyneuropathy, vasculitic neuropathy

Chemotherapeutics

Some of the chemotherapeutics that can cause DIPN include vinca alkaloids, platinum, bortezomib and thalidomide, epothilones, arsenic trioxides, and taxanes. Vinca alkaloids (i.e. vincristine, etc.) are used to treat gynecologic, lymphatic, and hematologic malignancies and solid tumors. They can cause distal lower extremity DIPN and it progresses proximally through microtubule-mediated axonal and cellular transport dysfunction [90]. Platinum drugs, such as cisplatin, irreversibly cross-links to DNA eventually causing apoptosis. This leads to chronic sensory neuropathy via accumulation in the dorsal root ganglia. Bortezomib and thalidomide, which are used to treat multiple myeloma, cause mitochondrial dysfunction in axons and calcium release leading to activation of the apoptosis cascade. Bortezomib can cause small fiber sensory neuropathy (i.e. c-fibers) leading to a burning sensation in the distal lower extremities [89]. Thalidomide can cause sensory neuropathy often leading to paresthesia in the distal extremities and mild numbness and motor dysfunction. Epothilones (i.e. ixabepilone), which are used to treat breast cancer, also cause microtubule dysfunction and cause predominantly sensory neuropathies but are also reversible. Arsenic trioxides (ATO) are frequently used to treat Acute Promyelocytic leukemia (APL). They can cause acute axonal damage and demyelination eventually leading to chronic motor and sensory polyneuropathy [90]. Taxanes (i.e. paclitaxel and docetaxel) have been frequently used to treat breast and ovarian cancer and interfere with metabolic calcium signaling which causes disruption of tubulin depolymerization in axonal transport [89]. This leads to predominantly sensory neuropathy but can also lead to motor loss if it is severe.

Antibiotics

Many antibiotics have been shown to cause peripheral neuropathy thus this is not an all-inclusive list, but rather a few select antimycobacterials that were chosen to highlight below [62]. A few of the drugs that are used to treat Tuberculosis and can cause DIPN include Isoniazid (INH), Ethambutol , and linezolid. INH interferes with vitamin B6 synthesis, which is the suspected pathophysiology for why INH and can cause sensory peripheral neuropathy. Ethambutol is suspected to chelate zinc, which affects metal-containing enzymes in mitochondria in the retinal ganglion neurons and excitotoxic pathway [91]. This leads to optic neuropathy. Linezolid is a bacterial protein synthesis inhibitor used to treat both MRSA and multi-drug resistant TB (MDR-TB). It is still unclear where linezolid alone can cause DIPN due to varying studies but is hypothesized to be related to mitochondrial toxicity and protein inhibition which can lead to sensory PN and optic neuropathy.

Cardiovascular Agents

Some cardiovascular agents that have been associated with DIPN include amiodarone and statins. Amiodarone is a class III anti-arrhythmic used to treat atrial and ventricular pathologies. Statins are universally given to reduce cardiovascular mortality and disease. Both of these drugs are not traditionally known to cause DIPN, but a growing number of studies indicate some type of association [89]. Amiodarone is theorized to cause demyelination and large axonal loss with lysosomal inclusions and degenerative processes, suggesting oxidative stress and impaired lysosomal degradation [89]. Further research into how both these drugs can possibly cause DIPN is needed to better understand the pathogenesis and clinical manifestations.

Immunosuppressants

Various immunosuppressants have been shown to induce DIPN but TNF-α inhibitors will be highlighted. TNF-α inhibitors such as adalimumab, etanercept, and infliximab are typically used to treat rheumatoid arthritis, inflammatory bowel disease, and other inflammatory conditions. However, they can cause immunosuppression and thus T-cell and humoral immune attacks on peripheral myelin, inhibition of axon signaling, and vasculitis-induced nerve ischemia [89]. This can lead to Guillain-Barré syndrome, chronic inflammatory demyelinating polyneuropathy, multifocal motor neuropathy, Miller fisher syndrome, and a whole host of other neuropathies. Interferons can also inhibit T-cell proliferation, decrease TNF-α, and increase anti-inflammatory cytokines. This can also cause a wide array of neuropathies including chronic inflammatory demyelinating polyneuropathy, acute axonal polyneuropathy, vasculitic neuropathy, and demyelinating polyneuropathy [89].

NRTIs

NRTIs (i.e. zalcitabine, didanosine, stavudine, lamivudine) can also cause PN. The incidence varies based on the specific drug and is often cited as one of the reasons for discontinuing use of NRTIs in therapy. The pathophysiology is still being studied, but it is commonly theorized to be due to inhibition of γ-DNA polymerase. This enzyme is responsible for replication of mitochondrial DNA and thus disruption can lead to mitochondrial dysfunction, increased lactate production, and accumulation of toxic metabolite [92]. This leads to a distal axonal-type sensory neuropathy that is difficult to distinguish from HIV-induced neuropathy [89].

Treatments of Painful Peripheral Neuropathies

As stated previously, treatment of PPNs and CPs should generally follow a multifactorial treatment plan to deliver optimal results for the patient and maximize function and quality of life. Thus, ideally less invasive and interventional techniques are preferred. However, since each patient's clinical presentation is unique, each treatment plan should be individually created for each patient's symptoms. General treatment includes pharmacotherapy and non-pharmacotherapy modalities, and interventional techniques.

Medications

Certain pharmacological medications are first-line treatment options and have been proven to be effective as listed in Table 1.6. The European Federation of Neurological Societies Task Force (EFNS) created a list of recommendations that guide treatment of PPNs. These include gabapentin, pregabalin, and TCAs as first-line, tramadol as second-line, and opioids as third-line treatments [93]. However, like most of the painful neuropathies whether central or peripheral, treatment varies and is individualized based on the neuropathic condition and specific patient presentation.

Table 1.6 Pharmacotherapy for painful peripheral neuropathy

Chemical regulator	Agent
Na+ channel antagonist	Gabapentin, carbamazepine, valproic acid, phenytoin
Alpha 2 agonist	Clonidine
Glutamate antagonist	Gabapentin
NE reuptake inhibitors	TCAs (i.e. duloxetine)
NDMA Ca channel antagonist	Ketamine, amantadine dextromethorphan
Non-NMDA Ca channel blocker	Nifedipine
GABA agonist	Baclofen

Anticonvulsants

As mentioned in CP disorders, anticonvulsants such as gabapentin and pregabalin are well supported for their tolerability and cost-effectiveness. They impact the voltage-gated calcium channels thereby reducing the release of the neurotransmitters and increasing the function of inhibitory GABA receptors [94]. They have been proven to treat many various forms of painful neuropathy. Typically, the number needed to treat is 7 and 8–9 for gabapentin and pregabalin, respectively [95]. Their primary adverse events include sedation, cerebellar symptoms (incoordination, tremor), nystagmus and some less common adverse events include cardiac arrhythmias and hematological changes [96]. Some key differences involve the pharmacokinetic profiles, saturability, and systems involved, and absorption rate. For example, pregabalin follows a linear pharmacokinetic profile and is unsaturable, whereas gabapentin follows a non-linear pharmacokinetic profile and is saturable [97].

Neuropathic agents such as carbamazepine and oxcarbazepine are used as first-line therapy for trigeminal neuralgia. Both block the voltage-gated sodium channels. Carbamazepine specifically only needs an NNT of 1.7, which renders it very effective. However, due to its effects on cardiac, liver, and renal systems, labs and EKG should be initially and periodically done to avoid adverse events [62]. Contraindications involve atrioventricular block, hypersensitivity, tricyclic antidepressants, bone marrow depression, and many others [62]. Side effects include rashes, nausea, diplopia, hyponatremia, hyperhydration edema, and memory issues. Some more severe side effects include teratogenicity during the first semester, Stevens-Johnson syndrome, hepatotoxicity, agranulocytosis, and aplastic anemia [98]. Initial dosing for acute treatment is 100–400 mg/day with a dosing recommendation of 2–4 divided doses per day depending on the preparation and is increased in increments of 200 mg/day every 1–4 days. Oxcarbazepine is given in 300–600 mg/day in 2 divided doses [98, 99].

Antidepressants

Tricyclic antidepressants (TCAs) such as amitriptyline and nortriptyline are the most studied antidepressants for neuropathic pain [100]. They are used as therapy for treating PPNs. However, their use is limited by adverse events and side effects. Their mechanism works by inhibiting the reuptake of norepinephrine and serotonin at the synapse. However, it differs based on chemical structure. The secondary amines (i.e. nortriptyline, desipramine) have inhibited norepinephrine more so than serotonin. In contrast, the tertiary amines (i.e. amitriptyline, imipramine, doxepin) have a greater effect on serotonin. Some argue that the two subclasses of TCAs have equal effects, while others say that tertiary amines are more effective [100]. Pain relief is uniquely not correlated with the primary antidepressant effects of the drugs and can be achieved at a lower clinical dose than that used in the therapeutic plan for depression. Despite this, their use is typically complicated by side effects such as weight gain, orthostatic hypotension, cardiovascular effects, anticholinergic effects, and lethality in overdose [100].

Other classes of antidepressants used include selective serotonin reuptake inhibitors (SSRIs), venlafaxine, and duloxetine. The mechanism of action for SSRIs and the others involves the reuptake inhibition of serotonin and norepinephrine, similar to that of TCAs. They have significantly lower affinity for other receptors though, leading to milder side effects. Venlafaxine is a unique mixed-action antidepressant that inhibits norepinephrine reuptake at high doses and serotonin reuptake at low dose doses. Thus, unlike SSRIs and like TCAs, they affect both neurotransmitters used in the regulation of PPNs. Duloxetine is also a dual-action drug (i.e. inhibits reuptake of serotonin and norepinephrine) that seems to have a higher binding affinity than venlafaxine. Side effects of these drugs can include constipation, somnolence, dry mouth, and decreased appetite [100].

Mirtazapine acts central alpha-2 adrenergic autoreceptors and heteroreceptors, resulting in increased norepinephrine and serotonin release while also blocking 5-HT2 and 5HT-3 receptors [101]. It has been studied in the treatment of phantom limb neuropathic pain and fibromyalgia. A case series suggests it may have some partial relief on postamputation limb pain, but the study was very limited and inconclusive [102]. No efficacy was found for the treatment of fibromyalgia because it had the same effect as that of the placebo [101]. Lastly, recent literature shows a partially beneficial effect in diabetes-induced hyperalgesia [102]. However, further research is needed to establish more conclusive evidence.

Cannabinoids

As mentioned before, medical cannabinoids and cannabis have increased in availability and popularity dramatically. Cannabidiol is the ligand in the cannabinoid receptors. It is present in both the CNS and PNS pain pathways. A numerous number of research studies have found the reduction of pain from use of medical cannabis [62]. Specifically, PPN induced from HIV-associated neuropathy has shown the greatest statistical benefit [62]. Classic side effects of cannabis include dry mouth, paranoid delusions, euphoria, anxiety, increase in appetite, hallucinations, conjunctival injection, impaired judgement, social withdrawal, tachycardia, and perception of slowed time. As more research is done, more information will be released to details the exact benefits and risks of using medical cannabis in the treatment of PPN.

Topical Medications

Local anesthetics (i.e. lidocaine), capsaicin, menthol products, and compounded topical medications are commonly used for PPN. Lidocaine is used as a medical patch or spreadable cream ointment. It is a sodium channel blocker which in turn blocks the increase in discharge threshold and reduces pain transduction [103]. In terms of treating localized neuropathic pain (LNP), it is Nav 1.7 and 1.8 are thought to be most important for inducing pain and have atypical and sensitized functions after nerve insults [103]. When applied as a 5% medical plaster, lidocaine has been shown to be effective in treating post-herpetic neuralgia and diabetic polyneuropathy.

Capsaicin is a natural vanilloid from the capsicum plant. It binds to the transient potential vanilloid receptor 1 (TRPV1) channels, which is a receptor expressed on Aδ and C-nerve fibers involved in pain. The mechanisms are not fully understood, but it is thought to release substance P and cause transient depolarization through sodium and calcium influx. Thus, it is counterintuitive, since, when initially applied, it causes pain. However, after repeated administration, chronic exposure will overstimulate and eventually desensitize its receptors causing defunctionalization and decrease in pain [104]. It has been used as both low concentration patches of 0.025 and 0.075% as well as 8%, which have been not particularly effective and much more efficacious, respectively [103]. In fact, the topical use of the 8% patch showed a 30–50% improvement in pain for patients with PHN and HIV-distal sensory polyneuropathy, which is an efficacy not achieved by the low-dose capsaicin patch [62].

Topical medications in combination have a large variety and are given based on a specific patient presentation and context. Some of these medications include ketamine, gabapentin, clonidine, baclofen, and clonidine. However, one study showed that compounded medications did not provide any additional benefit as compared to placebo [62]. To further complicate it these specific medications are often not included in health insurance coverage and are expensive. As such, other treatment options should be considered.

As mentioned before, cannabinoids are also increasing in extreme popularity. Topical cannabidiol (CBD) oils, specifically, are becoming much more widespread in pain management for not only patients experiencing PPN, but also for athletes. One group found a large reduction in pain with a 4-week application of CBD oil for lower extremity neuropathy. However, this was a small study with only 29 patients. Symptoms were looked at using a neuropathic pain scale [62]. Because there is still a lack of clinical studies, further research is needed to understand its true efficacy.

Infusion Medications

Intravenous (IV) administration of medications including ketamine and lidocaine have been used to treat many forms of neuropathic pain. IV ketamine is the most commonly used to treat patients with chronic pain [47]. It is an anesthetic induction agent that ranges in dosing levels from 1 to 4.5 mg kg [62]. As mentioned in the treatments for CP, ketamine is an NMDA-antagonist. At higher doses, ketamine acts at the opioid receptors. It is a phenylpiperidine derivative structure related to phencyclidine (PCP), which is colloquially known as "angel dust" and is a drug of abuse [62]. It was first synthesized in the early 1960s and was used during the Vietnam War because of its anesthetic effects and preservation of respiratory and hematological function. Of unique note, ketamine also impairs semantic memory, unlike other drugs. As noted earlier, ketamine has been extensively studied in treatment for

CRPS [105]. Typical literature shows the pain relief and benefits are achieved using doses at 100 mg over 4 h for 10 consecutive days [62]. Now, it varies widely and the optimal dose is not known. However, the efficacious pain relief found in most studies' follow-up time frames were 9–12 weeks [105].

There are many potential side effects, adverse events, and contraindications that accompany IV ketamine therapy. Side effects from clinical ketamine can generally be divided into CNS-related, cardiovascular, and hepatic. Some of the primary side effects can include psychedelic symptoms (panic attacks, hallucinations, memory defects), nausea/vomiting, somnolence, and cardiovascular stimulation. Further, the recreational use of ketamine is becoming increasingly popular and comes with additional risks such as bladder and renal complications, and persistent memory defects and psychotic behavior [105]. In clinical settings, ketamine can be well-tolerated if used with benzodiazepines to regulate the psychotropic side effects [105]. Further, clonidine may be used to counteract the increase in blood pressure of IV ketamine [62]. As with all levels of anesthesia, close monitoring of patients is critical to avoid unfavorable circumstances. They should be targeted toward CNS, hemodynamic, renal, and hepatic symptoms. This can include monitoring of blood pressure, electrocardiogram, pulse oximetry, respirations, and heart rate.

Intravenous lidocaine has also has also been used to treat PPN and chronic pain. It has been increased as an alternative to opioid use. As mentioned before, it is used to block sodium channels and reduce pain transduction. Literature indicates that it treats PPN conditions such as trigeminal neuralgia, PHN, and CRPS [106]. Some studies have shown that the effect of lidocaine on neuropathic pain is dose-related [106]. For example, one study shows doses comparing 1, 3, and 5 mg/kg suggest that doses less than 5 mg/kg is the same as placebo. Main side effects can include light-headedness, dizziness/vertigo, perioral numbness, speech disturbance, and nausea/vomiting [62].

Therapeutic Modalities

Many non-pharmacotherapy options are commonly used for treatment of PPN. These can include electrotherapeutic and physical agent modalities that use heat, cold, electricity, electromagnetic, water, and sound waves [107]. They are typically used in conjunction with other modes of treatment for neuropathic pain disorders. Transcutaneous electrical nerve stimulation (TENS), as previously mentioned in the treatments for CP, is one of the most commonly used treatments for neuropathic pain. One study by the Cochrane Library compared TENS to sham TENS in patients with neuropathic pain. It showed a mean postintervention difference in effect size favoring TENS of −1.58 (during TENS of −1.58, 95% confidence interval (CI) −2.08 to −1.09, $P < 0.00001$, $n = 207$) [108]. There were six comparisons from five studies and indicated very low-quality evidence. Despite meeting the pre-specified criteria, there was very low-quality evidence and thus the authors found this quality inconclusive. In fact, they mentioned that "the true effect is likely to be substantially different" from reported in the study [108]. As mentioned before, TENS has a theorized mechanism of activating large afferent nerve fibers, which then activates descending inhibitory fibers with the CNS to ultimately block the effects of small nociceptive c and A-delta fibers [108]. It is placed at the site where pain is located at or trigger points.

Temperature therapy involving cold and heat stimuli are typically not used in PPN because simultaneous decrease sensation is common and can lead to unfavorable skin injuries [62]. However, this treatment can provide some partial benefit in desensitization of hypersensitive neuropathic pain such as allodynia. For instance, patients with CRPS often have allodynia and/or erythromelalgia, and contrast baths can often be used to treat that. It is performed by using one bucket of moderately warm water and one bucket of cold water. Of note, each bucket should be extremely warm or extremely cold. The affected extremity with pain should be placed in one bucket for 2 min and/or until it adjusts, then switched immediately to the other bucket for the same length of time. This is repeated three times per day. Despite this benefit, there is still very limited research on the efficacy of this treatment [62]. Thus, more research is needed to establish the exact mechanisms and benefits in the treatment of PPNs.

Virtual reality is a growing and innovative field that has limited side effects and has recently been utilized in many pain pathologies. It is utilized as part of a larger effort to use visual feedback to regulate painful symptoms and processes. Treatments that have been leading up to this involve mirror visual feedback, which is a treatment that allows a clinician to create an illusion. When patients anticipate movements to be painful, mirrors help deceive their brains into thinking that there is no pain via dynamic feedback to their brains [109]. There are several working theories that are still being researched to determine how exactly this works.

Visual feedback is increasingly being used in treatment for PPN pathologies such as phantom limb pain, CRPS, and certain causes of SCI. For example, one case report showed extensive pain relief for a patient with chronic phantom limb pain when other conventional treatments such as pharmacotherapy, physical therapy, nerve blocks and nerve transformations did not work [110]. Another study found that the use of VR for patients with CRPS showed a 50% reduction in pain intensity scores [111]. Virtual reality has shown some advantages such as the ability to treat bilaterally, artificial and enhanced environments, and the option to customize [111]. However, this technology is extremely expensive. Some recent research has shown partial benefits for SCI patients experiencing PPN. However, this pain was short-lived, and more data is needed. Visual feedback treatments are a rapidly growing and innovative field of treatment modalities and can provide many benefits with minimal side effects and adverse events. Like all new treatments, however, more research is needed to determine the benefits.

Interventional

Various interventional procedures are used in the treatment of PPN. Neuromodulation and sympathetic ganglion blockade treatments are two examples that have been used to help manage the symptoms of PPN.

Neuromodulation

The use of neuromodulation with electrical stimulation can be traced back to the Romans, who used electric eels, a sea organism that can deliver electricity to stun prey, for the treatment of various pain conditions [112]. Now in modern times, Wall and Melzack's publication on the gate control theory of pain conceptualized neuromodulation for chronic pain [113]. Since then, it has been extensively studied in PPNs and CRPS. As already mentioned in the treatments for CP, spinal cord stimulation (or dorsal column stimulation) involves placing several electrical implanted devices with metal leads and a pulse generator into the spine or near the region that supplies the nerves to the pain area. Various waveforms have been utilized to deliver electrical impulses into the dorsal columns or dorsal root ganglions (DRGs) , but optimal waveforms are still yet to be determined. Many of these studies have shown that DRG stimulation is effective and frequently used as an interventional treatment [114–116]. In 2016, the FDA approved its use as a treatment option. It essentially functions similar as the dorsal column stimulation treatment, but instead places it over the spinal nerves instead of the spinal cord. It has been shown to provide significant efficacy in patients with CRPS in several studies [117, 118].

Sympathetic Ganglion Injections

Treating PPN through blocking sympathetic ganglia can be traced back to World War I. It has been shown to be effective in many pain conditions such as CRPS, cancer pain of different origins, and coccygodynia. Several mechanisms are proposed to be effective: the loss of regular inhibitory regulation on pain and adrenergic hypersensitivity. The therapeutic effects of the sympathetic injections typically outlast the original therapeutic duration of the agents that are applied [119]. This may suggest that the blocks disrupt the positive feedback mechanism and decrease the central hyperexcitability [119]. Some of the most common Sympathetic blocks include stellate (or cervicothoracic) ganglion block, lumbar sympathetic block, celiac block, superior hypogastric block and ganglion Impar block.

The stellate ganglion is part of the cervical sympathetic chain and is formed by the fusion of the first thoracic sympathetic ganglion and inferior cervical ganglion. Some structures that are close by involve the esophagus, scalene muscles, longus colli muscle, trachea, recurrent laryngeal nerve, and subclavian artery. The stellate ganglion provides sympathetic innervation to the ipsilateral head, face, chest, and upper extremity. Before, SGB was applied without any imaging guidance by palpating the C6 anterior transverse process and injecting slightly medial [119]. However now, it has now been done with imaging guidance such as computed tomography (CT) and ultrasound (US) [119]. The lumbar sympathetic ganglion is typically located anterolateral to the lumbar vertebral bodies [119]. They are typically blocked at the L2–L4 vertebrae with fluoroscopic guidance. It can also be blocked through utilizing neurolytic agents or radiofrequency ablation. It has been utilized for many clinical pathologies such as CRPS, herpes zoster, and amputation stump pain [119].

Peripheral Nerve Blocks and Hydrodissection

With the increase in advances in minimally invasive procedures and various surgical techniques, analgesic techniques must keep up with these advancements. These include peripheral nerve blocks which have been shown to be effective and well-tolerated to provide regional anesthesia that is superior to other methods such as general anesthesia and oral pain medications [120]. Generally, these are indicated once conservative treatments have been exhausted and failed or to avoid side effects of general anesthesia and oral medications [120]. For example, patients who are at high risk of respiratory depression related to general anesthesia, patients who want to avoid systematic medications, or patients who are intolerant to oral medications are all reasons that peripheral nerve blocks can be indicated. The mechanism of action remains unclear [120]. One theory is that repeated depolarization by a local anesthetic was proposed, but they have not been confirmed [120]. Another theory that emerged more recently is that fascial compression of nerves happens in various locations and a benefit of these blocks may be through partial improvement of fascial compression [120]. Some of the more common blocks include interscalene, supraclavicular, infraclavicular , axillary, intercostobrachial, radial nerve, median nerve, ulnar nerve, lumbar plexus, femoral nerve, fascia iliaca, obturator nerve, sciatic nerve, popliteal nerve, and saphenous nerve blocks.

Nerve Hydrodissection is a treatment method that involves the use of fluid injection under pressure to specifically target the separation of nerves from the surrounding tissue [121]. Oftentimes, ultrasound is also used to guide the fluid (hydro) and needles to separate and release (dissect) the nerves from the surrounding fascia. The pathophysiology of this method is also unclear but includes involvement of the reduction of TRPV1 receptors, hyperpolarizing normoglycemic C fibers and lowering their firing rates, and correction of local neural hypoglycemia [121].

Appendix

References

1. Szok D, Tajti J, Nyári A, Vécsei L. Therapeutic approaches for peripheral and central neuropathic pain. Behav Neurol. 2019;2019:8685954. https://doi.org/10.1155/2019/8685954.
2. Davidoff C, Leung E. Central pain syndromes. In: Pain care essentials and innovations. Amsterdam: Elsevier; 2021. p. 33–44.
3. Canavero S, Bonicalzi V. Central pain syndrome: pathophysiology, diagnosis and management, second edition. Cambridge: Cambridge University Press; 2011. https://doi.org/10.1017/CBO9780511845673.
4. Head H, Holmes G. Sensory disturbances from cerebral lesions. In: Brain. Oxford: Oxford University Press; 1911. https://doi.org/10.1093/brain/34.2-3.102.
5. Whitty CWM. Central pain: a neurosurgical survey. J Neurol Neurosurg Psychiatry. 1969;32(6):639. https://doi.org/10.1136/jnnp.32.6.639-c.

6. Ji R-R, Xu Z-Z, Wang X, Lo EH. MMP-2 and MMP-9—investigations in neuropathic pain phases. US Neurol; 2008. https://doi.org/10.17925/usn.2008.04.02.71.
7. Andersen G, Vestergaard K, Ingeman-Nielsen M, Jensen TS. Incidence of central post-stroke pain. Pain. 1995;61(2):187–93. https://doi.org/10.1016/0304-3959(94)00144-4.
8. Tasker RR, DeCarvalho GTC, Dolan EJ. Intractable pain of spinal cord origin: clinical features and implications for surgery. J Neurosurg. 1992;77(3):373–8. https://doi.org/10.3171/jns.1992.77.3.0373.
9. Watson JC, Sandroni P. Central neuropathic pain syndromes. Mayo Clin Proc. 2016;91(3):372–85. https://doi.org/10.1016/j.mayocp.2016.01.017.
10. Appelros P. Prevalence and predictors of pain and fatigue after stroke: a population-based study. Int J Rehabil Res. 2006;29(4):329–33. https://doi.org/10.1097/MRR.0b013e328010c7b8.
11. Bouhassira D, Attal N, Alchaar H, et al. Comparison of pain syndromes associated with nervous or somatic lesions and development of a new neuropathic pain diagnostic questionnaire (DN4). Pain. 2005;114(1–2):29–36. https://doi.org/10.1016/j.pain.2004.12.010.
12. Bouhassira D, Attal N, Fermanian J, et al. Development and validation of the neuropathic pain symptom inventory. Pain. 2004;108(3):248–57. https://doi.org/10.1016/j.pain.2003.12.024.
13. Finnerup NB, Haroutounian S, Kamerman P, et al. Neuropathic pain: an updated grading system for research and clinical practice. Pain. 2016;157(8):1599–606. https://doi.org/10.1097/j.pain.0000000000000492.
14. de Oliveira RAA, de Andrade DC, Machado AGG, Teixeira MJ. Central poststroke pain: somatosensory abnormalities and the presence of associated myofascial pain syndrome. BMC Neurol. 2012;12:89. https://doi.org/10.1186/1471-2377-12-89.
15. Widerström-Noga E, Loeser JD, Jensen TS, Finnerup NB. AAPT diagnostic criteria for central neuropathic pain. J Pain. 2017;18(12):1417–26. https://doi.org/10.1016/j.jpain.2017.06.003.
16. Huang-Lionnet JH, Brummett C, Raja SN. Central pain states. In: Essentials of pain medicine. Amsterdam: Elsevier; 2018. https://doi.org/10.1016/b978-0-323-40196-8.00030-9.
17. Lundström E, Smits A, Terént A, Borg J. Risk factors for stroke-related pain 1 year after first-ever stroke. Eur J Neurol. 2009;16(2):188–93. https://doi.org/10.1111/j.1468-1331.2008.02378.x.
18. Harrison RA, Field TS. Post stroke pain: identification, assessment, and therapy. Cerebrovasc Dis. 2015;39(3–4):190–201. https://doi.org/10.1159/000375397.
19. Harno H, Haapaniemi E, Putaala J, Haanpää M, Mäkelä JP, Kalso E, Tatlisumak T. Central poststroke pain in young ischemic stroke survivors in the Helsinki Young Stroke Registry. Neurology. 2014;83(13):1147–54. https://doi.org/10.1212/WNL.0000000000000818.
20. O'Donnell MJ, Diener HC, Sacco RL, Panju AA, Vinisko R, Yusuf S. Chronic pain syndromes after ischemic stroke: PRoFESS trial. Stroke. 2013;44(5):1238–43. https://doi.org/10.1161/STROKEAHA.111.671008.
21. Klit H, Finnerup NB, Jensen TS. Central post-stroke pain: clinical characteristics, pathophysiology, and management. Lancet Neurol. 2009;8(9):857–68. https://doi.org/10.1016/S1474-4422(09)70176-0.
22. Widar M, Samuelsson L, Karlsson-Tivenius S, Ahlström G. Long-term pain conditions after a stroke. J Rehabil Med. 2002;34(4):165–70. https://doi.org/10.1080/16501970213237.
23. Garcia-Larrea L. The posterior insular-opercular region and the search of a primary cortex for pain. Neurophysiol Clin. 2012;42(5):299–313. https://doi.org/10.1016/j.neucli.2012.06.001.
24. Bowsher D. Central pain: clinical and physiological characteristics. J Neurol Neurosurg Psychiatry. 1996;61(1):62–9. https://doi.org/10.1136/jnnp.61.1.62.
25. Hong JH, Choi BY, Chang CH, Kim SH, Jung YJ, Lee DG, Kwon YH, Jang SH. The prevalence of central poststroke pain according to the integrity of the spino-thalamo-cortical pathway. Eur Neurol. 2012;67(1):12–7. https://doi.org/10.1159/000333012.
26. Vestergaard K, Nielsen J, Andersen G, Ingeman-Nielsen M, Arendt-Nielsen L, Jensen TS. Sensory abnormalities in consecutive, unselected patients with central post-stroke pain. Pain. 1995;61(2):177–86. https://doi.org/10.1016/0304-3959(94)00140-A.

27. Kumar B, Kalita J, Kumar G, Misra UK. Central poststroke pain: a review of pathophysiology and treatment. Anesth Analg. 2009;108(5):1645–57. https://doi.org/10.1213/ane.0b013e31819d644c.
28. McCormick DA, Wang Z. Serotonin and noradrenaline excite GABAergic neurones of the Guinea-pig and cat nucleus reticularis thalami. J Physiol. 1991;442:235–55. https://doi.org/10.1113/jphysiol.1991.sp018791.
29. Willoch F, Schindler F, Wester HJ, Empl M, Straube A, Schwaiger M, Conrad B, Tölle TR. Central poststroke pain and reduced opioid receptor binding within pain processing circuitries: a [11C]diprenorphine PET study. Pain. 2004;108(3):213–20. https://doi.org/10.1016/j.pain.2003.08.014.
30. Treister AK, Hatch MN, Cramer SC, Chang EY. Demystifying poststroke pain: from etiology to treatment. PM R. 2017;9(1):63–75. https://doi.org/10.1016/j.pmrj.2016.05.015.
31. Bryce TN, Dijkers MPJM. Assessment of pain after SCI in clinical trials. Top Spinal Cord Inj Rehabil. 2006;11(3):50–68.
32. Siddall PJ, Taylor DA, Cousins MJ. Classification of pain following spinal cord injury. Spinal Cord. 1997;35(2):69–75. https://doi.org/10.1038/sj.sc.3100365.
33. Bryce TN, Biering-Sørensen F, Finnerup NB, et al. International spinal cord injury pain classification: part I. Background and description. Spinal Cord. 2012;50:413–7. https://doi.org/10.1038/sc.2011.156.
34. Finnerup NB, Jensen TS. Spinal cord injury pain—mechanisms and treatment. Eur J Neurol. 2004;11(2):73–82. https://doi.org/10.1046/j.1351-5101.2003.00725.x.
35. Hagen EM, Rekand T. Management of neuropathic pain associated with spinal cord injury. Pain Ther. 2015;4(1):51–65. https://doi.org/10.1007/s40122-015-0033-y.
36. Hulsebosch CE, Hains BC, Crown ED, Carlton SM. Mechanisms of chronic central neuropathic pain after spinal cord injury. Brain Res Rev. 2009;60(1):202–13. https://doi.org/10.1016/j.brainresrev.2008.12.010.
37. Hains BC, Waxman SG. Activated microglia contribute to the maintenance of chronic pain after spinal cord injury. J Neurosci. 2006;26(16):4308–17. https://doi.org/10.1523/JNEUROSCI.0003-06.2006.
38. Levendoğlu F, Öğün CÖ, Özerbil Ö, Öğün TC, Uğurlu H. Gabapentin is a first line drug for the treatment of neuropathic pain in spinal cord injury. Spine (Phila Pa 1976). 2004;29(7):743–51. https://doi.org/10.1097/01.BRS.0000112068.16108.3A.
39. Siddall PJ, Cousins MJ, Otte A, Griesing T, Chambers R, Murphy TK. Pregabalin in central neuropathic pain associated with spinal cord injury: a placebo-controlled trial. Neurology. 2006;67(10):1792–800. https://doi.org/10.1212/01.wnl.0000244422.45278.ff.
40. Cardenas DD, Nieshoff EC, Suda K, et al. A randomized trial of pregabalin in patients with neuropathic pain due to spinal cord injury. Neurology. 2013;80(6):533–9. https://doi.org/10.1212/WNL.0b013e318281546b.
41. Leijon G, Boivie J. Central post-stroke pain—a controlled trial of amitriptyline and carbamazepine. Pain. 1989;36(1):27–36. https://doi.org/10.1016/0304-3959(89)90108-5.
42. Cardenas DD, Warms CA, Turner JA, Marshall H, Brooke MM, Loeser JD. Efficacy of amitriptyline for relief of pain in spinal cord injury: results of a randomized controlled trial. Pain. 2002;96(3):365–73. https://doi.org/10.1016/S0304-3959(01)00483-3.
43. Shimodozono M, Kawahira K, Kamishita T, Ogata A, Tohgo SI, Tanaka N. Reduction of central poststroke pain with the selective serotonin reuptake inhibitor fluvoxamine. Int J Neurosci. 2002;112(10):1173–81. https://doi.org/10.1080/00207450290026139.
44. Vestergaard K, Andersen G, Gottrup H, Kristensen BT, Jensen TS. Lamotrigine for central poststroke pain: a randomized controlled trial. Neurology. 2001;56(2):184–90. https://doi.org/10.1212/WNL.56.2.184.
45. Cohen SP, Bhatia A, Buvanendran A, et al. Consensus guidelines on the use of intravenous ketamine infusions for chronic pain from the American Society of Regional Anesthesia and Pain Medicine, the American Academy of Pain Medicine, and the American Society

of Anesthesiologists. Reg Anesth Pain Med. 2018;43(5):521–46. https://doi.org/10.1097/AAP.0000000000000808.
46. Tajerian M, Leu D, Yang P, Huang TT, Kingery WS, Clark JD. Differential efficacy of ketamine in the acute versus chronic stages of complex regional pain syndrome in mice. Anesthesiology. 2015;123(6):1435–47. https://doi.org/10.1097/ALN.0000000000000889.
47. Amr YM. Multi-day low dose ketamine infusion as adjuvant to oral gabapentin in spinal cord injury related chronic pain: a prospective, randomized, double blind trial. Pain Physician. 2010;13(3):245–9. https://doi.org/10.36076/ppj.2010/13/245.
48. Whiting PF, Wolff RF, Deshpande S, et al. Cannabinoids for medical use. JAMA. 2015;313(24):2456–73. https://doi.org/10.1001/jama.2015.6358.
49. Grant LD, Haverkamp BE. A cognitive-behavioral approach to chronic pain management. J Couns Dev; 1995. https://doi.org/10.1002/j.1556-6676.1995.tb01818.x.
50. Santos ABO, Gozzani JL. Acupuncture as adjuvant therapy in thalamic syndrome: case report. Rev Bras Anesthesiol. 2011;61(1):88–94. https://doi.org/10.1016/s0034-7094(11)70010-1.
51. Vance CGT, Dailey DL, Rakel BA, Sluka KA. Using TENS for pain control: the state of the evidence. Pain Manag. 2014;4(3):197–209. https://doi.org/10.2217/pmt.14.13.
52. Park J, Chung ME. Botulinum toxin for central neuropathic pain. Toxins (Basel). 2018;10(6):224. https://doi.org/10.3390/toxins10060224.
53. Chun A, Levy I, Yang A, et al. Treatment of at-level spinal cord injury pain with botulinum toxin A. Spinal Cord Ser Cases. 2019;5:77. https://doi.org/10.1038/s41394-019-0221-9.
54. Ramachandran VS, McGeoch PD, Williams L, Arcilla G. Rapid relief of thalamic pain syndrome induced by vestibular caloric stimulation. Neurocase. 2007;13(3):185–8. https://doi.org/10.1080/13554790701450446.
55. Spitoni GF, Pireddu G, Galati G, Sulpizio V, Paolucci S, Pizzamiglio L. Caloric vestibular stimulation reduces pain and somatoparaphrenia in a severe chronic central post-stroke pain patient: a case study. PLoS One. 2016;11(3):e0151213. https://doi.org/10.1371/journal.pone.0151213.
56. Kanpolat Y. The surgical treatment of chronic pain: destructive therapies in the spinal cord. Neurosurg Clin N Am. 2004;15(3):307–17. https://doi.org/10.1016/j.nec.2004.02.013.
57. Sukul VV, Slavin KV. Deep brain and motor cortex stimulation. Curr Pain Headache Rep. 2014;18(7):427. https://doi.org/10.1007/s11916-014-0427-2.
58. Levy R, Deer TR, Henderson J. Intracranial neurostimulation for pain control: a review. Pain Physician. 2010;13(2):157–65. https://doi.org/10.36076/ppj.2010/13/157.
59. Nardone R, Höller Y, Leis S, Höller P, Thon N, Thomschewski A, Golaszewski S, Brigo F, Trinka E. Invasive and non-invasive brain stimulation for treatment of neuropathic pain in patients with spinal cord injury: a review. J Spinal Cord Med. 2014;37(1):19–31. https://doi.org/10.1179/2045772313Y.0000000140.
60. Tsubokawa T, Katayama Y, Yamamoto T, Hirayama T, Koyama S. Chronic motor cortex stimulation in patients with thalamic pain. J Neurosurg. 1993;78(3):393–401. https://doi.org/10.3171/jns.1993.78.3.0393.
61. Owen SLF, Green AL, Stein JF, Aziz TZ. Deep brain stimulation for the alleviation of post-stroke neuropathic pain. Pain. 2006;120(1–2):202–6. https://doi.org/10.1016/j.pain.2005.09.035.
62. Pang EK, Rudd-Barnard G. Neuropathic pain. In: Pain care essentials and innovations. Amsterdam: Elsevier; 2021. p. 59–71.
63. Mononeuropathy: what is it & how to treat it. https://my.clevelandclinic.org/health/diseases/16014-mononeuropathy. Accessed 15 May 2021.
64. Van Hecke O, Austin SK, Khan RA, Smith BH, Torrance N. Neuropathic pain in the general population: a systematic review of epidemiological studies. Pain. 2014;155(4):654–62. https://doi.org/10.1016/j.pain.2013.11.013.
65. Bouhassira D, Lantéri-Minet M, Attal N, Laurent B, Touboul C. Prevalence of chronic pain with neuropathic characteristics in the general population. Pain. 2008;136(3):380–7. https://doi.org/10.1016/j.pain.2007.08.013.

66. Woolf CJ, Mannion RJ. Neuropathic pain: aetiology, symptoms, mechanisms, and management. Lancet. 1999;353(9168):1959–64. https://doi.org/10.1016/S0140-6736(99)01307-0.
67. Gunthorpe MJ, Chizh BA. Clinical development of TRPV1 antagonists: targeting a pivotal point in the pain pathway. Drug Discov Today. 2009;14(1–2):56–67. https://doi.org/10.1016/j.drudis.2008.11.005.
68. Palazzo E, Rossi F, Maione S. Role of TRPV1 receptors in descending modulation of pain. Mol Cell Endocrinol. 2008;286(1–2 Suppl 1):S79–83. https://doi.org/10.1016/j.mce.2008.01.013.
69. Attal N, Bouhassira D. Mechanisms of pain in peripheral neuropathy. Acta Neurol Scand Suppl. 1999;173:12–24. https://doi.org/10.1111/j.1600-0404.1999.tb07386.x.
70. Jones RCW, Backonja MM. Review of neuropathic pain screening and assessment tools. Curr Pain Headache Rep. 2013;17(9):363. https://doi.org/10.1007/s11916-013-0363-6.
71. Baron R, Binder A, Wasner G. Neuropathic pain: diagnosis, pathophysiological mechanisms, and treatment. Lancet Neurol. 2010;9(8):807–19. https://doi.org/10.1016/S1474-4422(10)70143-5.
72. Mendell JR, Sahenk Z. Painful sensory neuropathy. N Engl J Med. 2003;348:1243–55. https://doi.org/10.1056/nejmcp022282.
73. Truini A, Biasiotta A, Di Stefano G, Leone C, La Cesa S, Galosi E, Piroso S, Pepe A, Giordano C, Cruccu G. Does the epidermal nerve fibre density measured by skin biopsy in patients with peripheral neuropathies correlate with neuropathic pain? Pain. 2014;155(4):828–32. https://doi.org/10.1016/j.pain.2014.01.022.
74. Backonja MM, Attal N, Baron R, et al. Value of quantitative sensory testing in neurological and pain disorders: NeuPSIG consensus. Pain. 2013;154(9):1807–19. https://doi.org/10.1016/j.pain.2013.05.047.
75. Arnold M. AIDP/CIDP part 1: evaluation and diagnosis—PM&R KnowledgeNow. 2013. https://now.aapmr.org/aidpcidp-part-1-evaluation-and-diagnosis/. Accessed 15 May 2021.
76. Liu J, Wang LN, Mcnicol ED. Pharmacological treatment for pain in Guillain-Barré syndrome. Cochrane Database Syst Rev. 2015;30(7):433–8. https://doi.org/10.1002/14651858.CD009950.pub3.
77. Guillain-Barre and CIDP. https://www.hopkinsmedicine.org/neurology_neurosurgery/centers_clinics/peripheral_nerve/conditions/guillain_barre_and_cidp.html. Accessed 15 May 2021.
78. Gruver C, Guthmiller KB. Postherpetic neuralgia. Orlando: StatPearls Publishing; 2021.
79. Gylfadottir SS, Christensen DH, Nicolaisen SK, et al. Diabetic polyneuropathy and pain, prevalence, and patient characteristics: a cross-sectional questionnaire study of 5,514 patients with recently diagnosed type 2 diabetes. Pain. 2020;161:574–83.
80. Diabetic Neuropathy | Johns Hopkins Medicine. https://www.hopkinsmedicine.org/health/conditions-and-diseases/diabetes/diabetic-neuropathy-nerve-problems. Accessed 15 May 2021.
81. Ratti C, Nordio A, Resmini G, Murena L. Post-traumatic complex regional pain syndrome: clinical features and epidemiology. Clin Cases Miner Bone Metab. 2015;12:11–6.
82. Harden RN. Complex regional pain syndrome. Br J Anaesth. 2001;87(1):99–106. https://doi.org/10.1093/bja/87.1.99.
83. Hammond N, Wang Y, Dimachkie MM, Barohn RJ. Nutritional neuropathies. Neurol Clin. 2013;31:477–89.
84. Zajaczkowską R, Kocot-Kępska M, Leppert W, Wrzosek A, Mika J, Wordliczek J. Mechanisms of chemotherapy-induced peripheral neuropathy. Int J Mol Sci. 2019;20(6):1451. https://doi.org/10.3390/ijms20061451.
85. Rudnik-Schöneborn S, Auer-Grumbach M, Senderek J. Charcot-Marie-tooth disease and hereditary motor neuropathies—update 2020. Medizinische Genet. 2020;32:207–19.
86. Schwartzlow C, Kazamel M. Hereditary sensory and autonomic neuropathies: adding more to the classification. Curr Neurol Neurosci Rep. 2019;19(8):52. https://doi.org/10.1007/s11910-019-0974-3.

87. Axelrod FB, Gold-Von Simson G. Hereditary sensory and autonomic neuropathies: types II, III, and IV. Orphanet J Rare Dis. 2007;2:1–12.
88. Brouwer BA, Merkies ISJ, Gerrits MM, Waxman SG, Hoeijmakers JGJ, Faber CG. Painful neuropathies: the emerging role of sodium channelopathies. J Peripher Nerv Syst. 2014;19(2):53–65. https://doi.org/10.1111/jns5.12071.
89. Jones MR, Urits I, Wolf J, Corrigan D, Colburn L, Peterson E, Williamson A, Viswanath O. Drug-induced peripheral neuropathy: a narrative review. Curr Clin Pharmacol. 2019;15:38–48.
90. Brewer JR, Morrison G, Dolan ME, Fleming GF. Chemotherapy-induced peripheral neuropathy: current status and progress. Gynecol Oncol. 2016;140(1):176–83. https://doi.org/10.1016/j.ygyno.2015.11.011.
91. Yoon YH, Jung KH, Sadun AA, Shin HC, Koh JY. Ethambutol-induced vacuolar changes and neuronal loss in rat retinal cell culture: mediation by endogenous zinc. Toxicol Appl Pharmacol. 2000;162(2):107–14. https://doi.org/10.1006/taap.1999.8846.
92. Weimer LH, Sachdev N. Update on medication-induced peripheral neuropathy. Curr Neurol Neurosci Rep. 2009;9(1):69–75. https://doi.org/10.1007/s11910-009-0011-z.
93. Attal N, Cruccu G, Baron R, Haanpää M, Hansson P, Jensen TS, Nurmikko T. EFNS guidelines on the pharmacological treatment of neuropathic pain: 2010 revision. Eur J Neurol. 2010;17:1113–e88.
94. Yu J, Wang DS, Bonin RP, Penna A, Alavian-Ghavanini A, Zurek AA, Rauw G, Baker GB, Orser BA. Gabapentin increases expression of δ subunit-containing GABA A receptors. EBioMedicine. 2019;42:203–13.
95. Finnerup NB, Haroutounian S, Baron R, et al. Neuropathic pain clinical trials: factors associated with decreases in estimated drug efficacy. Pain. 2018;159(11):2339–46. https://doi.org/10.1097/j.pain.0000000000001340.
96. Jensen TS. Anticonvulsants in neuropathic pain: rationale and clinical evidence. Eur J Pain. 2002;6:61–8.
97. Fudin J. Appropriate gabapentin dosing for neuropathic pain. https://www.pharmacytimes.com/view/appropriate-gabapentin-dosing-for-neuropathic-pain. Accessed 15 May 2021.
98. Al-Quliti KW. Update on neuropathic pain treatment for trigeminal neuralgia: the pharmacological and surgical options. Neurosciences. 2015;20(2):107–14. https://doi.org/10.17712/nsj.2015.2.20140501.
99. Spina A, Mortini P, Alemanno F, Houdayer E, Iannaccone S. Trigeminal neuralgia: toward a multimodal approach. World Neurosurg. 2017;103:220–30. https://doi.org/10.1016/j.wneu.2017.03.126.
100. Sansone RA, Sansone LA. Pain, pain, go away: antidepressants and pain management. Psychiatry (Edgmont). 2008;5:16–9.
101. Jilani TN, Gibbons JR, Faizy RM, Saadabadi A. Mirtazapine. Orlando: StatPearls Publishing; 2021.
102. Hirsch M, Birnbaum R. Atypical antidepressants: pharmacology, administration, and side effects—UpToDate. https://www.uptodate.com/contents/atypical-antidepressants-pharmacology-administration-and-side-effects?search=mirtazapine-&source=search_result&selectedTitle=2~83&usage_type=default&display_rank=2. Accessed 15 May 2021.
103. Casale R, Symeonidou Z, Bartolo M. Topical treatments for localized neuropathic pain. Curr Pain Headache Rep. 2017;21(3):15. https://doi.org/10.1007/s11916-017-0615-y.
104. Anand P, Bley K. Topical capsaicin for pain management: therapeutic potential and mechanisms of action of the new high-concentration capsaicin 8 patch. Br J Anaesth. 2011;107:490–502.
105. Niesters M, Martini C, Dahan A. Ketamine for chronic pain: risks and benefits. Br J Clin Pharmacol. 2014;77:357–67.
106. Hutson P, Backonja M, Knurr H. Intravenous lidocaine for neuropathic pain: a retrospective analysis of tolerability and efficacy. Pain Med (United States). 2015;16:531–6.
107. Braddom R. Physical medicine and rehabilitation fourth edition. Berlin: Springer; 2011.

108. Gibson W, Wand BM, O'Connell NE. Transcutaneous electrical nerve stimulation (TENS) for neuropathic pain in adults. Cochrane Database Syst Rev. 2017;9(9):CD011976. https://doi.org/10.1002/14651858.CD011976.pub2.
109. Mannino R. Using mirror therapy to reduce pain and improve movement. https://www.hss.edu/conditions_using-mirror-therapy-to-reduce-pain-and-improve-movement.asp. Accessed 16 May 2021.
110. Kim SY, Kim YY. Mirror therapy for phantom limb pain. Korean J Pain. 2012;25:272–4.
111. Li A, Montaño Z, Chen VJ, Gold JI. Virtual reality and pain management: current trends and future directions. Pain Manag. 2011;1:147–57.
112. Duarte RV, Nevitt S, McNicol E, Taylor RS, Buchser E, North RB, Eldabe S. Systematic review and meta-analysis of placebo/sham controlled randomised trials of spinal cord stimulation for neuropathic pain. Pain. 2020;161(1):24–35. https://doi.org/10.1097/j.pain.0000000000001689.
113. Katz J, Rosenbloom BN. The golden anniversary of Melzack and Wall's gate control theory of pain: celebrating 50 years of pain research and management. Pain Res Manag. 2015;20:285–6.
114. Duarte RV, Andronis L, Lenders MWPM, de Vos CC. Quality of life increases in patients with painful diabetic neuropathy following treatment with spinal cord stimulation. Qual Life Res. 2016;25(7):1771–7. https://doi.org/10.1007/s11136-015-1211-4.
115. Slangen R, Schaper NC, Faber CG, Joosten EA, Dirksen CD, Van Dongen RT, Kessels AG, Van Kleef M. Spinal cord stimulation and pain relief in painful diabetic peripheral neuropathy: a prospective two-center randomized controlled trial. Diabetes Care. 2014;37(11):3016–24. https://doi.org/10.2337/dc14-0684.
116. De Vos CC, Meier K, Zaalberg PB, Nijhuis HJA, Duyvendak W, Vesper J, Enggaard TP, Lenders MWPM. Spinal cord stimulation in patients with painful diabetic neuropathy: a multicentre randomized clinical trial. Pain. 2014;155(11):2426–31. https://doi.org/10.1016/j.pain.2014.08.031.
117. Levy RM, Mekhail N, Kramer J, et al. Therapy habituation at 12 months: spinal cord stimulation versus dorsal root ganglion stimulation for complex regional pain syndrome type I and II. J Pain. 2020;21(3–4):399–408. https://doi.org/10.1016/j.jpain.2019.08.005.
118. Deer TR, Levy RM, Kramer J, et al. Dorsal root ganglion stimulation yielded higher treatment success rate for complex regional pain syndrome and causalgia at 3 and 12 months: a randomized comparative trial. Pain. 2017;158(4):669–81. https://doi.org/10.1097/j.pain.0000000000000814.
119. Gunduz OH, Kenis-Coskun O. Ganglion blocks as a treatment of pain: current perspectives. J Pain Res. 2017;10:2815–26.
120. Pérez FAS, Sánchez GR. Peripheral nerve blocks. Rev Colomb Anestesiol. 2011;39:387–402.
121. Lam SKH, Reeves KD, Cheng AL. Transition from deep regional blocks toward deep nerve hydrodissection in the upper body and torso: method description and results from a retrospective chart review of the analgesic effect of 5% dextrose water as the primary hydrodissection injectate to enhance safety. Biomed Res Int. 2017;2017:7920438. https://doi.org/10.1155/2017/7920438.

Chapter 11
Chronic Neuropathic Pain: Fibromyalgia

Yasser El Miedany

Introduction

Chronic pain is a highly prevalent and onerous condition spanning the globe. Similar to other debilitating chronic disorders, chronic pain represents much more than a sequence of biological phenomena that impact people health. Chronic pain stems from and provokes several cognitive and emotional consequences. Therefore, a bio-psychosocial approach is highly required to understand and manage these conditions [1]. Whilst chronic pain disorders, presenting with a predominantly nociceptive/inflammatory or neuropathic component, tend to be appreciated by health care professionals; other chronic pain conditions with centralized phenomena are less well understood, especially in the context of a chronic pain continuum [2].

Fibromyalgia (FM) is a debilitating, widespread pain disorder that is assumed to originate from inappropriate pain processing in the central nervous system. However, accumulating evidence supports a peripheral neurological origin of the fibromyalgia symptoms too [3]. Fibromyalgia has a worldwide general population prevalence of 2–4%, hence, its importance. In addition to the chronic widespread pain, it is characterised by fatigue, unrefreshing sleep, and cognitive complications [4]. However, chronic widespread pain remains the most important defining feature of FM, though individual patients may also attribute variable weight to the other symptoms.

This chapter will discuss the debate of fibromyalgia as a bitterly controversial condition, the science of pain and where fibromyalgia fits in. It will then discuss fibromyalgia as a pain processing problem, different sources of pain in fibromyalgia patients and the wind-up theory. The chapter will expand to discuss Fibromyalgia

Y. El Miedany (✉)
Institute of Medical Sciences, Canterbury Christ Church University, Kent, England

Canterbury Christ Church University, Institute of Medical Sciences, Chatham, United Kingdom

© The Author(s), under exclusive license to Springer Nature Switzerland AG 2022

J. de Castro, Y. El Miedany (eds.), *Advances in Chronic and Neuropathic Pain*, Contemporary Rheumatology, https://doi.org/10.1007/978-3-031-10687-3_11

associated comorbidities, fibromyalgia pain in the clinical setting, fibromyalgianess, neuroimaging, as well as pain pathways and the pharmacotherapy of Fibromyalgia.

Fibromyalgia: The Debate

Despite considerable interest and investigations over the past 30 years, FM syndrome remains a "bitterly controversial condition" [5] which continues to provoke debate and raise challenges at variable levels [6, 7]. Fibromyalgia conflicts [5, 8] are fought on several fronts: the legitimacy and clinical utility of the diagnostic label FM, the nosological classification, diagnostic criteria, suggested aetiology and pathophysiology, "ownership", the preferred treatment options and long-term outcome [9–11].

Such controversy has reflected on the decision making of the FM diagnosis. It is often not diagnosed when it should be, and even more often, nowadays, it is diagnosed when it shouldn't be [12]. Furthermore, no specific medical speciality specializes in it. Rheumatologists and neurologists often feel "stuck" with fibromyalgia patients, and usually offer limited management options unless they've taken a special interest in the topic. Psychiatrists and psychologists prefer to diagnose patients who exhibit fibromyalgia-like symptoms with somatoform disorders (somatoform pain disorder or somatization disorder) [13]. Orthopedic surgeons, consider it a scape goat and excuse to refer the patient, either for physio or rheumatology, for having fibromyalgia symptoms, whereas, primary care physicians prefer to use the diagnostic label chronic widespread pain or chronic fatigue syndrome [14].

Over the past 30 years, there has also been controversy regarding the diagnosis of FM. In 1990, fibromyalgia was defined by the American College of Rheumatology (ACR) classification criteria as requiring multiple tender points (assessed during physical examination) and chronic widespread pain [15]. In 1994, the tenth revision of the International Classification of Diseases (ICD-10) listed fibromyalgia under 'diseases of the musculoskeletal system and connective tissue' [16]. However, the 2010 ACR preliminary diagnostic criteria [17] and its subsequent revisions in 2011 [18], and 2016 [19] which, briefly, ditched the "tender points" diagnostic approach and addressed important symptoms through which fibromyalgia could be identified and characterized in clinical settings, such as patient-reported somatic symptoms and cognitive difficulties [17].

Another major challenge is the lack of a specific medical consensus on how FM can be treated, which had a negative impact on health care professionals who are handling these cases with few information on identified treatment targets or outcomes. Consequently, it become a norm that no healthcare professional would feel bad about not knowing how to manage it, which made FM, literally, one of the hardest problems in medicine. This paved the way for alternative medicine, which rushed to fill this medical gap with a dizzying array of crackpot cures. Lastly, this uncertainty about how to diagnose and manage FM [20, 21], had a similar negative impact on the patients living with the condition. This medical uncertainty has translated into patient stress, anxiety, frustration and even dissatisfaction [22]. This has been attributed to the time taken to establish a definitive diagnosis of FM that often extends to many months or even years, with innumerable clinic visits, investigations and specialist consultations, all contributing to the FM personal and societal burden [21–23].

Therefore, greater understanding of the FM disorder and its management can enable clinicians to more effectively care for their patients and achieve better outcomes.

The Science of Pain

In normal pain processing path, the perception of pain involves two main groups of neural pathways: ascending and descending pathways [24]. Peripheral nerves transmit sensory signals, including nociceptive (pain-inducing) signals, to the spinal cord for transmission via the ascending nociceptive pathway to the brain for processing. Nociceptive signals are emitted when specialized receptors in the peripheral nerves called nociceptors are activated by stimuli such as temperature and physical pressure or impact. In the general population, perception of pain displays a normal distribution on a bell curve (Fig. 11.1)

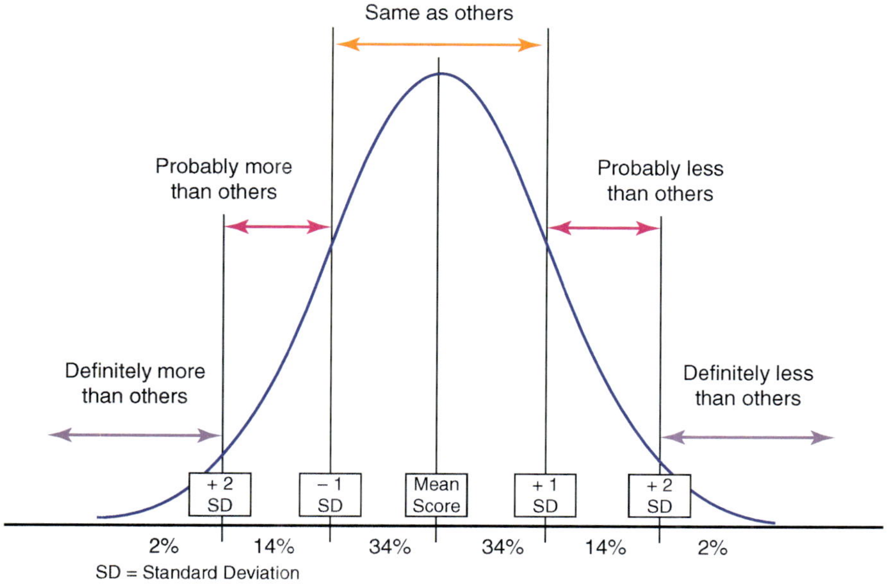

Fig. 11.1 Average is a range of scores in the middle of everyone else's scores. So, people in the middle (40–60th percentile) scored more than the people who scored less than the 40th percentile (the left hand side of the curve). However, the people in the middle scored less than the people on the right hand side of the curve. The processing of pain and other sensory information by the brain and spinal cord is governed by a "value control setting". The higher the volume control setting, the more pain experienced, irrespective of peripheral nociceptive input. (Quoted from at the top of the bell curve; under open access scheme. https://thinkingscifi.wordpress.com/2014/07/06/at-the-top-of-the-bell-curve/)

Descending pain modulatory pathways send both facilitatory and inhibitory signals from the brain to the spinal cord and to the periphery, either increasing or decreasing the "volume control" on incoming nociceptive signals reaching the brain. Signals in these pathways are mediated and propagated by a number of neurotransmitters and neurochemicals (e.g. norepinephrine, serotonin) [24–26].

Types of Pain and Where Fibromyalgia Fits in

Pain can be classified based on its acuity or chronicity, the pathophysiological mechanism, anatomic location and the presence of malignancy. Each classification is important and understanding those classifications and their definitions is vital to guide the process of diagnosis and management. However, fibromyalgia appears unique in this aspect too, as patients with fibromyalgia may present with different forms of pain including hyperalgesia, widespread soft tissue pain, joint pain, allodynia, neuropathic pain, headache as well as abdominal and pelvic pain (Fig. 11.2). The challenge with fibromyalgia pain, is that it is unpredictable, and varies in intensity from time to time; however, on the other hand, debilitating with significant negative impact on the patient's life.

Considering the variety of pain reported in fibromyalgia patients, it is evident that fibromyalgia doesn't seem to fit well into any of the two main pain categories:

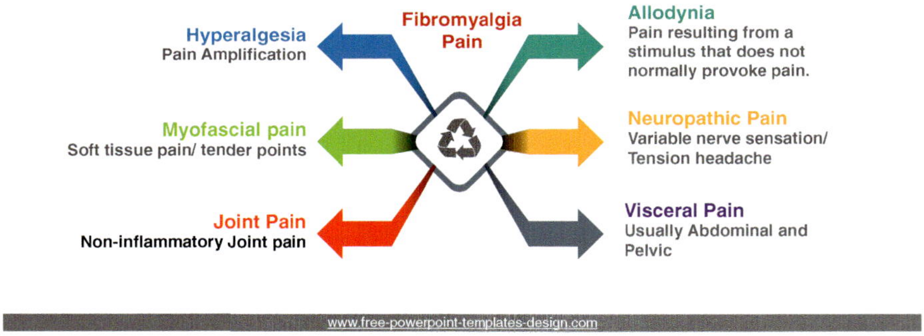

Fig. 11.2 The types of pain in fibromyalgia. Hyperalgesia: pain amplification in fibromyalgia (increased pain from a stimulus that normally provokes pain); Myofascial pain: soft tissue pain affecting different parts of the body manifest clinically as tender points, Joint pain: non-inflammatory joint pain; Allodynia: pain due to a stimulus that does not normally provoke pain. This hypersensitive reaction has been attributed to central sensitization (sensitization is increased responsiveness of nociceptive neurons to their normal input; and/or recruitment of a response to normally subthreshold inputs); neuropathic pain: variable nerve sensations such as tingling, burning which could be painful, despite normal neurological examination, headache: tension headache is the most common form; visceral pain: usually abdominal and pelvic, may present as irritable bowel syndrome, abdominal cramps, bloating, acid reflux, cystitis

nociceptive (the most common type of pain caused by damage to tissues and reported to the brain for assessment) and neuropathic (caused by a lesion or disease of the somatosensory system, including peripheral fibres [Aβ, Aδ and C fibres] as well as central neurons). As fibromyalgia does not involve confirmed damage to the somatosensory system or soft tissue, it may represent a third category, "a dysfunction". Dysfunction in pain modulation, demonstrated by allodynia and spontaneous pain, suggests that fibromyalgia could be a pain disease owing to an increase in pain sensitivity and decrease in pain inhibitory controls [27]. Such unique type of pain reported in fibromyalgia pain has also been described as a state of "algopathic" pain (Nociplastic/nocipathic) which describes pain that arises from altered nociception despite no clear evidence of actual or threatened tissue damage causing the activation of peripheral nociceptors or evidence of disease or lesion of the somatosensory system causing the pain.

Two international workgroups have recently released new classification criteria for chronic pain conditions [27, 28]. The International Association for the Study of Pain (in collaboration with World Health Organization) developed new ICD-11 codes that separate chronic pain conditions by whether or not the pain is secondary to another condition (e.g., osteoarthritis, diabetes, and cancer) [28]. The goal is to create a classification system that is applicable in primary care and in clinical settings for specialized pain management. Chronic primary pain is defined as pain in one or more anatomic regions that persists or recurs for longer than 3 months and is associated with significant emotional distress or significant functional disability (interference with activities of daily life and participation in social roles) and that cannot be better explained by another chronic pain condition. The new designation of chronic primary pain syndromes includes fibromyalgia in the chronic widespread pain category. The American Pain Society (in collaboration with multiple other groups) led the efforts to improve diagnostic classification criteria for chronic pain conditions [27]. The workgroup determined three dimensions for fibromyalgia: Dimension (1): the core diagnostic criteria for fibromyalgia are pain of at least 3 months duration occurring in at least six body sites (using the nine-site Manikin) that is accompanied by fatigue (physical or mental) or sleep disturbances judged to be of at least moderate severity by a clinician [29]. Dimension (2): include tenderness (widespread heightened sensitivity to pressure), executive functioning deficits (disorganized/slow thinking, difficulty concentrating, forgetfulness), and sensory intolerance (heightened sensitivity to lights, sounds, odours, or cold). Dimension (3): common comorbidities include several psychiatric conditions (major mood disorders, anxiety disorders, substance use disorders) [29].

Fibromyalgia: A Pain Processing Problem

The pathophysiologic sequence of events that leads to the development of fibromyalgia is not well elucidated; however, a number of discrete cellular and biochemical abnormalities have been identified. The volume of abnormalities discovered in patients with fibromyalgia is high enough to substantiate the claim that it is not a subjective pain condition. When viewed collectively, these abnormalities suggest that fibromyalgia is a disorder of central sensitization or abnormal central processing of nociceptive pain input.

Fibromyalgia Is a Brain Disease-Central Sensitization

Central sensitization is considered the best-established pathophysiological feature of FM. This has been described as augmented pain and sensory processing in the brain, with increased functional connectivity to pro-nociceptive brain regions and decreased connectivity to anti-nociceptive regions, together with associated changes in the central nervous system neurotransmitters, as well as in the size and shape of brain regions (Fig. 11.3). This was endorsed by the findings of earlier studies which noted that when these central nervous system changes were targeted with pharmacologic or nonpharmacologic therapies known to influence central nervous system function, improvement in the cardinal fibromyalgia symptoms has been reported in a subset of the patients. The improvement in functional, chemical, and structural

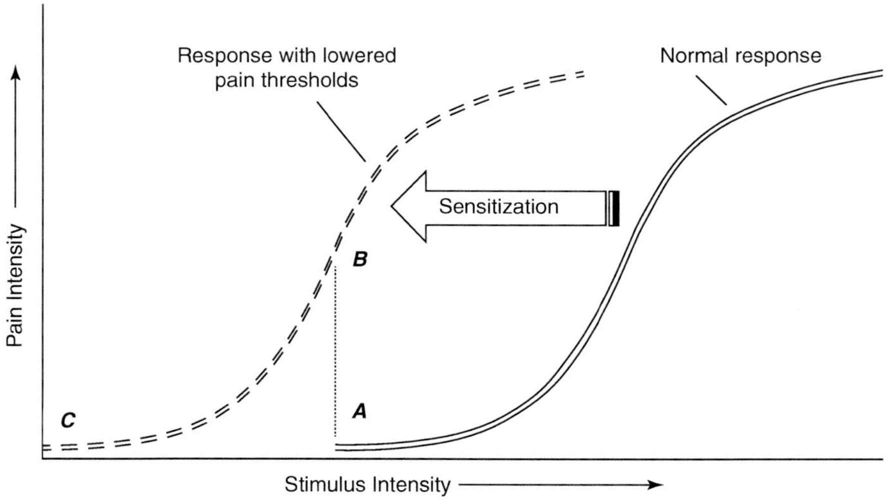

Fig. 11.3 Hypothesized sensitization process. The normal response curve (double line) portrays the relationship between pain perception and stimulus intensity. In the presence of sensitization, this curve shifts to the left (double dashed line). (A) Represents pain onset in the normal response condition; (B) represents hyperalgesia, in which a stimulus intensity that causes pain onset in the normal condition is perceived as more painful after sensitization; (C) represents allodynia, in which a stimulus intensity below that of normal onset is now perceived as painful. (Copied from Borstad J, Woeste C. The role of sensitization in musculoskeletal shoulder pain. Braz J Phys Ther. 2015;19(4):251–257. https://doi.org/10.1590/bjpt-rbf.2014.0100, under via license: CC BY 4.0, open access scheme)

neuroimaging findings in association with these therapies, supported the concept that fibromyalgia is a brain disease [27].

However, these changes are not unique or distinct to fibromyalgia. Findings of central nervous system alterations that are used to support the idea of pain centralization also support other central nervous system-based hypotheses, including the consequences of personality traits (such as pain catastrophizing), sympathetic nervous system dysfunction, the evolutionary stress response, and the activation of homeostatic neural programs [30, 31].

Fibromyalgia Is a Small Fiber Neuropathy

The identification of small-nerve-fiber pathology in some fibromyalgia patients, paved the way to the hypotheses that fibromyalgia is a neurological disease (small fiber neuropathy) [32]. However, such small fiber pathology findings could not be detected in all patients meeting the established fibromyalgia criteria [33]. Furthermore, some small-pathology findings, such as decreased intraepidermal nerve fiber density (IENFD) have been reported in in most of the other chronic pain conditions and also in other conditions not normally associated with pain, such as postural tachycardia syndrome and amyotrophic lateral sclerosis [33, 34]. Finally, the classic clinical picture of patients living with small fiber neuropathy differs considerably from that seen in most fibromyalgia patients [6, 33].

Mechanisms Underlying Abnormal Pain Sensitivity

The mechanisms underlying the central sensitization that occurs in patients with FM is based on the hyperexcitability of spinal dorsal horn neurons that transmit nociceptive input to the brain. As a consequence, high levels of nociceptive input to the brain are generated in response to low intensity stimuli delivered to the skin or deep muscle tissue generate giving the perception of pain. In his article, Staud [35] assessed the biology of pain in FM. Impulses from peripheral nociceptors are transmitted to the CNS by myelinated A-δ (first pain) and unmyelinated C-fibers (second pain). A-δ mediated pain signals are rapidly conducted to the CNS (at about 10 m/s), whereas C-fiber impulses travel relatively slowly (at about 1.6 m/s). Specifically, intense or prolonged impulse input from A-δ and C afferents sufficiently depolarizes the dorsal horn neurons and results in the removal of the Mg^{2+} block of *N*-methyl D-aspartate, NMDA-gated, ion channels. This is followed by the influx of extracellular Ca^{2+} and production of nitric oxide, which diffuses out of the dorsal horn neurons. Nitric oxide, in turn, promotes the exaggerated release of excitatory amino acids and substance P from presynaptic afferent terminals and causes the dorsal horn neurons to become hyperexcitable. Subsequently, low intensity stimuli evoked by minor physical activity may be amplified in the spinal cord resulting in painful sensations.

Muscle Tissue as a Source of Nociceptive Input

Muscle tissue is considered a potential source of nociceptive input that might be linked to FM pain [36]. Several forms of muscle abnormalities have been described in FM patients. These include the appearance of inflammatory infiltrates, ragged red fibers, as well as moth-eaten fibers [37–39]. Such muscle changes have been attributed to repetitive muscle microtrauma, which could explain the post-exertional pain as well as some of the other painful symptoms reported by these patients. In addition, prolonged muscle tension and ischemia have been reported in FM patients' muscles [40, 41]. Changes in the pH of the muscles induced by ischemia [42] might give an explanation for the sensitization of spinal and supraspinal pain pathways [43]. The study carried out by Park et al., revealed that assessment using ^{31}P nuclear magnetic resonance spectroscopy have demonstrated that FM patients display significantly lower phosphorylation potential and total oxidative capacity in the quadriceps muscle during rest and exercise [44]. Significantly lower levels of muscle phosphocreatine and ATP, as well as a lower phosphocreatine/inorganic phosphate ratio were also reported in FM patients [37, 38]. Furthermore, magnetic resonance imaging of FM patients' muscles revealed increased prevalence of phosphodiester peaks, which have been associated with sarcolemmal membrane damage [44, 45].

Focal muscle abnormalities, in particular the well-known trigger points, frequently detectable in FM patients, may act as pain generators. Using sensitive techniques such as microdialysis revealed significantly higher concentrations of bradykinin, protons, calcitonin gene-related peptide, substance P, tumor necrosis factor-α, IL-1b, serotonin, and norepinephrine in the trigger points than normal muscle tissue [46, 47]. Furthermore, other studies have shown that advanced glycation end products might also play a role that is relevant for FM pain. These can trigger the synthesis of cytokines, particularly IL-1b and tumor necrosis factor-α. A study carried out by Rust et al revealed the detection of elevated advanced glycation end product levels in interstitial connective tissue of the muscles as well as the serum of FM patients [48]. All these biochemical mediators are able to sensitize muscle nociceptors and thus indirectly contribute to central sensitization and chronic pain. Because nociceptive input from muscles is very powerful in inducing and maintaining central sensitization [49], FM muscle abnormalities may strongly contribute to pain through important mechanisms of pain amplification.

The Windup and Fibromyalgia Pain

The windup The temporal summation of second pain (windup) was first described by Mendell and Wall in 1965 [50]. The theory is based on the finding that repetitive C-fiber stimulation can result in a progressive increase of electrical discharges from second order neurons in the spinal cord [50] leading to pain amplification. This process which take place in the dorsal horn neurons of the spinal cord, results in temporal summation of the second pain. Whilst the first pain, which is described as sharp or lancinating in character, is conducted by the myelinated A-δ pain fibers, the second pain is most frequently reported as dull, aching, or burning in character, and is linked to chronic pain states; is transmitted by unmyelinated C-fibers. When painful stimuli are applied more often than once every 3 s, this increases the intensity of the second pain. This progressive increase, which results from central rather than a peripheral nervous system mechanism, represents the temporal summation or windup (Fig. 11.4).

Similar windup of C afferent-mediated responses of dorsal horn nociceptive neurons was reported in animal studies. This summation has been found to involve *N*-methyl D-aspartate (NMDA) receptor mechanisms. Interestingly, the second pain (windup) was reported to be inhibited by NMDA receptor antagonists, including dextromethorphan and ketamine [51–53].

The windup abnormality in fibromyalgia patients The prominent secondary hyperalgesia and allodynia in fibromyalgia patients attracted the attention to the central sensitization and windup process [54]. Several studies depicted psychophysical evidence suggestive of abnormal input to central nociceptive pathways in fibromyalgia patients [55–59]. In contrast to normal controls, when windup pain is evoked in fibromyalgia patients, the perceived pain increase by experimental stimuli (mechanical, heat, cold, or electricity) is greater for fibromyalgia patients. These results provide convincing evidence for a role for central sensitization in the patho-

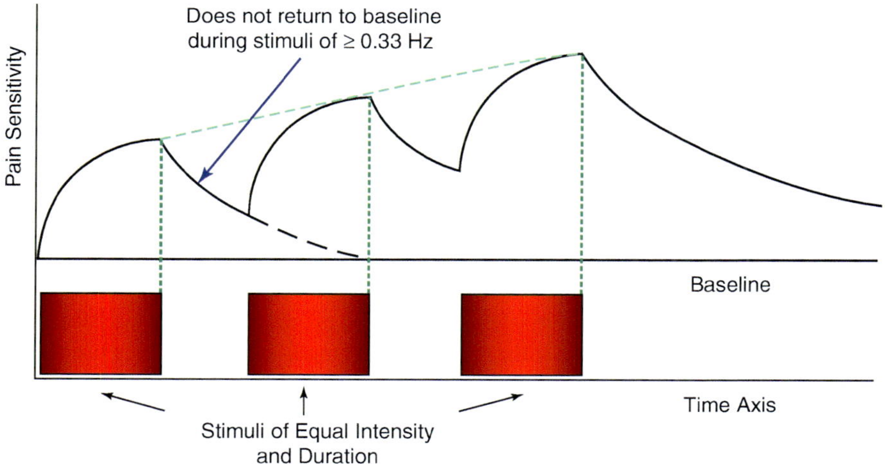

Fig. 11.4 Temporal summation of second pain (windup). When identical stimuli are applied to normal subjects at frequencies of ≥0.33 Hz, pain sensations will not return to baseline during the interstimulatory interval. Windup is strongly dependent on stimulus frequency and is inversely correlated with interstimulatory interval. In contrast to normal subjects, FM patients windup at frequencies of <0.33 Hz and require lower stimulus intensities. (Quoted from: Staud, R. Biology and therapy of fibromyalgia: pain in fibromyalgia syndrome. Arthritis Res Ther 8, 208 (2006); under open access scheme)

genesis of this syndrome. However, when central sensitization occurs in chronic pain patients, including FM patients, little additional nociceptive input is needed to maintain the sensitized state. Consequently, innocuous daily activities may contribute to the maintenance process of the chronic pain status. In addition, the prolonged decay of painful sensations in fibromyalgia patients explains why there are no significant changes reported in their pain levels during brief therapeutic interventions. This would clarify why the most commonly used analgesic medications do not improve central sensitization, and even some other potent medications, including opioids, have been shown to maintain or even worsen this CNS phenomenon. Sustained administration of opioids in rodents over one week can not only elicit hyperalgesia but also induce neurochemical CNS changes commonly seen with inflammatory pain [60]. Thus, long-term analgesic therapy may sometimes result in unintended worsening of the targeted pain processing abnormalities.

Fibromyalgia and Associated Comorbidities

Whether fibromyalgia is indeed a sole pain disorder remains contested. As early as 1989, Turk and Flor [61] stated that fibromyalgia is more than chronic widespread pain and tender points. Tender points can be regarded as the "sedimentation rate" of somatic and psychological distress [62, 63]. The new diagnostic criteria for fibromyalgia give unrefreshed sleep and fatigue a nearly equal weight for diagnosis and even include depression as a minor symptom [18, 63, 64].

The composite of symptoms that occur in patients with fibromyalgia raises the question of whether these various other symptoms are merely the consequence of chronic pain or whether they occur uniquely as a critical component of this disorder. Individual patients may also attribute variable weight to the comorbid symptoms of fibromyalgia, although chronic widespread pain remains the defining feature of fibromyalgia [19].

Generally, pain has two emotional components, including the unpleasantness of the sensation (primary pain affect) as well as negative feelings like depression, anger and fear (secondary pain affect). This relationship of emotions with pain is bidirectional because modulation of negative feelings can powerfully alter the pain experience [65]. Due to the fact that pain is a personal experience it can only be partially captured by definitions. The International Association for the Study of Pain has defined pain as an "unpleasant sensory and emotional experience associated with actual and potential tissue damage or described in terms of such damage" [66]. This definition of pain, however, has significant shortcomings because it does not encompass all aspects of pain.

The pain associated with fibromyalgia is typically described as radiating diffusely from the axial skeleton over large areas of the body, predominantly involving the muscles and joints. Patients also present with various additional complaints.

Fatigue and poor sleep are nearly universal, and most patients with fibromyalgia also meet the classification for chronic fatigue syndrome (CFS). Cognitive problems ("fibro fog") produce impairments in memory and thinking [67]. Other, less commonly reported symptoms of fibromyalgia have also been reported. There is a significant amount of overlap among chronic pain disorders (Fig. 11.5), central sensitivity syndromes (e.g. chronic fatigue syndrome, irritable bowel syndrome [IBS], and posttraumatic stress disorder [PTSD]), and anxiety disorders. Systemic inflammatory illnesses (e.g. rheumatoid arthritis, chronic hepatitis C, and systemic lupus erythematosus [SLE]) may be complicated by fibromyalgia. Patients with fibromyalgia typically suffer for many years before diagnosis and sometimes receive unnecessary, expensive, or needlessly invasive procedures or medication before fibromyalgia is recognized.

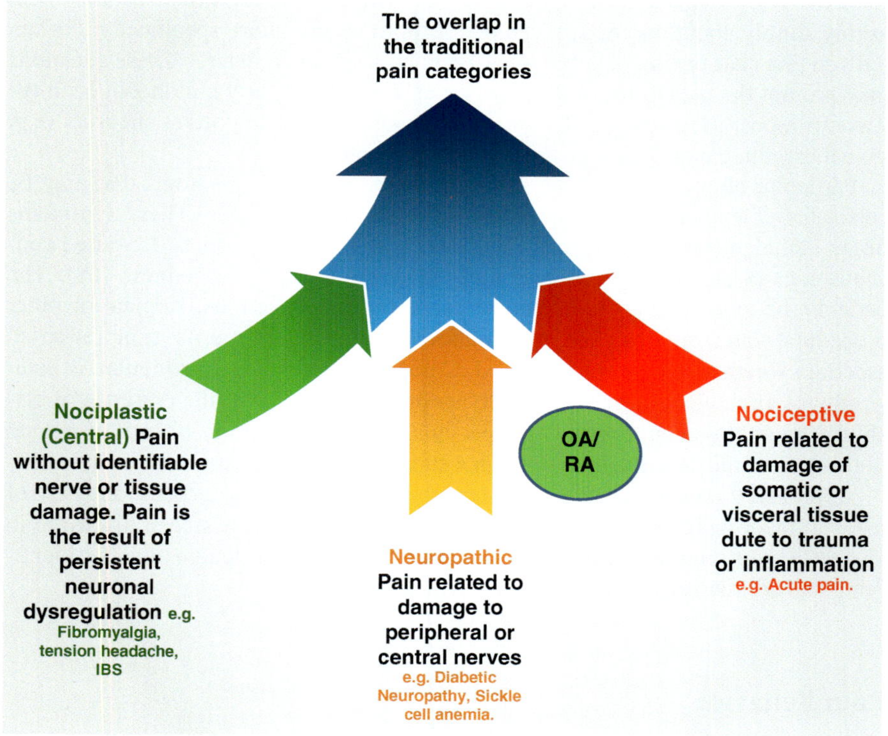

Fig. 11.5 The overlap in the traditional pain categories: some common or highly prevalent chronic pain conditions tend to coexist. This would have implications on the variable diseases' diagnosis and classification

Fibromyalgia Pain in the Clinical Setting

On several occasions, fibromyalgia patients have usually undergone multiple medical evaluations; consequently most if not all, have often developed a highly medicalized personal story, dominated by a reporting of procedures and test results. Some have even settled on a diagnosis and want the clinician to perform a desired test or treat it with a specific intervention. Traditional open-ended questions in this setting may be resisted as the patient prefers a shortcut to the test or treatment as opposed to further dialogue. Other patients may present equivalent challenges to the usual open-ended question technique by virtue of cultural differences, educational levels, maladaptive personality styles, or co-morbid illnesses. Given the usual time constraints, however, more directive interviewing must occur so as to determine quickly the most salient historical data.

In this regard, understanding the timing of symptom onset is crucial. Rather than asking simply about duration, it can be useful to inquire more specifically: "When did you first start having pain? Grade school, high school, or later?" These questions may prompt the patient to recall forgotten episodes from early childhood, or in the wake of a past illness (e.g. infectious mononucleosis), or important stressors (e.g. sexual assault, car accident, death of a family member).

Particular attention should be given to the reporting of symptoms that may be correlates of unpleasant and unacknowledged emotional states. These symptoms might include neuropsychiatric problems such as sleep disturbance, decreased concentration, poor memory, "mental fog," tremors, and lightheadedness [68]. The patient's history of drug trials, chronic narcotic use, injections, surgical or other procedural interventions, and non-traditional approaches merits exploration to ascertain whether benefit was achieved. Chronic narcotic use, in particular, is noteworthy as an inducer of unremitting hyperalgesia [17]. Lastly, the presence of disability, unemployment, drug or interpersonal abuse, or a family history of mental illness can usually be obtained through a standard patient questionnaire.

Approach to evaluate FM and related symptoms, including a focused review of medical records, interviewing techniques, and observations, has been discussed in an article published by Fleming and Volcheck [69], giving valuable tools for identifying and addressing the most relevant symptoms.

Pain Behavior

During the clinical consultation fibromyalgia patients may exhibit notable pain behaviors which have been described as communicative or protective (Fig. 11.6). Communicative pain behaviors include non-verbal facial expressions such as grimacing, wincing, or crying, as well as verbal or paraverbal pain expressions such as words, grunts, sighs, and moans. Protective pain behaviors include touch avoidance, anticipatory flinches, and movements such as guarding or holding the painful area.

"Protective" also entails therapeutic maneuvers, such as moving or rubbing the painful area of the body, rocking, weight shifting, or repeatedly standing up, arching the back, walking around, or even lying on the exam floor (Fig. 11.7) [70].

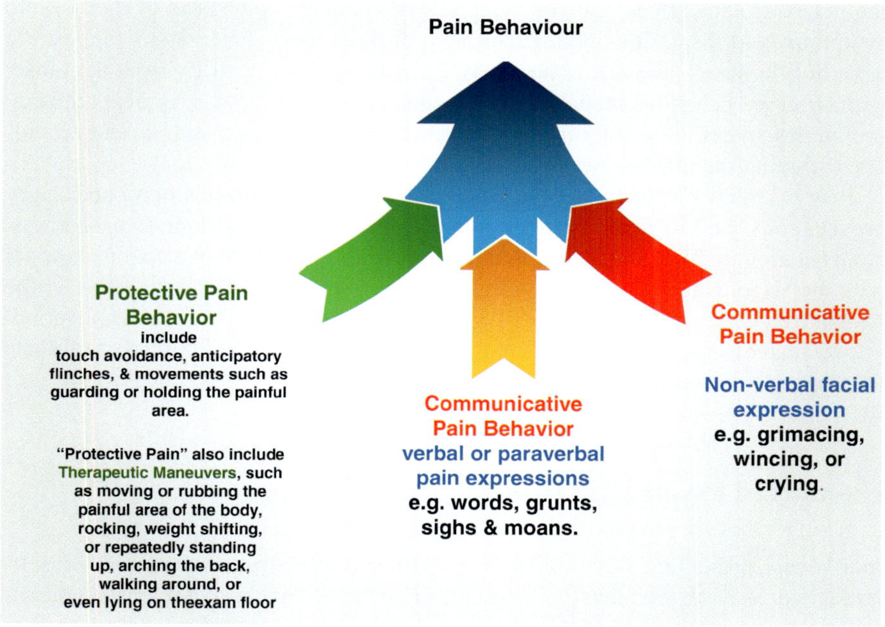

Fig. 11.6 Variable types of pain behaviour in fibromyalgia patients

Fig. 11.7 Verbal and non-verbal communication red flags

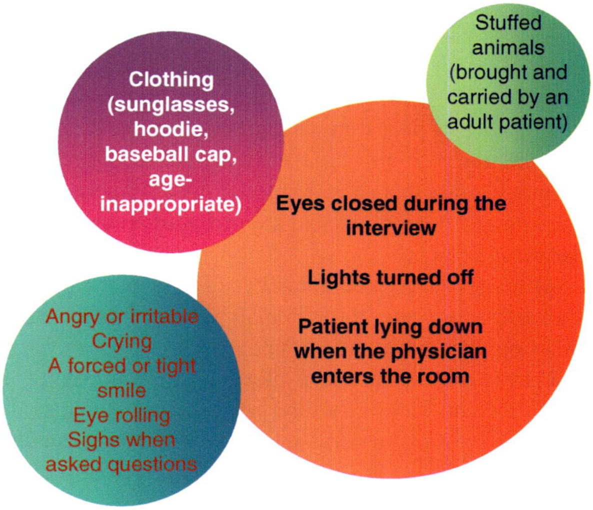

Emotional Behaviour

Fibromyalgia patients may exhibit also emotional behavior ranging from apathy to anger. Neutral, virtually expressionless postures may be maintained while discussing issues of pain, stress, loss, or trauma. Some patients may speak of their severe symptoms and disabilities with such inappropriate nonchalance as to suggest "la belle indifference" [71, 72]. Others may act with anger or hostility from the outset with observed behaviors including: curt responses, frowns, scowls, cynical remarks, profanities, eye rolling, and direct criticism of the skills of past and present providers, including the interviewer.

It is essential to maintain equanimity in the face of both apathetic and angry provocations, and to exhibit empathy and forbearance rather than defensiveness, confrontation, or rejection. Confronting the frustration of a patient's apathy or anger with the same usually exacts an enormous cost in time and emotional effort. If the patient cannot be effectively engaged or redirected, the clinician must avoid responding defensively, focus on completing the clinic consultation, and possibly terminate the session if behavior(s) prevent further dialogue [73].

Co-morbid Psychiatric Disorders and Trauma

Individuals presenting with fibromyalgia often demonstrate high levels of self-critical perfectionistic behavior. This chronic form of psychosocial stress includes an internalized sense of helplessness or hopelessness and ultimately increases fatigue, depression, and pain awareness while diminishing health and longevity [74–76]. Fibromyalgia patients frequently suffer anxiety disorders, sleep disorders, and personality disorders as well [77–80].

Additionally, there is a tendency for FM patients to share histories of early life physical or sexual abuse [81]; of assault, neglect, alcoholic parents, and physical trauma [82, 83]; and of various catastrophic events such as war, torture, floods, and other causes of post-traumatic stress disorder [84–86]. Indeed, several studies have reported that patients who have a history of adverse childhood experiences or post-traumatic stress disorder or are victims of intimate partner violence often have multiple somatic complaints and an increased prevalence of both functional and chronic illnesses [87–95].

Although the connection between trauma and fibromyalgia or somatic symptoms is an important one, the clinician must be judicious when approaching this topic. Many patients have already undergone considerable psychological work in efforts to address these issues and quite reasonably balk at the idea of resurrecting these memories and feelings with a newly encountered clinician. Even if no such treatment has yet been undertaken, an initial visit is usually not the time to search fully for this possibility. Instead, it is better to revisit this arena during a later appointment, or to defer it to other clinicians further on in the evaluation process when the patient will more likely feel safer and assured of the team's good intention. In the first visit, it is sufficient for a physician to be aware that the story behind any patient with fibromyalgia is almost always "fraught with background" [96].

Notably, fibromyalgia patients with multiple unexplained symptoms must be evaluated without an expectation of attributing their difficulties to mental illness. The recently updated Diagnostic and Statistical Manual of Mental Disorders (DSM-V) has replaced the previous edition's (DSM-IV) somatoform disorders grouping with the current somatic symptom and related disorders section [97]. The stated intent of this change was to avoid a mental disorder diagnosis only on the basis of undiagnosed somatic symptoms. Instead, an emphasis upon abnormal patient responses to positive symptoms and signs, whether explained or not, is their critical feature [97].

Brain/Mental Fog

Fibromyalgia patients often complain of cognitive difficulties. This may even be observed in the initial clinic consultation. These states are characterized as sensations of being in a daze or mental fog, sometimes referred to as "fibrofog". Patients may report forgetting conversations, phone numbers, plans, and activities. They may note feeling lost in familiar places, being unable to carry out simple tasks like grocery shopping; or finding complex tasks like driving almost impossible [98]. Formal cognitive testing in these patients is often within normal limits overall but also may reveal patchy attention deficits. It is a situation in which impaired mental function appears mostly to come from a compromised capacity for focusing attention, for processing and remembering new sensory data, and for then performing complex tasks. This patchy attention focus impairs memory formation since new data are not collected with clarity or stored reliably [99]. Clinician awareness and recognition of this phenomenon can further support consideration of central sensitization during initial contacts with FM patients.

Centralized Pain Processing and Neuroimaging

The presence of elevated sensitivity to other types of sensory input (e.g., everyday sounds, sights, and odors) in fibromyalgia patients supports the recently proposed theory of generalized or global state of sensory amplification as a result of "top-down" central mechanisms [100]. Although the regions commonly activated by painful stimuli have been historically referred to as the pain matrix, there is considerable evidence that these areas cannot be considered pain-specific [101–104].

In a functional MRI (fMRI) case-control study, a lower pressure stimulus was required to produce similar central somatosensory cortical activation in fibromyalgia patients than that was required for the same level of activation in the healthy control brains [105]. This was supported by subsequent studies [106] which provided objective evidence of an increased CNS set point for experimental pain in fibromyalgia. Co-morbid psychological factors, such as catastrophizing or depression, which are present in a subset of patients, can amplify these abnormalities, and this can be seen in neuroimaging studies with increases in activity in limbic regions in individuals with these co-morbidities [106].

MRI studies have used voxel-based morphometry to identify differences in regional brain volumes between fibromyalgia and healthy control groups [107–109]. Two meta-analyses of such studies reported similar areas of decreased volume in anterior and posterior cingulate cortices [110, 111]. Of these meta-analyses, one has also identified other areas of decreased (parahippocampal/fusiform cortex) and increased (cerebellum) volume in fibromyalgia [110]. Single studies have reported differences in multiple other regions (thalamus, pons, precuneus, and basal ganglia) [108–111]. A longitudinal study in fibromyalgia patients with insomnia assessed regional cortical thickness in areas previously identified as altered in either condition before as well as after treatment [112]. Finding support the potential reversibility of some of these differences.

Resting-state connectivity analysis is a more-recent advance that has been helpful in studying CNS activity in fibromyalgia. Increased connectivity between the default mode network and insula was related to spontaneous pain intensity [113, 114] as well as decreased connectivity between pain-inhibitory areas [115]. Thus, fibromyalgia is associated with objective signs of altered connectivity, which might serve as both a biomarker and a tool to direct rational treatment development.

Proton magnetic resonance spectroscopy has shown increased glutamate activity and decreased insular levels of γ-aminobutyric acid (GABA) [116]. The assumption that GABA plays a pathophysiological part has been supported by the finding that GABA agonists, for example, γ-hydroxybutyrate and even low amounts of alcohol [78], can lead to symptomatic improvements in some patients with fibromyalgia.

From the clinical perspective, the most intriguing may be the few longitudinal studies in fibromyalgia patients that incorporated both resting state fMRI functional connectivity metrics and clinical measures before and after treatment [117, 118]. Studies using a variety of interventions (medications, acupuncture, exercise therapy, transcranial direct current stimulation, and cognitive-behavioral therapy) have demonstrated treatment-related changes in functional connectivity, most of which correlated with improvement in clinical metrics [119–124]. One group of investigators explored the potential of pre-treatment functional connectivity to predict treatment response [120, 122, 123]. Although these studies indicate potential for identifying resting state fMRI-based biomarkers for tracking treatment-induced normalization of function and for treatment selection, a great deal more will be required for clinical validation [125, 126].

Diagnosis and Screening

The diagnosis of fibromyalgia is currently made based on the history of fibromyalgia-like symptoms and the exclusion of another somatic condition that sufficiently explains the symptoms [127]. However, the criteria for fibromyalgia have undergone numerous revisions since first reported.

No confirmatory blood tests (biomarkers), imaging or histological analysis have been identified for fibromyalgia. However, for the initial assessment of a patient with chronic widespread pain, guidelines have proposed diagnostic workups, including obtaining a history of pharmacological drug use, complete medical assessment and some laboratory tests (including complete blood count, C-reactive protein levels, serum calcium levels, creatine phosphokinase levels, serum vitamin D and thyroid-stimulating hormone levels [9, 87]) to screen for medical conditions that can mimic fibromyalgia symptoms. Particular concerns are widespread metastatic cancer and statin-induced muscle pain [127, 128]. In addition, the diagnosis of other medical conditions that contribute to widespread pain is important for the management of the patient, as, for example, osteoarthritis of the knee as a cause of knee pain would require treatment strategies other than those for fibromyalgia.

2010 ACR Preliminary Diagnostic Criteria

The ACR preliminary diagnostic criteria [129] addressed several challenges with the 1990 ACR criteria. First, the 2010 ACR preliminary criteria excluded the tender point examination, which was replaced by the Widespread Pain Index (WPI). The WPI is a 0–19 count of the number of body regions that are reported as painful or sensitive to pressure ('tender') by the patient. Second, the criteria assessed on a 0–3 severity scale a series of symptoms that were defined as additional key symptoms of fibromyalgia: fatigue, unrefreshing sleep, cognitive problems and the extent of somatic symptom reporting. The items were combined into a 0–12-point Symptom Severity (SS) Scale. Lastly, the WPI and SS Scale could be combined. In addition, the diagnostic criteria require that the patient has had symptoms present at a similar level for ≥3 months and the patient does not have another disorder that would otherwise sufficiently explain the pain.

Modified 2010 ACR diagnostic criteria In concordance with the 1990 ACR classification criteria, the modified 2010 ACR diagnostic criteria assessment in the clinical setting was reported to be at least as time consuming. Some challenges have been reported [129] including, (1) the WPI and SS Scale items require a thorough and meticulous interview of the patient; (2) Symptom assessment carried out by the treating physician is fundamentally subjective. A self-reported questionnaire, the Fibromyalgia Survey Questionnaire (FSQ; also known as the Fibromyalgia Symptom Scale and the Polysymptomatic Distress Scale) was developed to be completed by the patient. The questionnaire involves evaluation of the key fibromyalgia symptoms. The questionnaire would assess the number of pain sites and extent of somatic symptom intensity and replace the step of the FSQ completed by the treating physician. Patients who meet the research criteria (consequently the diagnosis of fibromyalgia can be made) meet the following criteria: the patient has a WPI of ≥7 out of 19 pain sites and an SS score of ≥5 out of 12, or a WPI of between 3 and 6 pain sites and an SS score of ≥9. The symptoms should be present for at least 3 months [129–132].

Fibromyalgianess

The concept of fibromyalgianess or subsyndromal fibromyalgia has been first suggested by Wolfe in 2009 [133]. Fibromyalgianess appear to have high clinical relevance. In the studies by Brummett and colleagues, they noted that amongst the individuals who were scheduled for either lower extremity joint replacement or hysterectomy, those who achieved relatively higher FM scores on the 2011 FM survey criteria [134] would predict increased opioid requirements in the inpatient admission following surgery, as well as long-term postsurgical pain outcomes. Whilst the fibromyalgia measure is scored from 0 to 31, with a score of 13 typically used as the diagnostic cut-off point for fibromyalgia, the authors noted that for each 1-point increase in this measure from 0 to 31, individuals needed an adjusted 7–9 mg more oral morphine equivalents to control their pain in the first 24–48 h following surgery, and were 15–20% less likely to show pain improvement following surgery [135–138].

These findings were independent of a number of preoperative characteristics, including age, sex, anxiety, depression, catastrophizing, and opioid use. More importantly, these findings were linear, and the same incremental increase in opioid requirements and surgery non-responsiveness was observed both in individuals well below the threshold to diagnose fibromyalgia, and in individuals exceeding this threshold. The findings of suggest that a degree of central sensitization is reflected in this fibromyalgia measure, which would help to identify those patients who did not meet the fibromyalgia criteria but do present different points along the fibromyalgianess continuum. This was supported by the significant difference in opioid responsiveness and improvement in pain following arthroplasty that these two individuals would experience. These data suggest also that the degree of central sensitization reflected in this measure may help identify individuals in perioperative or other settings who are less likely to respond to peripherally directed treatments such as surgery [133].

Management of Pain in the Fibromyalgia Syndrome

Understanding the fibromyalgia syndrome and how to manage the pain experienced by FM patients remains a challenge. This could be attributed to the multifaceted psychosomatic nature of the FM pains and its significant negative impact on the patients and their lives. Another challenge is that FM patients typically present with several key clinical manifestations (also called comorbidities or domains). Pain is one of them, but treatments which focus on the pain alone will likely fail [139]. It is currently believed that optimal treatment of FM will involve a combination of a one or more pharmacologic (Fig. 11.8) and a one or more complementary interventions. Whilst several medications which offer benefits of relatively small effect sizes have been extensively studied by the pharmaceutical industry, studies of complementary

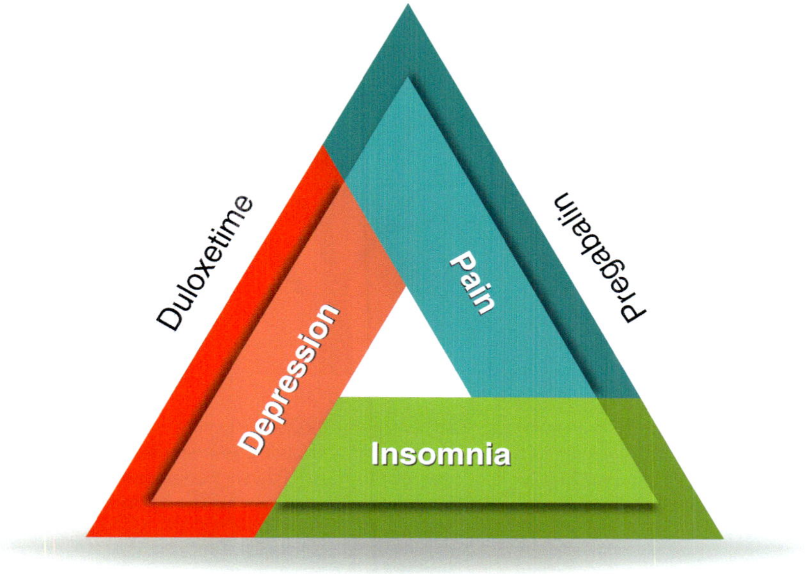

Fig. 11.8 Triangle method for conceiving strategic polypharmacy for the management of fibromyalgia syndrome

therapies have disclosed larger effect sizes, generally but based upon with lower quality data. A better approach to FM management will likely be based on the disordered biology of FM. This will be discussed in this section.

Pharmacologic vs. Complementary Interventions

Whilst pharmacologic therapy refers to the use of one or more medications to manage a medical problem, the term "complementary" or "alternative" therapy refers to the use of one or more nonpharmaceutical interventions [140]. Examples of complementary interventions that have been studied in FM include education, peer group support, aerobic exercises, hydrotherapy, electrical stimulation, and cognitive behavioral therapy. It should be recognized that intentionally-prescribed therapy of any kind is probably not pure in the "real world". Prescribed complementary therapy may be accompanied by over-the-counter medications, that are taken by the patient without informing the treating clinician. In concordance, patients taking a prescribed pharmacotherapy may be simultaneously trying a variety of complementary interventions on the advice of family, acquaintances, media advertisements, or internet sources. Therefore, a frank and completely open relationship between the patient and the treating health care professional is expected to help to ensure that therapies actually being used by the patient are accurately documented in the medical record, so they can have been professionally cross-examined to ensure safety and efficacy, while the assumed goal is efficacy.

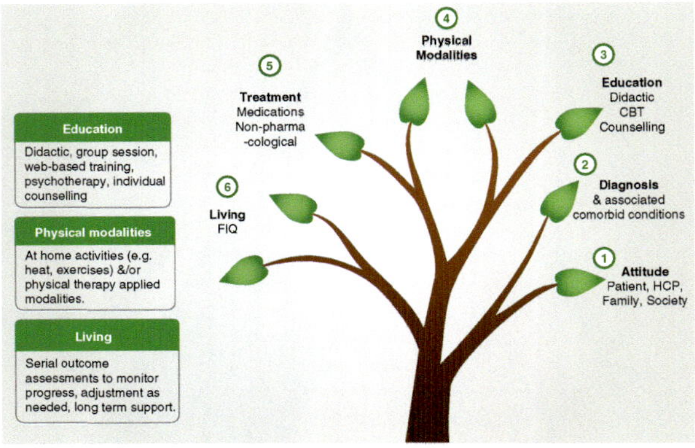

Fig. 11.9 Fibromyalgia management: The acronym "ADEPT Living" stands for Attitude, Diagnosis, Education, Physical modalities, Treatments, and Living assessments to document clinical improvement. It is recommended that each of the ADEPT Living components be considered and initiated soon after the diagnosis of FM is made and contemporaneously with prescription of medications

An earlier attempt to organize the management of FM for easy clinician memory resulted in the development of a six-step approach (Fig. 11.9), symbolized by the acronym "ADEPT Living" [141]. The acronym "ADEPT Living" stands for Attitude, Diagnosis, Education, Physical modalities, Treatments, and Living assessments to document clinical improvement. It is recommended that each of the ADEPT Living components be considered and initiated soon after the diagnosis of FM is made and contemporaneously with prescription of medications. The critical principle of this concept is that complementary medications would address the same symptomatic domain (e.g. pain, insomnia, or depression) with different mechanisms of action or address different domains in the same affected individual.

Biology and Therapy of Fibromyalgia

Based on the suggestion that neural over-sensitization, or "central sensitization", (meaning that the CNS interprets benign stimulations as unpleasant), has been identified as the main pathophysiological change in FM [142–144], CNS involvement has been considered to be a key element in FM management. This principal was demonstrated by an increased CNS response to stimulation and decreased conditioned pain modulation (CPM). Conditioned pain modulation is a neural process of sensitization modulation, which involves activation of specific neurotransmitters including serotonin and noradrenaline. Thus, it has been suggested that medications that modulate levels of these neurotransmitters in the CNS, can have the potential to improve the conditioned pain modulation (CPM) and reduce central sensitization [145, 146].

Other neurotransmitters, including GABA, cannabinoid receptors, substance P, nerve growth factor (NGF), and opioid receptors participate in this complex modulation of pain transmission [147], therefore functioning as optional therapeutic targets. There is also evidence that glial cells may play a role in maintaining central sensitization and contribute to chronic pain production by producing IL-6, IL-8, and other cytokines, which are found to be at high levels in FM patients' sera [148].

Comorbid conditions, including mood disorders, anxiety, headaches, irritable bowel syndrome, sleep disturbances, and chronic fatigue syndrome, are found in a large percentage of FM patients [149, 150]. Accordingly, medications which improve sleep disorders, as well as those that improve daytime alertness, could be useful for FM management. From a neurobiological perspective, sensory, affective, and cognitive centers within the brain interact in producing the final pain experience. Indeed, increased connectivity between different brain areas is a known phenomenon in FM [43]. Increased connectivity has also been demonstrated between various other areas participating in pain processing, alertness, and cognition [151]. By perceiving brain function in general, and specifically the pathophysiology of FM, new targets for medication development for the syndrome can be found [152], which was reviewed in a recent article on current and emerging pharmacotherapy for fibromyalgia [153].

Pain Pathways and the Pharmacotherapy of Fibromyalgia

Over the past years, FM pharmacotherapy has seen significant developments. Inspite of the fact that a discrete cause for FM has yet to be identified [154], a leap has been reported in the understanding of the underlying cellular, molecular and pathophysiologic mechanisms which contribute to its neuropathic pain component. These include dopaminergic, opioidergic, and serotoninergic abnormalities [155], hypothalamic-pituitary-adrenal (HPA) axis dysfunction [156–159] as well as defective nocioceptive input [160, 161]. Linking pharmacotherapy to the FM pain mechanism pathways, appear to be a reasonable approach to the management of these patients [162].

Activated Ca^{2+} Channels

High-voltage-activated (HVA) Ca^{2+} channels are widely expressed in the nervous system. They play an important role in pain conduction by participating in various physiological processes such as synaptic transmission, changes in synaptic plasticity, and neuronal excitability. Available evidence suggests that the HVA channel is an important therapeutic target for pain management [153]. Gabapentinoids are synthetic molecules that are structurally related to γ-aminobutyric acid (GABA) The two main members of this family of medications, pregabalin and gabapentin, act by binding to the alpha2-delta subunit of voltage-gated calcium channels in the CNS. Originally used as anticonvulsants, they are currently used for the treatment of chronic pain [163]. Pregabalin has FDA approval for the treatment of FM, and its use is recommended in the American guidelines [164–167].

A series of placebo-controlled clinical trials showed pregabalin to improve pain and sleep disturbances. However, compared to placebo, it was not found to significantly improve complaints of fatigue in some trials, and none of the trials indicated any improvement in depressive symptoms [168, 169]. A meta-analysis of randomized controlled trials regarding both pregabalin and gabapentin further emphasized their effect in improving pain, fatigue, sleep, and overall quality of life, in addition to their lack of effect on depressive symptoms and relatively non-substantial effect on anxiety [170]. A series of placebo-controlled clinical trials showed pregabalin to improve pain and sleep disturbances. However, compared to placebo, it was not found to significantly improve complaints of fatigue in some trials, and none of the trials indicated any improvement in depressive symptoms [168, 169]. A meta-analysis of randomized controlled trials regarding both pregabalin and gabapentin further emphasized their effect in improving pain, fatigue, sleep, and overall quality of life, in addition to their lack of effect on depressive symptoms and relatively non-substantial effect on anxiety [170].

Kim et al. demonstrated that low-to-moderate alcohol consumption was associated with an improvement in FM symptoms, namely, pain level, physical and social function, general health perception, and general quality of life. However, this association was not observed in heavy drinkers [56]. It was assumed that the effect might be centrally mediated through ethanol enhancement of GABA release in the CNS [171, 172].

K^+ Channel Modulation

Voltage-gated sodium (Na_V) and potassium (K_V) channels are critical components of neuronal action potential generation and propagation. The delayed rectifier K^+ channels belonging to the K_v1 family, and in particular, $K_v1.1$ and Kv7.2/$K_v7.3$, have been implicated in neuronal excitability [173]. In vitro studies revealed that $K_v1.1$ and $K_v7.2$/$K_v7.3$ channels play a significant role in regulating the excitatory nocioceptive pathway common to pain-sensing neurons. Furthermore, these K^+ channels appear to be the likely molecular mechanism that is affected in vivo by amitriptyline. In a recent study [174], amitriptyline was shown to inhibit $K_v.1.1$ and $K_v7.2$/$K_v7.3$ channels in a dose-dependent and toxicologically relevant manner in human embryonic kidney 293 cells and in Chinese hamster ovary cells [174, 175].

Although different Tricyclic Antidepressants have been used in the treatment of chronic pain, the largest body of evidence on therapeutic utility in FM exists regarding amitriptyline. It is recommended by all various clinical practice guidelines [176–178]. Amitriptyline was found to reduce the Fibromyalgia Impact Questionnaire (FIQ) results from baseline to endpoint by over 30% [45–47]. It was found to improve pain, fatigue, sleep, and quality of life [179].

Voltage-Gated Sodium (Na_V) Channels Modulation

Voltage-gated sodium (Na_V) channels are a family of transmembrane ion channel proteins. They function by forming a gated, water-filled pore to help establish and control cell membrane potential via control of the flow of ions between the intracellular and the extracellular environments. Blockade of Na_Vs has been successfully accomplished in the clinic to enable control of pathological firing patterns that occur in a diverse range of conditions such as chronic pain, epilepsy, and cardiac arrhythmias [180].

Lidocaine, a drug that exerts analgesic and anti-inflammatory effects by blocking sodium channels in the neuronal cell membrane, was used for refractory FM symptoms. Also, intravenous magnesium has shown a beneficial impact on neuropathic back pain and post-herpetic neuralgia. On these premises, a study aimed to establish an effective dose of intravenous (IV) lidocaine in FM treatment, with magnesium added to the highest dose of lidocaine [181]. A total of 74 FM patients received a lidocaine infusion once every 2 months. During the first infusion, every patient received 5 mg/kg of lidocaine. After that, if the patient had >25% pain relief for less than 2 weeks, the dose was escalated, reaching 7.5 mg/kg, or magnesium (2.5 mg magnesium sulfate) added up to 7.5 mg/kg of lidocaine. This study showed that lidocaine infusions were able to reduce safely and effectively the pain in a significant number of FM patients who were refractory to other conventional therapies, with higher dosage producing a greater analgesic response. The adjunct of magnesium sulfate did not seem to have a clear statistically significant benefit [182].

N-Methyl-D-Aspartate (NMDA) Antagonists

Glutamate is the most abundant excitatory neurotransmitter in the nervous system. Central sensitization of pain transmission pathways is associated with hyperexcitability of the glutamatergic system, which leads symptoms observed in persons suffering from chronic pain [183].

The *N*-methyl-D-aspartate (NMDA) receptors are one of three subgroups of glutamate receptors. *N*-methyl D-aspartate (NMDA) receptors are ligand-gated cation channels activated by an excitatory neurotransmitter, glutamate. These receptors are located mostly at excitatory synapses, and thereby, participate in excitatory neurotransmission in the central nervous system. Activated by a variety of agonists, including substance P and neurokinin, it is known to be involved in the pathogenesis of central sensitization [184], a trait for which efforts were made to develop NMDA antagonists as therapeutic options for FM, as well as other disorders resulting from central sensitization.

In their study, Palucha et al. [185] presented evidence that blockade of the NMDA subtype of ionotropic glutamate receptors with 3-(2-methyl-1,3 thiazol-4-yl) ethynylpyridine (MTEP) reduced glutamatergic activity and produced anti-depressant effects in Wistar rats. These results suggested that NMDA antagonists might be useful for suppressing nocioceptive input as well as being considered efficacious for reducing the clinical signs of depressive illness that is often a co-morbid condition in FM [166].

Ketamine, an NMDA antagonist, was found to reduce muscular and referred pain in FM patients [186]. Memantine, another receptor antagonist, was suggested to be useful because of its ability to reduce neurotoxicity caused by high levels of glutamate found in different brain areas of FM patients [187, 188]. These high glutamate levels were found to be related to the severity of FM symptoms [189]. A double-blind, randomized-controlled trial published in 2014 found memantine to achieve a significant reduction in pain [190], with another hypothesis suggesting the combined use of pregabalin and memantine to concomitantly affect voltage-gated calcium channels and NMDA receptors, as a possible therapeutic approach [184]. A recent meta-analysis of 15 studies regarding the benefit of memantine in treating chronic pain (either neuropathic or FM) concluded that the current evidence regarding memantine for chronic pain is limited and reported an increase in dizziness as a side effect of the medication [191].

Serotonergic Circuitry

In the brain, serotonin (5-hydroxytryptamine, 5-HT) controls a multitude of physiological and behavioral functions. Serotonergic neurons in the raphe nuclei give rise to a complex and extensive network of axonal projections throughout the whole brain. Brain serotonergic circuitries interact with other neurotransmitter systems on a multitude of different molecular levels [192]. A major challenge in the analysis of these circuits is to understand how the serotonergic networks are linked to the numerous functions of this neurotransmitter. Among the large variety of chemical messengers acting in nerve cell signaling, 5-HT is the focus of much interest due to its implication in almost every physiological function (eating, reward, thermoregulation, cardiovascular regulation, locomotion, pain, reproduction, sleep-wake cycle, memory, cognition, aggressiveness, responses to stressors, emotion, and mood) and in several human pathologies.

Agomelatine is a melatonin and serotonin 5-HT_{2c} receptor antagonist which was shown to improve sleep quality by shortening the sleep latency period [193]. These findings suggested that a 5-HT_{2c} antagonist might have some efficacy in treating the sleep quality disturbances common to many FM patients.

Cyclobenzaprine is a 5-HT_2 receptor blocker, which acts on a subfamily of serotonin receptors, and causes muscle relaxation. It resembles amitriptyline in structure and is commonly used in FM patients. A systematic review of the literature reported that it has a moderate benefit in improving sleep disturbances and only a mild improvement in pain [194]. Moldofsky et al. have previously shown that bedtime very low doses of cyclobenzaprine were shown to significantly improve pain and sleep in patients with a specific sleep pattern (architecture) [195]. A sublingual formulation of low-dose cyclobenzaprine (TNX102SL, 2.8 mg) has been reported to improve nonrestorative sleep in FM patients [196]; however, this formulation has subsequently failed to reach primary pain-related endpoints, and its development has been stopped.

Mirtazapine is an atypical antidepressant with noradrenergic and specific serotonergic activity. It is not licensed for use in FM. A meta-analysis held by Welsch et al. did not find the drug effective for pain relief in FM nor for any other associated mental or functional symptoms related to it (depression, sleep problems, fatigue, etc.) [197].

The serotonin 5-HT_3 pathway was shown to be permissive for gabapentin in Sprague-Dawley rats treated by substance-P/saporin ablation [198]. The activity of gabapentin in these animals was found to be dependent on neurokinin-1 and the 5-HT_3 receptor. As was previously mentioned, gabapentin has shown efficacy in modulating the neuropathic pain of FM [168, 169].

Serotonin/Norepinephrine Reuptake Inhibition (SNRI)

The human serotonin transporter (SERT) and norepinephrine transporter (NET) are membrane transport proteins that are responsible for the reuptake of serotonin and norepinephrine from the synaptic cleft back into the presynaptic nerve terminal. Serotonin and norepinephrine have long been implicated in modulating the central nervous system descending inhibitory pain pathways [199]. Dual inhibition of serotonin and norepinephrine reuptake can offer advantages over other antidepressant drugs by treating a wider range of symptoms.[1] They can be especially useful in concomitant chronic or neuropathic pain.[200]

The SNRIs duloxetine and milnacipran have been approved by the US Food and Drug Administration (FDA). Various clinical trials published evaluating duloxetine showed a significant improvement in FM-associated pain. The effect of duloxetine, an SNRI, on FM pain was reviewed based on the results of two randomised, placebo-controlled double-blind parallel group clinical trials [201]. A critical assessment of both clinical trial studies indicated a palliative effect of duloxetine on FM persistent pain, especially in women.

Milnacipran, a non-tricyclic compound was studied in a double-blind placebo-controlled clinical trial involving 125 FM patients. In that study, Vitton et al. [202] showed that 75% of milnacipran-treated patients had an overall clinical improvement compared to 38% in the placebo-treated group ($p < 0.01$). Furthermore, 37% of the twice-daily milnacipran-treated group reported at least a 50% reduction in pain intensity compared to the placebo group ($p < 0.05$) and 84% of all milnacipran-treated subjects escalated to the highest dose (200 mg/day) with no tolerability issues or mild to moderate side-effects.

A meta-analysis reviewing five different studies regarding duloxetine and five different studies regarding and milnacipran showed that these drugs had positive effects on pain and patient-perceived clinical improvement [203].

Selective Serotonin Reuptake Inhibitors (SSRIs)

Among the SSRIs investigated for the treatment of FM were citalopram, escitalopram, fluoxetine, paroxetine, and sertraline. Despite the theoretical assumption, that the combined inhibition of serotonin and noradrenaline is more efficacious than selective serotonin augmentation vis-a-vis for the inhibition of pain [204], the use of this class of drugs is recommended in some practice guidelines [176, 178, 205, 206]. According to the results of a meta-analysis performed by Hauser et al., SSRIs improve pain, depression, and overall quality of life, but to a small extent. The effect size for improvement in sleep disorders was found to be non-substantial [207].

Dopamine Receptor Agonists

Earlier data indicated the involvement of dopaminergic pathways in FM pathophysiology [208]. This has led to attempts to develop medications intervening with dopaminergic metabolism. Bearing in mind the sporadic evidence about the benefit of dopaminergic agonists, it is worth mentioning, a randomized, double-blind placebo-controlled trial, which evaluated terguride (a serotonin receptor antagonist and dopamine receptor agonist) in FM patients. Results revealed improvement of the FM symptoms in a subgroup of patients with spinal stenosis (as opposed to all the other terguride-assigned patients as well as the placebo group, where no significant improvement was noted) [209]. Despite the EULAR recommendations for management of FM from 2008, recommending the consideration of dopamine agonists [176], a meta-analysis conducted by Sommer et al. did not find them of proven benefit [210], and hence, they have not been included in the revised 2016 EULAR recommendations [211].

Opioids

Endogenous descending antinociceptive activity has been suggested to be reduced in FM patients [59]. In humans, there are two descending pain inhibitory pathways: the noradrenaline/serotonin-mediated pathway and the opioid-mediated one [212]. Baraniuk et al. suggested an excess of endogenous opioids in FM [213]. Following these data, Harris et al. used positron emission tomography (PET) technology to show that the availability of μ-opioid receptors in FM patients is reduced in certain areas of the brain, possibly as a result of receptor downregulation secondary to their increased levels. Reduced availability was inversely correlated with clinical pain ratings [214].

Following these findings, naltrexone, a competitive opioid receptor antagonist, was suggested as potential new means of treating chronic pain. The beneficial effect of naltrexone on fibromyalgia symptoms was reported, in a pilot study, by Youner and Mackey [215]. This was a randomized controlled trial published in 2013, finding it to be superior to placebo in reducing pain and associated depressive symptoms [216].

Apart from its opioid receptor antagonist activities, naltrexone also has antagonist activity to other nonopioid receptors (toll-like receptor 4) expressed on activated microglia cells, which are specialized macrophages involved in neuroinflammatory processes. Overactivation of microglia cells in the cerebral cortex of FM patients was demonstrated by Albrecht et al. using PET [217]. Inhibition of microglial activation by naltrexone or naloxone therefore has an anti-inflammatory effect through the decrease in production of neurotoxic chemicals [218, 219], which is suggested to contribute to its analgesic effect [216].

There is no evidence from clinical trials that opioids are effective in treating FM, and the EULAR guidelines discourage the use of opioid analgesics. Only tramadol (a relatively weak opioid with mild SNRI activity), administered alone, or together with paracetamol, is currently supported by the EULAR recommendations and was found to reduce pain by 30%. Generally, it is believed that only short-term use of opioids may be appropriate in carefully selected patients, particularly those with severe FM [211].

Cannabinoids

There are two major active components in cannabinoids: tetrahydrocannabinol (THC) and cannabidiol (CBD). The former is the psychoactive component, which affects pain (as well as emotions) and works through CB1 and CB2 receptors. The latter has anti-inflammatory and analgesic traits. The THC:CBD therefore determines the product's overall effect [220]. CB1 cannabinoid receptors are found predominantly in the CNS and peripheral nervous system. Their agonists act along sensory pathways as modulators of pain [221]. With regard to the complex function of the endocannabinoid system in pain modulation, FM is hypothesized to be induced, among other factors, by a lack of endocannabinoid activity [222].

The main cannabinoids studied were nabilone and dronabinol, with conflicting results. Three randomized controlled studies have been published regarding cannabinoid treatment for FM: Fiz et al. reported a significant relief in pain 2 h after consumption [223]. Skrabek et al. reported a reduction in pain, as well as level of anxiety, and an improved quality of life when using nabilone in comparison with placebo [224]. Ware et al. found a moderate effect on insomnia when using nabilone versus amitriptyline but no proven effect on pain or general quality of life [225]. However, a systematic review by Walitt et al. concluded that no convincing evidence suggests that nabilone is useful in treating people with FM [226].

Cannabinoids have been offered by the Canadian guidelines for the management of FM as a therapeutic option for FM patients with prominent sleep abnormalities [178]. However, more controlled studies are needed to clarify the role of cannabinoids in this syndrome. Furthermore, research is called for focusing on the effects of various cannabinoids (as well as their combinations) on the basic neurophysiological aspects of FM such as altered CNS connectivity patterns.

Manipulating the endocannabinoid system is gradually emerging as another fascinating strategy for treating pain [227]. Endocannabinoids such as anandamide are metabolized by specific enzymes including fatty acid amide hydrolase (FAAH) and monoacylglycerol lipase (MAGL), and agents capable of inhibiting these enzymes are being tested as novel analgesic targets [228]. Future research into the clinical utility of endocannabinoid metabolism manipulation in FM is expected [153].

Tables 11.1 and 11.2 show a summary of the significant effect sizes from meta-analyses on fibromyalgia core domain variables resulting from both pharmaco- as well as complementary therapies for fibromyalgia syndrome patients.

Table 11.1 Pharmacotherapy for fibromyalgia: significant effect sizes from meta-analysis on fibromyalgia core domain variables [Quoted from Russell [139] under open access scheme under the terms of the Creative Commons Attribution License]

Treatment	Pain	Sleep disturbance	Fatigue	Depression and/or anxiety	Physical dysfunction	Cognitive dysfunction
Amitriptyline	+	+	+	–	–	*
Citalopram	–	–	–	–	*	*
Duloxetine	+	+	+	+	+	+
Fluoxetine	+	–	–	+	–	*
Growth hormone	+	*	*	*	–	*
Milnacipran	+	–	+	+	+	+
Pregabalin	–	+	*	*	–	*
Oxybate	+	+	+	*	*	*

[+] available data met significance criteria
[–] failure to meet significance criteria
[*] inadequate data for analysis

Table 11.2 Complementary therapy for fibromyalgia: significant effect sizes from meta-analyses on core domain variables [Quoted from Russell [139] under open access scheme under the terms of the Creative Commons Attribution License]

Treatment	Pain	Sleep disturbance	Fatigue	Depression and/or anxiety	Physical dysfunction	Cognitive dysfunction
Acupuncture	–	–	–	*	–	*
Balneotherapy	+	*	*	+	+	*
Cognitive behavioural therapy	+	+	+	–	+	+
Exercise	+	+	+	+	+	+
Education	+	–	+	+	–	*
Exercise/education	–	–	+	–	–	*
Homeopathy	+	*	–	–	+	*
Magnetic cerebral stimulation	+	–	+	–	+	*
Massage	+	–	*	*	–	*
Neurotherapy	+	–	–	–	–	–
Pool/water	+	+	+	+	+	–
UV/bright light	–	–	–	–	–	*

[+] available data met significance criteria
[–] failure to meet significance criteria
[*] inadequate data for analysis

Conclusion

In conclusion, Fibromyalgia (FM) is a chronic pain syndrome characterised by widespread musculoskeletal pain, extreme fatigue and sleep disturbances. It affects at least 1 in 40 people worldwide, although some estimates suggest nearly 1 in 20 people may be affected to some degree. The associated crippling fatigue—paved the way for its nick name "fibro fog". Over the past few years, the attention towards FM has focused on the diagnostic, pathogenetic and therapeutic aspects of this syndrome. Current treatment tends to focus on gentle aerobic exercise, as well as medication(s) and psychological therapies designed to manage pain. However, in many patients, these have proven ineffective and have left behind an enormous unmet clinical need.

References

1. Arnold LM, Choy E, Clauw DJ, Goldenberg DL, Harris RE, Helfenstein M Jr, Jensen TS, Noguchi K, Silverman SL, Ushida T, Wang G. Fibromyalgia and chronic pain syndromes: a white paper detailing current challenges in the field. Clin J Pain. 2016;32(9):737–46.
2. Phillips K, Clauw DJ. Central pain mechanisms in the rheumatic diseases: future directions. Arthritis Rheum. 2013;65:291–302.
3. Hulens M, Dankaerts W, Stalmans I, Somers A, Vansant G, Rasschaert R, Bruyninckx F. Fibromyalgia and unexplained widespread pain: the idiopathic cerebrospinal pressure dysregulation hypothesis. Med Hypotheses. 2018;110:150–4.
4. Talotta R, Bassichi L, Di Franco M, et al. One year in review 2017: fibromyalgia. Clin Exp Rheumatol. 2017;35(Suppl 105):S6–12.
5. Wolfe F. Fibromyalgia wars. J Rheumatol. 2009;36(4):671–8.
6. Häuser W, Fitzcharles MA. Facts and myths pertaining to fibromyalgia. Dialogues Clin Neurosci. 2018;20:53–62.
7. Talotta R, Bazzichi L, Di Franco M, et al. One year in review 2017: fibromyalgia. Clin Exp Rheumatol. 2017;35(Suppl 105):S6–12.
8. Wolfe F. Criteria for fibromyalgia? What is fibromyalgia? Limitations to current concepts of fibromyalgia and fibromyalgia criteria. Clin Exp Rheumatol. 2017;35(Suppl 105):S3–5.
9. Agarwal A, Oparin Y, Glick L, et al. Attitudes toward and management of fibromyalgia: a national survey of Canadian rheumatologists and critical appraisal of guidelines. J Clin Rheumatol. 2018;24:243–9.
10. Häuser W, Ablin J, Fitzcharles MA, et al. Fibromyalgia. Nat Rev Dis Primers. 2015;1:15022.
11. Shir Y, Fitzcharles MA. Should rheumatologists retain ownership of fibromyalgia? J Rheumatol. 2009;36:667–70.
12. Wolfe F. www.fmperplex.com [Internet]. 75% of persons in the general population diagnosed with fibromyalgia don't have it, but it is worse than that ... – the fibromyalgia perplex; 2017 January 11 [cited 11 April 2021].
13. Bass C, Henderson M. Fibromyalgia: an unhelpful diagnosis for patients and doctors. BMJ. 2014;348:2168.
14. Kroenke K. A practical and evidence-based approach to common symptoms: a narrative review. Ann Intern Med. 2014;161:579–86.
15. Wolfe F, Smythe HA, Yunus MB, et al. The American College of Rheumatology 1990 criteria for the classification of fibromyalgia. Report of the Multicenter Criteria Committee. Arthritis Rheum. 1990;33(2):160–72.

16. World Health Organization. International Classification of Diseases (ICD). WHO [online]. 2015. http://www.who.int/classifications/icd/en/.
17. Wolfe F, Clauw DJ, Fitzcharles MA, et al. The American College of Rheumatology preliminary diagnostic criteria for fibromyalgia and measurement of symptom severity. Arthritis Care Res (Hoboken). 2010;62(5):600–10.
18. Wolfe F, Clauw DJ, Fitzcharles MA, et al. Fibromyalgia criteria and severity scales for clinical and epidemiological studies: a modification of the ACR Preliminary Diagnostic Criteria for Fibromyalgia. J Rheumatol. 2011;38(6):1113–22.
19. Wolfe F, Clauw DJ, Fitzcharles MA, et al. 2016 revisions to the 2010/2011 fibromyalgia diagnostic criteria. Semin Arthritis Rheum. 2016;46(3):319–29.
20. Perrot S, Choy E, Petersel D, Ginovker A, Kramer E. Survey of physician experiences and perceptions about the diagnosis and treatment of fibromyalgia. BMC Health Serv Res. 2012;12:356.
21. Briones-Vozmediano E, Vives-Cases C, Ronda-Pérez E, Gil-González D. Patients' and professionals' views on managing fibromyalgia. Pain Res Manag. 2013;18:19–24.
22. Choy E, Perrot S, Leon T, et al. A patient survey of the impact of fibromyalgia and the journey to diagnosis. BMC Health Serv Res. 2010;10:102.
23. Häuser W, Zimmer C, Felde E, Köllner V. [What are the key symptoms of fibromyalgia? Results of a survey of the German Fibromyalgia Association]. Schmerz. 2008;22:176–83.
24. Russell IJ, Larson AA. Neurophysiopathogenesis of fibromyalgia syndrome: a unified hypothesis. Rheum Dis Clin North Am. 2009;35(2):421–35.
25. Williams DA, Clauw DJ. Understanding fibromyalgia: lessons from the broader pain research community. J Pain. 2009;10(8):777–91.
26. Clauw DJ, Arnold LM, McCarberg BH, FibroCollaborative. The science of fibromyalgia. Mayo Clin Proc. 2011;86(9):907–11.
27. Clauw DJ. Fibromyalgia: a clinical review. JAMA. 2014;311(15):1547–55.
28. Dworkin RH, Bruehl S, Fillingim RB, et al. Multidimensional diagnostic criteria for chronic pain: introduction to the ACTTION-American Pain Society Pain Taxonomy (AAPT). J Pain. 2016;17(Suppl):T1–9.
29. Treede RD, Rief W, Barke A, et al. Chronic pain as a symptom or a disease: the IASP Classification of Chronic Pain for the International Classification of Diseases (ICD-11). Pain. 2019;160:19–27.
30. Hâuser W, Ablin J, Fitzcharles MA, et al. Fibromyalgia. Nat Rev Dis Primers. 2015;1:15022.
31. Walitt B, Ceko M, Gracely JL, Gracely RH. Neuroimaging of central sensitivity syndromes: key insights from the scientific literature. Curr Rheumatol Rev. 2016;12(1):55–87.
32. Oaklander AL, Herzog ZD, Downs HM, Klein MM. Objective evidence that small-fiber polyneuropathy underlies some illnesses currently labeled as fibromyalgia. Pain. 2013;154(11):2310–236.
33. Üçeyler N, Burgmer M, Friedel E, et al. Etiology and pathophysiology of fibromyalgia syndrome: updated guidelines 2017, overview of systematic review articles and overview of studies on small fiber neuropathy in FMS subgroups. Schmerz. 2017;31(3):239–45.
34. Clauw DJ. What is the meaning of "small fiber neuropathy" in fibromyalgia? Pain. 2015;156(11):2115–6.
35. Staud R. Biology and therapy of fibromyalgia: pain in fibromyalgia syndrome. Arthritis Res Ther. 2006;8:208–15.
36. Henriksson KG. Is fibromyalgia a distinct clinical entity? Pain mechanisms in fibromyalgia syndrome. A myologist's view. Best Pract Res Clin Rheumatol. 1999;13:455–61.
37. Bengtsson A, Henriksson KG, Larsson J. Muscle biopsy in primary fibromyalgia. Light-microscopical and histochemical findings. Scand J Rheumatol. 1986;15:1–6.
38. Bengtsson A, Henriksson KG, Jorfeldt L, Kagedal B, Lennmarken C, Lindstrom F. Primary fibromyalgia. A clinical and laboratory study of 55 patients. Scand J Rheumatol. 1986;15:340–7.
39. Pongratz DE, Spath M. Morphologic aspects of fibromyalgia. Z Rheumatol. 1998;57:47–51.

40. Bennett RM, Clark SR, Goldberg L, Nelson D, Bonafede RP, Porter J, Specht D. Aerobic fitness in patients with fibrositis. A controlled study of respiratory gas exchange and 133xenon clearance from exercising muscle. Arthritis Rheum. 1989;32:454–60.
41. Lund N, Bengtsson A, Thorborg P. Muscle tissue oxygen pressure in primary fibromyalgia. Scan J Rheumatol. 1986;15:165–73.
42. de Kerviler E, Leroy-Willig A, Jehenson P, Duboc D, Eymard B, Syrota A. Exercise-induced muscle modifications: study of healthy subjects and patients with metabolic myopathies with MR imaging and P-31 spectroscopy. Radiology. 1991;181:259–64.
43. Sluka KA, Kalra A, Moore SA. Unilateral intramuscular injections of acidic saline produce a bilateral, long-lasting hyperalgesia. Muscle Nerve. 2001;24:37–46.
44. Park JH, Phothimat P, Oates CT, Hernanz-Schulman M, Olsen NJ. Use of P-31 magnetic resonance spectroscopy to detect metabolic abnormalities in muscles of patients with fibromyalgia. Arthritis Rheum. 1998;41:406–13.
45. Jubrias SA, Bennett RM, Klug GA. Increased incidence of a resonance in the phosphodiester region of 31P nuclear magnetic resonance spectra in the skeletal muscle of fibromyalgia patients. Arthritis Rheum. 1994;37:801–7.
46. Shah JP, Phillips TM, Danoff JV, Gerber LH. An in vivo microanalytical technique for measuring the local biochemical milieu of human skeletal muscle. J Appl Physiol. 2005;99:1977–84.
47. Rosendal L, Kristiansen J, Gerdle B, Sogaard K, Peolsson M, Kjaer M, Sorensen J, Larsson B. Increased levels of interstitial potassium but normal levels of muscle IL-6 and LDH in patients with trapezius myalgia. Pain. 2005;119:201–9.
48. Ruster M, Franke S, Spath M, Pongratz DE, Stein G, Hein GE. Detection of elevated N-epsilon-carboxymethyllysine levels in muscular tissue and in serum of patients with fibromyalgia. Scand J Rheumatol. 2005;34:460–3.
49. Wall PD, Woolf CJ. Muscle but not cutaneous C-afferent input produces prolonged increases in the excitability of the flexion reflex in the rat. J Physiol Lond. 1984;356:443–58.
50. Mendell LM, Wall PD. Responses of single dorsal cord cells to peripheral cutaneous unmyelinated fibres. Nature. 1965;206:97–9.
51. Price DD, Mao J, Frenk H, Mayer DJ. The N-methyl-D-aspartate receptor antagonist dextromethorphan selectively reduces temporal summation of second pain in man. Pain. 1994;59:165–74.
52. Staud R, Vierck CJ, Robinson ME, Price DD. Effects of the NDMA receptor antagonist dextromethorphan on temporal summation of pain are similar in fibromyalgia patients and normal controls. J Pain. 2005;6:323–32.
53. Vierck CJ, Cannon RL, Fry G, Maixner W, Whitsel BL. Characteristics of temporal summation of second pain sensations elicited by brief contact of glabrous skin by a preheated thermode. J Neurophysiol. 1997;78:992–1002.
54. Woolf CJ, Costigan M. Transcriptional and posttranslational plasticity and the generation of inflammatory pain. Proc Natl Acad Sci USA. 1999;96:7723–30.
55. Staud R, Domingo M. Evidence for abnormal pain processing in fibromyalgia syndrome. Pain Med. 2001;2:208–15.
56. Staud R, Domingo M. New Insights into the pathogenesis of fibromyalgia syndrome. Med Aspects Hum Sex. 2001;1:51–7.
57. Vierck CJ, Staud R, Price DD, Cannon RL, Mauderli AP, Martin AD. The effect of maximal exercise on temporal summation of second pain (wind-up) in patients with fibromyalgia syndrome. J Pain. 2001;2:334–44.
58. Staud R. Evidence of involvement of central neural mechanisms in generating fibromyalgia pain. Curr Rheumatol Rep. 2002;4:299–305.
59. Price DD, Staud R, Robinson ME, Mauderli AP, Cannon RL, Vierck CJ. Enhanced temporal summation of second pain and its central modulation in fibromyalgia patients. Pain. 2002;99:49–59.
60. King T, Gardell LR, Wang RZ, Vardanyan A, Ossipov MH, Malan TP, Vanderah TW, Hunt SP, Hruby VJ, Lai J, et al. Role of NK-1 neurotransmission in opioid-induced hyperalgesia. Pain. 2005;116:276–88.

61. Turk DC, Flor H. Primary fibromyalgia is greater than tender points: toward a multiaxial taxonomy. J Rheumatol Suppl. 1989;19:80–6.
62. Wolfe F. The relation between tender points and fibromyalgia symptom variables: evidence that fibromyalgia is not a discrete disorder in the clinic. Ann Rheum Dis. 1997;56(4):268–71.
63. McBeth J, Macfarlane GJ, Benjamin S, Morris S, Silman AJ. The association between tender points, psychological distress, and adverse childhood experiences: a community-based study. Arthritis Rheum. 1999;42(7):1397–404.
64. Wolfe F, Clauw DJ, Fitzcharles MA, et al. The American College of Rheumatology preliminary diagnostic criteria for fibromyalgia and measurement of symptom severity. Arthritis Rheum. 2010;62(5):600–10.
65. Rainville P, Bao QV, Chretien P. Pain-related emotions modulate experimental pain perception and autonomic responses. Pain. 2005;118:306–18.
66. Raja SN, Carr DB, Cohen M, Finnerup NB, Flor H, Gibson S, Keefe FJ, Mogil JS, Ringkamp M, Sluka KA, Song XJ, Stevens B, Sullivan MD, Tutelman PR, Ushida T, Vader K. The revised International Association for the Study of Pain definition of pain: concepts, challenges, and compromises. Pain. 2020;161(9):1976–82.
67. Walitt B, Čeko M, Khatiwada M, Gracely JL, Rayhan R, VanMeter JW, Gracely RH. Characterizing "fibrofog": subjective appraisal, objective performance, and task-related brain activity during a working memory task. Neuroimage Clin. 2016;11:173–80.
68. Zimmermann C, Del Piccolo L, Bensing J, et al. Coding patient emotional cues and concerns in medical consultations: the Verona coding definitions of emotional sequences (VR-CoDES). Patient Educ Couns. 2011;82:141–8.
69. Fleming KC, Volcheck MM. Central sensitization syndrome and the initial evaluation of a patient with fibromyalgia: a review. Rambam Maimonides Med J. 2015;6(2):e0020.
70. Gauthier N, Thibault P, Adams H, Sullivan MJ. Validation of a French-Canadian version of the Pain Disability Index. Pain Res Manag. 2008;13:327–33.
71. Bengtzen R, Woodward M, Lynn MJ, Newman NJ, Biousse V. The "sunglasses sign" predicts nonorganic visual loss in neuro-ophthalmologic practice. Neurology. 2008;70:218–21.
72. Morrison JR. The first interview. 3rd ed. New York, NY: Guilford Press; 2008. p. 124.
73. Valliant G. The beginning of wisdom is never calling a patient a borderline or, the clinical management of immature defenses in the treatment of individuals with personality disorders. In: Adshead G, Jacob C, editors. Personality disorder: the definitive reader. Philadelphia, PA: Jessica Kingsley Publishers; 2009. p. 104–30.
74. Molnar DS, Flett GL, Sadava SW, Colautti J. Perfectionism and health functioning in women with fibromyalgia. J Psychosom Res. 2012;73:295–300.
75. Kempke S, Luyten P, Claes S, et al. Self-critical perfectionism and its relationship to fatigue and pain in the daily flow of life in patients with chronic fatigue syndrome. Psychol Med. 2013;43:995–1002.
76. Luyten P, Kempke S, Van Wambeke P, Claes S, Blatt SJ, Van Houdenhove B. Self-critical perfectionism, stress generation, and stress sensitivity in patients with chronic fatigue syndrome: relationship with severity of depression. Psychiatry. 2011;74:21–30.
77. Uguz F, Ciçek E, Salli A, et al. Axis I and Axis II psychiatric disorders in patients with fibromyalgia. Gen Hosp Psychiatry. 2010;32:105–7.
78. Arnold LM, Hudson JI, Keck PE, Auchenbach MB, Javaras KN, Hess EV. Comorbidity of fibromyalgia and psychiatric disorders. J Clin Psychiatry. 2006;67:1219–25.
79. Sansone RA, Sansone LA. Chronic pain syndromes and borderline personality. Innov Clin Neurosci. 2012;9:10–4.
80. Hooley JM, Wilson-Murphy M. Adult attachment to transitional objects and borderline personality disorder. J Pers Disord. 2012;26:179–91.
81. Hauser W, Kosseva M, Uceyler N, Klose P, Sommer C. Emotional, physical, and sexual abuse in fibromyalgia syndrome: a systematic review with meta-analysis. Arthritis Care Res (Hoboken). 2011;63:808–20.

82. Buskila D, Neumann L, Vaisberg G, Alkalay D, Wolfe F. Increased rates of fibromyalgia following cervical spine injury: a controlled study of 161 cases of traumatic injury. Arthritis Rheum. 1997;40:446–52.
83. Ashenberg Straussner SL, Fewell CH. Children of substance-abusing parents: dynamics and treatment. New York, NY: Springer; 2011.
84. Ablin JN, Buskila D, Van Houdenhove B, Luyten P, Atzeni F, Sarzi-Puttini P. Is fibromyalgia a discrete entity? Autoimmun Rev. 2012;11:585–8.
85. Ablin JN, Cohen H, Eisinger M, Buskila D. Holocaust survivors: the pain behind the agony. Increased pre-valence of fibromyalgia among Holocaust survivors. Clin Exp Rheumatol. 2010;28(6 Suppl 63):S51–6.
86. Katon W, Sullivan M, Walker E. Medical symptoms without identified pathology: relationship to psychiatric disorders, childhood and adult trauma, and personality traits. Ann Intern Med. 2001;134(9 Pt 2):917–25.
87. Cleary BS, Keniston A, Havranek EP, Albert RK. Intimate partner violence in women hospitalized on an internal medicine service: prevalence and relationship to responses to the review of systems. J Hosp Med. 2008;3:299–307.
88. Felitti VJ, Anda RF, Nordenberg D, et al. Relationship of childhood abuse and household dysfunction to many of the leading causes of death in adults: the Adverse Childhood Experiences (ACE) Study. Am J Prev Med. 1998;14:245–58.
89. McCauley J, Kern DE, Kolodner K, et al. The "battering syndrome": prevalence and clinical characteristics of domestic violence in primary care internal medicine practices. Ann Intern Med. 1995;123:737–46.
90. Ouimette P, Cronkite R, Henson BR, Prins A, Gima K, Moos RH. Posttraumatic stress disorder and health status among female and male medical patients. J Trauma Stress. 2004;17:1–9.
91. Kramer A, Lorenzon D, Mueller G. Prevalence of intimate partner violence and health implications for women using emergency departments and primary care clinics. Womens Health Issues. 2004;14:19–29.
92. Campbell J, Jones AS, Dienemann J, et al. Intimate partner violence and physical health consequences. Arch Intern Med. 2002;162:1157–63.
93. Seng JS, Graham-Bermann SA, Clark MK, McCarthy AM, Ronis DL. Posttraumatic stress disorder and physical comorbidity among female children and adolescents: results from service-use data. Pediatrics. 2005;116:e767–76.
94. Coker AL, Smith PH, Bethea L, King MR, McKeown RE. Physical health consequences of physical and psychological intimate partner violence. Arch Fam Med. 2000;9:451–7.
95. Drossman DA, Leserman J, Nachman G, et al. Sexual and physical abuse in women with functional or organic gastrointestinal disorders. Ann Intern Med. 1990;113:828–33.
96. Auerbach E. Mimesis: the representation of reality in Western Literature. Trask WR, trans. Princeton, NJ: Princeton University Press; 1973.
97. Dimsdale J, Creed F. The proposed diagnosis of somatic symptom disorders in DSM-V to replace somatoform disorders in DSM-IV—a preliminary report. J Psychosom Res. 2009;66:473–6.
98. Stahl SM. Fibromyalgia—pathways and neurotransmitters. Hum Psychopharmacol. 2009;24(Suppl 1):S11–7.
99. Glass JM. Review of cognitive dysfunction in fibromyalgia: a convergence on working memory and attentional control impairments. Rheum Dis Clin North Am. 2009;35:299–311.
100. Harte SE, Harris RE, Clauw DJ. The neurobiology of central sensitization. J Appl Behav Res. 2018;23:e12137.
101. Salomons TV, Iannetti GD, Liang M, et al. The "pain matrix" in pain-free individuals. JAMA Neurol. 2016;73:755–6.
102. Geha P, Waxman SG. Pain perception: multiple matrices or one? JAMA Neurol. 2016;73:628–30.
103. Archibald J, Warner FM, Ortiz O, et al. Recent advances in objectifying pain using neuroimaging techniques. J Neurophysiol. 2018;120:387–90.

104. Reddan MC, Wager TD. Modeling pain using fMRI: from regions to biomarkers. Neurosci Bull. 2018;34:208–15.
105. Gracely RH, Petzke F, Wolf JM, Clauw DJ. Functional magnetic resonance imaging evidence of augmented pain processing in fibromyalgia. Arthritis Rheum. 2002;46:1333–43.
106. Cook DB, et al. Functional imaging of pain in patients with primary fibromyalgia. J. Rheumatol. 2004;31:364–78.
107. Martucci KT, Mackey SC. Neuroimaging of pain: human evidence and clinical relevance of central nervous system processes and modulation. Anesthesiology. 2018;128:1241–54.
108. Cagnie B, Coppieters I, Denecker S, et al. Central sensitization in fibromyalgia? A systematic review on structural and functional brain MRI. Semin Arthritis Rheum. 2014;44:68–75.
109. Walitt B, Ceko M, Gracely JL, et al. Neuroimaging of central sensitivity syndromes: key insights from the scientific literature. Curr Rheumatol Rev. 2016;12:55–87.
110. Shi H, Yuan C, Dai Z, et al. Gray matter abnormalities associated with fibromyalgia: a meta-analysis of voxel-based morphometric studies. Semin Arthritis Rheum. 2016;46:330–7.
111. Lin C, Lee SH, Weng HH. Gray matter atrophy within the default mode network of fibromyalgia: a meta-analysis of voxel-based morphometry studies. BioMed Res Int. 2016;2016:7296125.
112. McCrae CS, Mundt JM, Curtis AF, et al. Gray matter changes following cognitive behavioral therapy for patients with comorbid fibromyalgia and insomnia: a pilot study. J Clin Sleep Med. 2018;14:1595–603.
113. Napadow V, et al. Intrinsic brain connectivity in fibromyalgia is associated with chronic pain intensity. Arthritis Rheum. 2010;62:2545–55.
114. Napadow V, Kim J, Clauw DJ, Harris RE. Decreased intrinsic brain connectivity is associated with reduced clinical pain in fibromyalgia. Arthritis Rheum. 2012;64:2398–403.
115. Jensen KB, et al. Patients with fibromyalgia display less functional connectivity in the brain's pain inhibitory network. Mol Pain. 2012;8:32.
116. Foerster BR, et al. Reduced insular γ-aminobutyric acid in fibromyalgia. Arthritis Rheum. 2012;64:579–83.
117. Napadow V, Harris RE. What has functional connectivity and chemical neuroimaging in fibromyalgia taught us about the mechanisms and management of centralized pain? Arthritis Res Ther. 2014;16:425.
118. Thorp SL, Suchy T, Vadivelu N, et al. Functional connectivity alterations: novel therapy and future implications in chronic pain management. Pain Physician. 2018;21:E207–14.
119. Lazaridou A, Kim J, Cahalan CM, et al. Effects of cognitive-behavioral therapy (CBT) on brain connectivity supporting catastrophizing in fibromyalgia. Clin J Pain. 2017;33:215–21.
120. Cummiford CM, Nascimento TD, Foerster BR, et al. Changes in resting state functional connectivity after repetitive transcranial direct current stimulation applied to motor cortex in fibromyalgia patients. Arthritis Res Ther. 2016;18:40.
121. Napadow V, Kim J, Clauw DJ, et al. Decreased intrinsic brain connectivity is associated with reduced clinical pain in fibromyalgia. Arthritis Rheum. 2012;64:2398–403.
122. Harris RE, Napadow V, Huggins JP, et al. Pregabalin rectifies aberrant brain chemistry, connectivity, and functional response in chronic pain patients. Anesthesiology. 2013;119:1453–64.
123. Schmidt-Wilcke T, Ichesco E, Hampson JP, et al. Resting state connectivity correlates with drug and placebo response in fibromyalgia patients. Neuroimage Clin. 2014;6:252–61.
124. Flodin P, Martinsen S, Mannerkorpi K, et al. Normalization of aberrant resting state functional connectivity in fibromyalgia patients following a three month physical exercise therapy. Neuroimage Clin. 2015;9:134.
125. Reckziegel D, Vachon-Presseau E, Petre B, et al. Deconstructing biomarkers for chronic pain: context- and hypothesis-dependent biomarker types in relation to chronic pain. Pain. 2019;160(Suppl 1):S37–48.
126. Richard JY, Hurley RA, Taber KH. Fibromyalgia: centralized pain processing and neuroimaging. J Neuropsychiatry Clin Neurosciences. 2019;31(3):A6–187.
127. Häuser W, Ablin J, Fitzcharles MA, Littlejohn G, Luciano JV, Usui C, Walitt B. Fibromyalgia. Nat Rev Dis Primers. 2015;1:15022.

128. Fitzcharles M-A, et al. Classification and clinical diagnosis of fibromyalgia syndrome: recommendations of recent evidence-based interdisciplinary guidelines. Evid Based Complement Alternat Med. 2013;2013:528952.
129. Wolfe F, et al. The American College of Rheumatology preliminary diagnostic criteria for fibromyalgia and measurement of symptom severity. Arthritis Care Res (Hoboken). 2010;62:600–10.
130. Wolfe F, et al. Fibromyalgia criteria and severity scales for clinical and epidemiological studies: a modification of the ACR preliminary diagnostic criteria for fibromyalgia. J Rheumatol. 2011;38:1113–22.
131. Wolfe F, Häuser W. Fibromyalgia diagnosis and diagnostic criteria. Ann Med. 2011;43:495–502.
132. Wolfe F. Editorial: the status of fibromyalgia criteria. Arthritis Rheumatol. 2015;67:330–3.
133. Wolfe F. Fibromyalgianess. Arthritis Rheum. 2009;61(6):715–6.
134. Woolf CJ. Central sensitization: implications for the diagnosis and treatment of pain. Pain. 2011;152(3 Suppl):S2–S15.
135. Brummett C, Clauw D, Harris R, Harte S, Hassett A, Williams D. We agree with the need for a new term but disagree with the proposed terms. Pain. 2016;157(12):2876.
136. Brummett CM, Janda AM, Schueller CM, Tsodikov A, Morris M, Williams DA, Clauw DJ. Survey criteria for fibromyalgia independently predict increased postoperative opioid consumption after lower-extremity joint arthroplasty: a prospective, observational cohort study. Anesthesiology. 2013;119(6):1434–43.
137. Brummett CM, Urquhart AG, Hassett AL, Tsodikov A, Hallstrom BR, Wood NI, Clauw DJ. Characteristics of fibromyalgia independently predict poorer long-term analgesic outcomes following total knee and hip arthroplasty. Arthritis Rheumatol. 2015;67(5):1386–94.
138. Janda AM, As-Sanie S, Rajala B, Tsodikov A, Moser SE, Clauw DJ, Brummett CM. Fibromyalgia survey criteria are associated with increased postoperative opioid consumption in women undergoing hysterectomy. Anesthesiology. 2015;122(5):1103–11.
139. Russell I. Management of pain in the fibromyalgia syndrome. Arthritis. 2018;7:4.
140. Russel IJ. Fibromyalgia syndrome: approaches to management. Bull Rheum Dis. 1996;45:1–4.
141. Russell IL. Fibromyalgia syndrome: approach to management. Prim Psychol. 2006;13(9):76–84.
142. Clauw DJ, Arnold LM, McCarberg BH. The science of fibromyalgia. Mayo Clinic Proc. 2011;86(9):907–11.
143. Woolf CJ. Evidence for a central component of post-injury pain hypersensitivity. Nature. 1983;306(5944):686–8.
144. Yunus MB. Central sensitivity syndromes: a new paradigm and group nosology for fibromyalgia and overlapping conditions, and the related issue of disease versus illness. Semin Arthritis Rheum. 2008;37(6):339–52.
145. Yarnitsky D. Conditioned pain modulation (the diffuse noxious inhibitory control-like effect): its relevance for acute and chronic pain states. Curr Opin Anaesthesiol. 2010;23(5):611–5.
146. Atzeni F, Gerardi MC, Masala IF, Alciati A, Batticciotto A, Sarzi-Puttini P. An update on emerging drugs for fibromyalgia treatment. Expert Opin Emerg Drugs. 2017;22(4):357–67.
147. Abeles AM, Pillinger MH, Solitar BM, Abeles M. Narrative review: the pathophysiology of fibromyalgia. Ann Intern Med. 2007;146(10):726–34.
148. Uçeyler N, Häuser W, Sommer C. "Systematic review" with meta-analysis: cytokines in fibromyalgia syndrome. BMC Musculoskelet Disord. 2011;12(1):245.
149. Aaron LA, Buchwald D. Chronic diffuse musculoskeletal pain, fibromyalgia and co-morbid unexplained clinical conditions. Baillieres Best Pract Res Clin Rheumatol. 2003;17(4):563–74.
150. White LA, Birnbaum HG, Kaltenboeck A, Tang J, Mallett D, Robinson RL. Employees with fibromyalgia: medical comorbidity, healthcare costs, and work loss. J Occup Environ Med. 2008;50(1):13–24.
151. Napadow V, LaCount L, Park K, As-Sanie S, Clauw DJ, Harris RE. Intrinsic brain connectivity in fibromyalgia is associated with chronic pain intensity. Arthritis Rheum. 2010;62(8):2545–55.

152. Napadow V, Kim J, Clauw DJ, Harris RE. Brief report: decreased intrinsic brain connectivity is associated with reduced clinical pain in fibromyalgia. Arthritis Rheum. 2012;64(7):2398–403.
153. Tzadok R, Ablin J. Current and emerging pharmacotherapy for fibromyalgia. Pain Res Manag. 2020;2020:6541798. https://doi.org/10.1155/2020/6541798.
154. Crofford LJ. Pharmaceutical treatment options for fibromyalgia. Curr Rheumatol Rep. 2004;6:274–80.
155. Schweinhardt P, Sauro KM, Bushnell MC. Fibromyalgia: a disorder of the brain? Neuroscientist. 2008;14:415–21.
156. Denko CW, Malemud CJ. Role of the growth hormone/insulin-like growth factor-1 paracrine axis in rheumatic diseases. Semin Arthritis Rheum. 2005;35:24–34.
157. Vierck CJ Jr. Mechanisms underlying development of spatially distributed chronic pain. Pain. 2006;124:242–63.
158. Staud R. Treatment of fibromyalgia and its symptoms. Expert Opin Pharmacother. 2007;8:1629–42.
159. Wingenfeld K, Wagner D, Schmidt I, Meinischmidt G, Hellhammer DH, Heim C. The low dose dexamethasone suppression test in fibromyalgia. J Psychosom Res. 2007;62:85–91.
160. Staud R, Rodriguez ME. Mechanisms of disease: pain in fibromyalgia syndrome. Nat Clin Pract Rheumatol. 2006;2:90–8.
161. Nielsen LA, Henriksson KG. Pathophysiological mechanisms in chronic musculoskeletal pain (fibromyalgia): the role of central and peripheral sensitization and pain disinhibition. Best Pract Res Clin Rheumatol. 2007;21:465–80.
162. Malemud CJ. Focus on pain mechanisms and pharmacotherapy in the treatment of fibromyalgia syndrome. Clin Exp Rheumatol. 2009;27(5 Suppl 56):S86–91.
163. Landis CA, Lentz MJ, Rothermel J, Buchwald D, Shaver JL. Decreased sleep spindles and spindle activity in midlife women with fibromyalgia and pain. Sleep. 2004;27:741–50.
164. Price DD, Staud R. Neurobiology of fibromyalgia syndrome. J Rheumatol. 2005;75(Suppl):22–8.
165. Chakrabarty S, Zoorob R. Fibromyalgia. Am Fam Physician. 2007;76:247–54.
166. Buskila D, Cohen H. Comorbidity of fibromyalgia and psychiatric disorders. Curr Pain Headache Rep. 2007;11:333–8.
167. Bennett R, Nelson D. Cognitive behavioral therapy for fibromyalgia. Nat Clin Pract Rheumatol. 2006;8:416–24.
168. Crofford LJ, Rowbotham MC, Mease PJ, et al. Pregabalin for the treatment of fibromyalgia syndrome: results of a randomized, double-blind, placebo-controlled trial. Arthritis Rheum. 2005;52(4):1264–73.
169. Ohta H, Oka H, Usui C, Ohkura M, Suzuki M, Nishioka K. A randomized, double-blind, multicenter, placebo-controlled phase III trial to evaluate the efficacy and safety of pregabalin in Japanese patients with fibromyalgia. Arthritis Res Ther. 2012;14(5):R217.
170. Häuser W, Bernardy K, Uçeyler N, Sommer C. Treatment of fibromyalgia syndrome with gabapentin and pregabalin—a meta-analysis of randomized controlled trials. Pain. 2009;145(1–2):69–81.
171. Kelm MK, Criswell HE, Breese GR. Ethanol-enhanced GABA release: a focus on G protein-coupled receptors. Brain Res Rev. 2011;65(2):113–23.
172. Gordon ER. The effect of ethanol on the concentration of c-aminobutyric acid in the rat brain. Can J Physiol Pharmacol. 1967;45(5):915–8.
173. Hatton WJ, Mason HS, Carl A, et al. Functional and molecular expression of a voltage-dependent K+ channel (Kv1.1) interstitial cells of Cajal. J Physiol. 2001;533:315–27.
174. Punke MA, Friederich P. Amitryptyline is a potent blocker of human Kv1.1 and Kv7.2/7.3 channels. Anesth Analg. 2007;104:1256–64.
175. Wuttke TV, Seebohm G, Bail S, Maljevic S, Lerche H. The new anticonvulsant retigabine favors voltage-dependent opening of the Kv7.2 (KCNQ2) channel by binding to its activation gate. Mol Pharmacol. 2005;67:1009–17.

176. Carville SF, Arendt-Nielsen S, Bliddal H, et al. EULAR evidence-based recommendations for the management of fibromyalgia syndrome. Ann Rheum Dis. 2008;67(4):536–41.
177. Häuser W, Arnold B, Eich W, et al. Management of fibromyalgia syndrome—an interdisciplinary evidence-based guideline. German Med Sci. 2008;6:Doc14.
178. Fitzcharles M-A, Ste-Marie PA, Goldenberg DL, et al. 2012 Canadian guidelines for the diagnosis and management of fibromyalgia syndrome: executive summary. Pain Res Manag. 2013;18(3):119–26.
179. Calandre EP, Rico-Villademoros F, Slim M. An update on pharmacotherapy for the treatment of fibromyalgia. Expert Opin Pharmacother. 2015;16(9):1347–68.
180. Bagal SK, Marron BE, Owen RM, Storer RI, Swain NA. Voltage gated sodium channels as drug discovery targets. Channels (Austin). 2015;9(6):360–6.
181. Wilderman I, Pugacheva O, Perelman VS, Wansbrough MCT, Voznyak Y, Zolnierczyk L. Repeated intravenous lidocaine infusions for patients with fibromyalgia: higher doses of lidocaine have a stronger and longer-lasting effect on pain reduction. Pain Med. 2020;21:1230–9.
182. Alciati A, Nucera V, Masala IF, Giallanza M, La Corte L, Giorgi V, Sarzi-Puttini P, Atzeni F. One year in review 2021: fibromyalgia. Clin Exp Rheumatol. 2021;39(Suppl 130):S3–S12.
183. Pereira V, Goudet C. Emerging trends in pain modulation by metabotropic glutamate receptors. Front Mol Neurosci. 2019;11:464.
184. Dougherty P, Palecek J, Paleckova V, Sorkin L, Willis W. The role of NMDA and non-NMDA excitatory amino acid receptors in the excitation of primate spinothalamic tract neurons by mechanical, chemical, thermal, and electrical stimuli. J Neuroscience. 1992;12(8):3025–41.
185. Palucha A, Brański P, Szewczyk B, et al. Potential anti-depressant-like effects of MTEP, a potent and highly specific mGlu5R antagonist. Pharmacol Biochem Behav. 2005;81:901–6.
186. Cohen SP, Verdolin MH, Chang AS, Kurihara C, Morlando BJ, Mao J. The intravenous ketamine test predicts subsequent response to an oral dextromethorphan treatment regimen in fibromyalgia patients. J Pain. 2006;7(6):391–8.
187. Johnson J, Kotermanski S. Mechanism of action of memantine. Curr Opin Pharmacol. 2006;6(1):61–7.
188. Harris RE, Sundgren PC, Craig AD, et al. Elevated insular glutamate in fibromyalgia is associated with experimental pain. Arthritis Rheum. 2009;60(10):3146–52.
189. Harris RE, Sundgren PC, Pang Y, et al. Dynamic levels of glutamate within the insula are associated with improvements in multiple pain domains in fibromyalgia. Arthritis Rheum. 2008;58(3):903–7.
190. Olivan-Blázquez B, Herrera-Mercadal P, Puebla-Guedea M, et al. Efficacy of memantine in the treatment of fibromyalgia: a double-blind, randomised, controlled trial with 6-month follow-up. Pain. 2014;155(12):2517–25.
191. Kurian R, Raza K, Shanthanna H. A systematic review and meta-analysis of memantine for the prevention or treatment of chronic pain. Eur J Pain. 2019;23(7):1234–50.
192. Charnay Y, Léger L. Brain serotonergic circuitries. Dialogues Clin Neurosci. 2010;12(4):471–87.
193. Quera-Salva M-A, Lemoine P, Guilleminault C. Impact of the novel antidepressant agomelatine on disturbed sleep–wake cycles in depressed patients. Hum Psychopharmacol Clin Exp. 2010;25:222–9.
194. Mestres J, Seifert SA, Oprea TI. Linking pharmacology to clinical reports: cyclobenzaprine and its possible association with serotonin syndrome. Clin Pharmacol Ther. 2011;90(5):662–5.
195. Moldofsky H, Inhaber NH, Guinta DR, Alvarez-Horine SB. Effects of sodium oxybate on sleep physiology and sleep/wake-related symptoms in patients with FM syndrome: a double-blind, randomized, placebo-controlled study. J Rheumatol. 2010;37:2156–66.
196. Gendreau R, Clauw D, Gendreau J, et al. THU0322 TNX-102 SL for treatment of fibromyalgia: approaches to pain measurement. Ann Rheum Dis. 2015;74:312.
197. Welsch P, Bernardy K, Derry S, Moore RA, Häuser W. Mirtazapine for fibromyalgia in adults. Cochrane Database Syst Rev. 2018;8(8):CD012708.

198. Hu WP, You XH, Guan BC, Ru LQ, Chen JG, Li ZW. Substance P potentiates 5-HT3 receptor-mediated current in rat trigeminal ganglion neurons. Neurosci Lett. 2004;365(2):147–52.
199. Cashman JR, Ghirmai S. Inhibition of serotonin and norepinephrine reuptake and inhibition of phosphodiesterase by multi-target inhibitors as potential agents for depression. Bioorg Med Chem. 2009;17(19):6890–7.
200. Wright ME, Rizzolo D. An update on the pharmacologic management and treatment of neuropathic pain. JAAPA. 2017;30(3):13–7.
201. Arnold LM. Duloxetine and other antidepressants in the treatment of patients with fibrmyalgia. Pain Med. 2007;8(Suppl 2):S63–74.
202. Vitton O, Gendreau M, Gendreau J, Kranzler J, Rao SG. A double-blind placebo-controlled trial of milnacipran in the treatment of fibromyalgia. Hum Psychopharmacol. 2004;19(Suppl 1):S27–35.
203. Hauser W, Urrútia G, Tort S, Uçeyler N, Walitt B. Serotonin and noradrenaline reuptake inhibitors (SNRIs) for fibromyalgia syndrome. Cochrane Database Syst Rev. 2018;(2):CD010292.
204. Marks D, Shah M, Patkar A, Masand P, Park G-Y, Pae C-U. Serotonin-norepinephrine reuptake inhibitors for pain control: premise and promise. Curr Neuropharmacol. 2009;7(4):331–6.
205. Häuser W, Arnold B, Eich W, et al. Management of fibromyalgia syndrome-an interdisciplinary evidence-based guideline. German Med Sci. 2008;6:Doc14.
206. Ablin J, Fitzcharles M-A, Buskila D, Shir Y, Sommer C, Häuser W. Treatment of fibromyalgia syndrome: recommendations of recent evidence-based interdisciplinary guidelines with special emphasis on complementary and alternative therapies. Evid Based Complement Altern Med. 2013;2013:485272. , 7 pages.
207. Häuser W, Wolfe F, Tölle T, Uçeyler N, Sommer C. The role of antidepressants in the management of fibromyalgia syndrome. CNS Drugs. 2012;26(4):297–307.
208. Wood PB, Schweinhardt P, Jaeger E, et al. Fibromyalgia patients show an abnormal dopamine response to pain. Eur J Neurosci. 2007;25(12):3576–82.
209. Distler O, Eich W, Dokoupilova E, et al. Evaluation of the efficacy and safety of terguride in patients with fibromyalgia syndrome: results of a twelve-week, multicenter, randomized, double-blind, placebo-controlled, parallel-group study. Arthritis Rheum. 2010;62(1):291–300.
210. Sommer C, Häuser W, Alten R, et al. Drug therapy of fibromyalgia syndrome: systematic review, meta-analysis and guideline. Schmerz. 2012;26(3):297–310.
211. Macfarlane GJ, Kronisch C, Dean LE, et al. EULAR revised recommendations for the management of fibromyalgia. Ann Rheum Dis. 2017;76(2):318–28.
212. Julien N, Goffaux P, Arsenault P, Marchand S. Widespread pain in fibromyalgia is related to a deficit of endogenous pain inhibition. Pain. 2005;114(1):295–302.
213. Baraniuk JN, Whalen G, Cunningham J, Clauw DJ. Cerebrospinal fluid levels of opioid peptides in fibromyalgia and chronic low back pain. BMC Musculoskelet Disord. 2004;5(1):48.
214. Harris RE, Clauw DJ, Scott DJ, McLean SA, Gracely RH, Zubieta J-K. Decreased central-opioid receptor availability in fibromyalgia. J Neurosci. 2007;27(37):10000–6.
215. Younger J, Mackey S. Fibromyalgia symptoms are reduced by low-dose naltrexone: a pilot study. Pain Med. 2009;10(4):663–72.
216. Younger J, Noor N, McCue R, MacKey S. Low-dose naltrexone for the treatment of fibromyalgia: findings of a small, randomized, double-blind, placebo-controlled, counterbalanced, crossover trial assessing daily pain levels. Arthritis Rheum. 2013;65(2):529–38.
217. Albrecht DS, Forsberg A, Sandstrom A, et al. Brain glial activation in fibromyalgia—a multi-site positron emission tomography investigation. Brain Behav Immun. 2019;75:72–83.
218. Liu B, Du L, Hong JS. Naloxone protects rat dopaminergic neurons against inflammatory damage through inhibition of microglia activation and superoxide generation. J Pharmacol Exp Ther. 2000;293(2):607–17.
219. Chang RCC, Rota C, Glover RE, Mason RP, Hong JS. A novel effect of an opioid receptor antagonist, naloxone, on the production of reactive oxygen species by microglia: a study by electron paramagnetic resonance spectroscopy. Brain Res. 2000;854(1–2):224–9.

220. MacCallum CA, Russo EB. Practical considerations in medical cannabis administration and dosing. Eur J Intern Medicine. 2018;49:12–9.
221. Cravatt BF, Lichtman AH. The endogenous cannabinoid system and its role in nociceptive behavior. J Neurobiol. 2004;61(1):149–60.
222. Smith SC, Wagner MS. Clinical endocannabinoid deficiency (CECD) revisited: can this concept explain the therapeutic benefits of cannabis in migraine, fibromyalgia, irritable bowel syndrome and other treatment-resistant conditions? Neuroendocrinol Lett. 2014;35(3):198–201.
223. Fiz J, Duran M, Capella D, Carbonell J, Farre M. Cannabis use in patients with fibromyalgia: effect on symptoms relief and health-related quality of life. PLoS One. 2011;6(4):e18440.
224. Skrabek RQ, Galimova L, Ethans K, Perry D. Nabilone for the treatment of pain in fibromyalgia. J Pain. 2008;9(2):164–73.
225. Ware MA, Fitzcharles MA, Joseph L, Shir Y. The effects of nabilone on sleep in fibromyalgia: results of a randomized controlled trial. Anesth Analg. 2010;110(2):604–10.
226. Walitt B, Klose P, Fitzcharles MA, Phillips T, Hauser W. Cannabinoids for fibromyalgia. Cochrane Database Syst Rev. 2016;7(7):CD011694.
227. Hohmann AG. In: Farquhar-Smith P, Beaulieu P, Jagger S, editors. Control of pain initiation by endogenous cannabinoids, vol. 1. Oxford: Oxford University Press; 2018.
228. Adamson Barnes NS, Mitchell VA, Kazantzis NP, Vaughan CW. Actions of the dual FAAH/MAGL inhibitor JZL195 in a murine neuropathic pain model. Br J Pharmacol. 2016;173(1):77–87.

Part V
Clinical Matters

Chapter 12
Diagnostic Testing of Neuropathic Pain

Eman A. Tawfik

Introduction

Neuropathic pain is currently defined as 'pain arising as a direct consequence of a lesion or disease affecting the somatosensory system' [1]. Further, neuropathic pain is graded as 'possible' probable' or 'definite' based on the history, the distribution of clinical symptoms, the clinical signs, and the results of the diagnostic tests. To diagnose a patient as having 'definite neuropathic pain', confirmation of a lesion in the somatosensory system by objective diagnostic tests is required [1, 2].

Neuropathic pain is not a simple symptom. It is a complex clinical condition that can be caused by various disorders of the peripheral or the central parts of the somatosensory system. Thus, it can be classified into central and peripheral neuropathic pain. Central neuropathic pain results from brain or spinal cord lesions like stroke, spinal cord injury, syringomyelia, and multiple sclerosis. Peripheral neuropathic pain may involve the large and myelinated A-alpha and A-beta fibers or may involve the small, myelinated A-delta and unmyelinated C-fibers. The peripheral nerve disorders that may present with neuropathic pain include entrapment neuropathies, traumatic nerve injuries, post herpetic neuralgia, polyneuropathies, plexopathies, radiculopathies, and trigeminal neuralgia. Given the extensive list of the central and peripheral nerve disorders that can cause neuropathic pain, defining its cause is challenging.

Various diagnostic tests are available to assess neuropathic pain and its underlying cause. The optimum approach is to perform the least number of the diagnostic tests rather than requesting all available tests. Although objective diagnostic tests

E. A. Tawfik (✉)
Department of Physical Medicine & Rehabilitation, Faculty of Medicine, Ain-Shams University, Cairo, Egypt
e-mail: Eman_Tawfik@med.asu.edu.eg

© The Author(s), under exclusive license to Springer Nature Switzerland AG 2022

J. de Castro, Y. El Miedany (eds.), *Advances in Chronic and Neuropathic Pain*, Contemporary Rheumatology, https://doi.org/10.1007/978-3-031-10687-3_12

are important, the diagnosis of neuropathic pain relies on the interpretation of the results of these diagnostic tests in the context of the clinical data.

This chapter focuses on the most important and valuable diagnostic tests for neuropathic pain. They are categorized under six headings: quantitative sensory testing, neurophysiological tests, microstructural testing, neuroimaging, laboratory and genetic testing, and other tests. Neurophysiological tests provide functional assessment and include nerve conduction studies, cutaneous silent period, somatosensory evoked potentials, laser evoked potentials, trigeminal reflexes, and microneurography. Microstructure tests include skin and nerve biopsy. Neuroimaging tools allows structural/anatomical assessment and include functional neuroimaging, neuromuscular ultrasound, and magnetic resonance neurography.

The chapter provides a general overview of each diagnostic tool, its value, utilities, and limitations. The full technical details of the tests are beyond the scope of the chapter and the reader can refer to dedicated technical textbooks addressing each category of the diagnostic tests.

At the end of the chapter, a flow chart is provided showing a general diagnostic approach to neuropathic pain (Fig. 12.12).

Quantitative Sensory Testing

Quantitative sensory testing is a reliable psychophysical sensory test that complements the neurological clinical examination. It involves testing patient's perception to various external stimuli applied to the skin in a graded order to determine the sensory threshold. Sensitivity to tactile, painful, vibration, and thermal stimuli can be tested using plastic filaments, weighted needles, electronic vibrameter, and thermode, respectively [3]. As a result, quantitative sensory testing allows the assessment of all types of fibers including large myelinated, small myelinated, and unmyelinated fibers [4]. Elevated painful and or thermal sensory threshold denotes small fiber dysfunction or loss. On the other hand, low threshold denotes hyperalgesia [5]. Hence, the test can quantify negative as well as positive sensory signs as hyperalgesia and allodynia and thus can be used to monitor treatment effect especially in clinical trials [6, 7]. The European Federation of Neurological societies recommends the use of simple tools such as a brush and at least one high-intensity weighted pinprick or von Frey filament to assess mechanical hyperalgesia and allodynia. However, the federation does not recommend systematic assessment of thermal stimuli except in pathophysiological research and treatment trials [8]. Two methods of stimulus application are commonly used: Method of limits and Method of levels. Getting accurate results from the test requires standardization of the application method, clearly defined stimulus intensity and physical properties, and full cooperation of the patient.

Quantitative sensory testing is mainly used to evaluate peripheral nerve disorders although it can be abnormal in patients with neuropathic pain secondary to central nervous system disorder and in patients with non-neuropathic pain [9].

The main clinical application of quantitative sensory testing is diabetic neuropathy. Given its validity, the Peripheral Neuropathy Association, and the American Diabetes Association included quantitative sensory testing in the neurophysiologic workup of diabetic neuropathy [10]. The test can also be used for early diagnosis of small fiber neuropathy [11]. However, skin biopsy and quantification of the intraepidermal nerve fiber density represent the gold standard for the diagnosis of small fiber neuropathy.

Although the test allows quantitative assessment of the somatosensory deficits, it depends on patient's perception to the stimuli and his/her full cooperation which makes it a relatively subjective test. Moreover, the test is unable to localize the lesion because abnormal tests can be caused by central or peripheral nervous system disorders [12]. Being time consuming and not readily available in all neurological centers add to the limitations of the test.

Neurophysiological Tests

Neurophysiological tests allow objective assessment of the functional status of the somatosensory system. Hence, it can provide the evidence for a lesion in the somatosensory system which is required to reach the 'definite' diagnosis of neuropathic pain. The neurophysiological tests that can used to assess neuropathic pain are numerous. They include nerve conduction studies, cutaneous silent periods, somatosensory evoked potentials, laser- and contact heat- evoked potentials, trigeminal reflexes, and microneurography.

Nerve Conduction Studies

Nerve conduction studies remain an important cornerstone in the diagnostic workup of neuropathic pain and is considered the most useful tool for the assessment of peripheral neuropathies as per the European Federation of Neurological Societies (EFNS) guidelines [10]. At first glance, it may seem logical to overview only the sensory nerve conduction studies since we address neuropathic pain in this chapter, but motor nerve conduction studies are equally important as part of the electrodiagnostic protocols to reach the final diagnosis. Nerve conduction studies are indicated in any suspected nerve disorder including entrapment neuropathies, polyneuropathies, plexopathies, and radiculopathies. Although needle electromyography does not test sensation, it complements the nerve conduction studies and is often required to reach a final diagnosis.

It should be noted that nerve conduction studies assess the non-nociceptive pathway namely type A-beta fibers. This means that the responses obtained in sensory and motor nerve conduction studies reflect only the function of the largest and fastest conducting fibers. As a result, normal nerve conduction studies do not exclude peripheral nerve dysfunction, but only exclude large fiber involvement. Although it is generally known that neuropathic pain is mainly associated with dysfunction of the nociceptive pathway rather than being associated with non-nociceptive pathway dysfunction, nerve conduction studies remain important cornerstone in the diagnostic workup of neuropathic pain because they evaluate the peripheral part of the leminscal system which is one of the somatosensory pathways.

Valuable information can be obtained from nerve conduction studies. The tests together with needle electromyography can localize the lesion, provide a diagnosis in many instances, determine the underlying pathology and the type of fibers involved, and assess severity and chronicity. The main limitations of nerve conduction and electromyography studies are their inability to evaluate the small myelinated and unmyelinated nerve fibers, and inability to differentiate between severe axonotemesis and neurotmesis in the first several weeks of nerve trauma. Moreover, they do not give a clue on the structural and anatomical aspects of the neuromuscular system. Hence, the importance of neuroimaging to complement the functional information obtained via nerve conduction studies and electromyography. In addition, both nerve conduction and needle electromyography studies are painful and can be time consuming.

Nerve conduction studies include motor nerve conduction studies, sensory nerve conduction studies, and late responses. The late responses include F-wave study and H-reflex. In motor nerve conduction studies, the resultant compound muscle action potential is analyzed as regards distal motor latency, amplitude, and conduction velocity. In sensory nerve conduction, peak latency, amplitude, and conduction velocity of the sensory nerve action potential are the typically evaluated parameters. F-wave assessment include calculation of the minimum F-wave latency, mean F-wave latency, chronodispersion, persistence, and F-estimate in some cases. H-reflex involves mainly evaluation of H-wave latency.

In general, pure demyelinating lesions are characterized by delayed sensory or motor latencies and/or slowing of the conduction velocities. Additionally, focal demyelination may manifest as partial or complete conduction block. On the other hand, pure axonal lesions are characterized by reduced sensory and/or motor amplitudes in addition to acute or chronic axonal changes in the relevant muscles on needle electromyography. These typical demyelinating and axonal patterns may differ with the chronicity and severity of the lesions. Moreover, severe axonal lesions usually lead to secondary demyelinating features due to loss of the fastest conducting fibers and severe demyelinating lesions may be associated with secondary axonal features.

The examination protocol depends on the provisional diagnosis. In suspected entrapment neuropathies, motor and sensory nerve conduction studies and F-wave study of the nerve under investigation should be performed in addition to examining at least another nerve in the same limb to exclude generalized nerve disorders such as polyneuropathies, plexopathies and radiculopathies. In suspected polyneuropathy, motor and sensory nerve conduction studies, and late responses of the main lower and upper limb nerves should be performed on one side in addition to at least one motor and sensory study on the other side [13]. An alternative approach is to follow a stepwise strategy starting with sural sensory and tibial motor nerve conduction studies as the first tests then procced to other nerves according to the findings [14]. The aforementioned general protocols may need to be modified or extended based on the initial findings. Also, more sensitive nerve conduction tests may be needed if the routine tests are negative to detect subtle abnormalities. Needle EMG is indicated if the muscles are clinically wasted or weak, or if there is evidence of axonal affection in motor nerve conduction studies.

In the following section, the general electrodiagnostic features of common nerve disorders that can present with neuropathic pain are briefly discussed. Purely motor nerve disorders are not addressed because they do not present with neuropathic pain.

Entrapment Neuropathies

The aims of the nerve conduction studies in entrapment neuropathies are to confirm the entrapment and localize its site, determine the type of the fibers involved, the underlying pathology, severity, and chronicity, and exclude more widespread or superimposed lesions.

Carpal tunnel syndrome is the most common entrapment neuropathy. Because the entrapment involves the sensory fibers early in the course of the disease, the patient usually presents with neuropathic pain and paresthesia in the hand which typically take the distribution of the median nerve but can occasionally refer to forearm, arm, or even the shoulder. The typical electrodiagnostic abnormalities encountered in carpal tunnel syndrome include delayed peak sensory and distal motor latencies of the median nerve (Fig. 12.1). Chronic entrapment may lead to

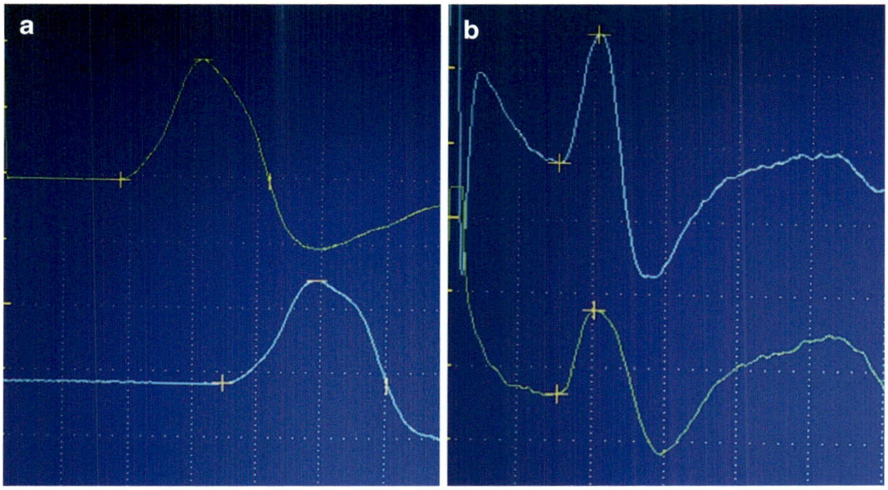

Fig. 12.1 Nerve conduction studies of the median nerve in patient with carpal tunnel syndrome showing delayed distal motor latency (**a**), latency = 5.5 ms, and delayed peak sensory latency (**b**) with recording from the index (upper trace) and the middle finger (lower trace)

axonal injury which is reflected as reduced sensory and motor amplitudes in addition to axonal changes in the thenar muscles. F-wave latency is usually delayed due to conduction delay in the distal nerve segment. In some instances, the routine median nerve conduction studies are normal despite the highly suggestive clinical picture. In such cases, the abnormalities may appear in other tests like inching, mid-palmar stimulation, median-versus-radial, and median-versus-ulnar sensory comparison studies.

In contrast to carpal tunnel syndrome, many patients with ulnar neuropathy at the elbow present with motor symptoms rather than sensory symptoms. The neuropathic pain and the sensory symptoms when present involve the little and ring fingers. The electrodiagnostic hallmark of ulnar neuropathy at the elbow is focal conduction block and/or focal slowing across the elbow. However, in many cases nerve conduction studies reveal diffuse axonal lesion without any localizing features. Such cases of non-localizing diffuse axonal ulnar neuropathy benefit from neuromuscular ultrasound which can easily identify the entrapment site.

Similar to ulnar neuropathy at the elbow, the symptoms in radial neuropathy at the axilla or the spiral groove are predominately motor. The main complaint driving the patient to seek medical advice is the wrist and/or finger drop., but it may be associated with sensory symptoms and neuropathic pain along the distribution of the superficial radial nerve. Isolated superficial radial neuropathy can occur as well and in such cases, the patient's complaint is entirely sensory in nature. Conduction block across the spiral groove is commonly found in radial neuropathy at the elbow. The nerve conduction studies in isolated superficial radial neuropathies usually reveal isolated abnormalities of the radial nerve sensory studies with normal motor nerve conduction studies. It should be noted here that although electrodiagnostic tests can diagnose isolated superficial radial neuropathy with confidence, it cannot localize the exact entrapment site. In these situations, nerve ultrasonography can help by its ability to visualize the superficial small nerves and trace them along their entire courses.

As regards lower limb entrapment, proximal fibular neuropathy causes foot drop and neuropathic pain along the distribution of the superficial fibular nerve, but pure fibular sensory neuropathy is rare. On the other hand, tarsal tunnel syndrome can present with neuropathic pain along the sole of the foot. Proximal fibular neuropathy usually manifests as conduction block proximal to the fibular head (Fig. 12.2). In contrast, axonal lesion is the most common abnormality seen in tarsal tunnel syndrome.

Polyneuropathy

The typical distal sensorimotor neuropathy like the diabetic polyneuropathy starts with sensory symptoms and neuropathic pain at the feet and/or hands. Motor weakness may eventually develop with the progression of the disease.

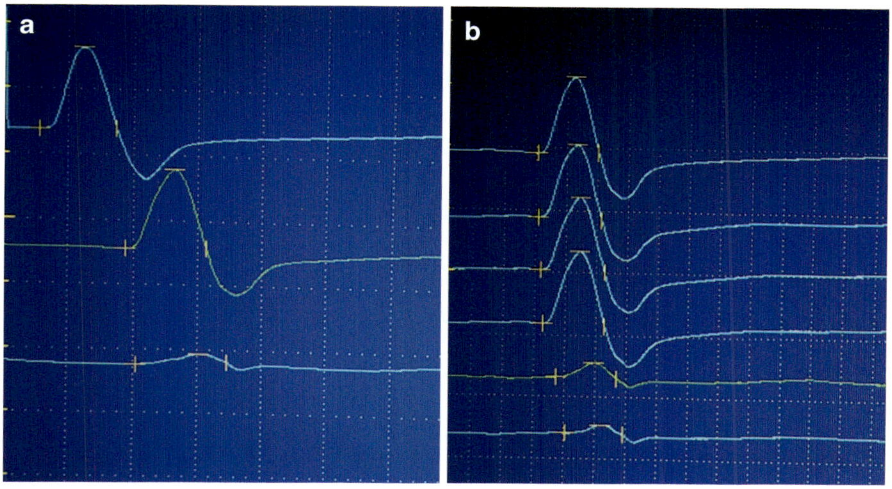

Fig. 12.2 Nerve conduction study of the right common fibular nerve in a patient presented with weak ankle dorsiflexion and evertors and neuropathic pain along the lateral leg. (**a**) motor nerve conduction study with recording from the extensor digitorum brevis showing abrupt drop in amplitude upon stimulation at the lateral popliteal fossa denoting partial conduction block and indicating proximal fibular focal neuropathy. (**b**) motor inching study localizing the conduction block at a level 1 cm proximal to the fibular head

The electrodiagnostic criteria of polyneuropathy relies on documenting symmetrical sensorimotor axonal, or demyelinating, or mixed axonal/demyelinating features in a length-dependent pattern (Fig. 12.3). Asymmetrical findings may raise the suspicion of mononeuritis multiplex or a superimposed lesion on top of the polyneuropathy.

Other polyneuropathies may present with neuropathic pain including acute inflammatory demyelinating polyneuropathy (AIDP) and its acute motor and sensory axonal neuropathy (AMSAN), a rare variant, and chronic inflammatory demyelinating polyneuropathy (CIDP). The diagnosis of AIDP or CIDP requires finding features of acquired demyelination affecting two or more nerves in the form of delayed latencies and slowing of the conduction velocities at non-entrapment sites, conduction block or temporal dispersion, and prolonged F-wave latencies [15]. In the first few weeks of AIDP, sural sparing can be seen in about half of the patients and is considered characteristic of the disease [16, 17]. A simple, graded diagnostic criteria of AIDP incorporating the sural sparing phenomena has been recently proposed [18]. On the other hand, the diagnostic criteria of AMSAN are reduced sensory amplitude <50% of the lower limit of normal and reduced motor amplitude <80% of the lower limit of normal in at least two nerves with no evidence of demyelination [19].

Sensory neuronopathy or what is known as sensory ganglionopathy are rare group of neuropathies caused by primary degeneration of dorsal root ganglion and trigeminal ganglion sensory neurons. An underlying malignancy or autoimmune

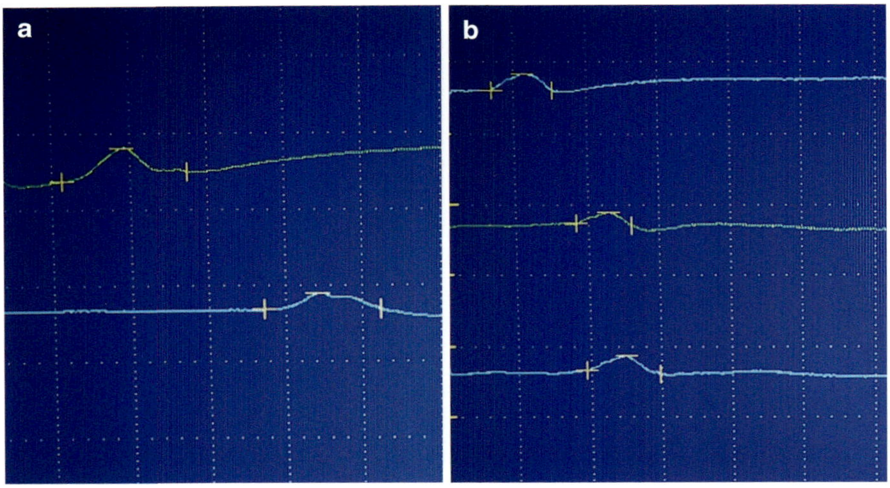

Fig. 12.3 Motor nerve conduction studies of the tibial (**a**) and common fibular nerve (**b**) showing markedly reduced amplitudes of the compound muscle action potentials in patient presented with neuropathic pain along the feet and lower legs. The findings were symmetrical and bilateral, with lost sural sensory responses denoting axonal sensorimotor polyneuropathy

disease is usually encountered in patients with these group of ganglionopathies. Sensory ataxia, positive sensory symptoms as burning sensation and allodynia, and patchy asymmetric non-length dependent sensory deficit are the classical features [20, 21]. The electrodiagnostic features include markedly reduced sensory amplitudes or absent sensory responses with normal or minimally reduced sensory conduction velocities and normal motor nerve conduction studies [22]. These findings are usually more evident in the upper limb nerves and acquire an asymmetric pattern. It is differente from the classical symmetric length-dependent pattern of the axonal sensorimotor polyneuropathies [22].

Additionally, nerve conduction studies are typically normal in small fiber neuropathy because as previously mentioned, nerve conduction studies evaluate only the large, myelinated fibers. Hence, normal nerve conduction studies in a patient with clinical picture of peripheral neuropathy should raise the suspicion of small fiber neuropathy and necessitates skin biopsy as will be discussed in one of the next sections of the chapter.

Radiculopathy and Plexopathy

Radiculopathy and plexopathies can present with neuropathic pain in addition to muscle weakness. Both are considered mimics from the electrodiagnostic point of view. Sensory nerve conduction studies and needle electromyography of the paraspinal muscles are crucial to differentiate between root and plexus lesions. In radiculopathies, the lesion is proximal to the dorsal root ganglion, thus sensory nerve conduction studies are typically normal despite the sensory symptoms and signs. In contrast, plexus or peripheral nerve lesions lead to abnormal sensory responses because the lesion is distal to the dorsal root ganglion.

The main aims of electrodiagnosis in radiculopathies and plexopathies are to localize the lesion, determine its severity and chronicity, and exclude polyneuropathy. The workup of radiculopathy and plexopathy requires extensive nerve conduction and EMG studies to localize the lesion. Electrodiagnosis of radiculopathy is best established on needle electromyography by searching for abnormalities in muscles belonging to the same myotome although innervated by different peripheral nerves. Nerve conduction studies may reveal abnormalities in multiple motor nerves innervated by same nerve root. On the other hand, plexopathies are diagnosed based on abnormalities in multiple nerves and muscles belonging to the same plexus.

Cutaneous Silent Period

Cutaneous silent period is one of the cutaneous reflexes. It refers to transient silence in voluntary muscle contraction in response to a strong electrical stimulation of a cutaneous nerve. The clinical usefulness of the reflex lies in its ability to evaluate the small-diameter A-delta nerve fibers that cannot be evaluated using the routine nerve conduction studies. The electrical stimulation of a cutaneous nerve stimulates A-delta nerve fibers and causes temporary inhibition of the voluntary muscle contraction in the muscles ipsilateral and contralateral to the stimulated side.

The technique of the test is simple and is performed using the standard Electromyography (EMG) machine. To elicit the reflex, digital nerves or cutaneous nerves are electrically stimulated while the patient maintains moderately strong and steady contraction [23]. In the upper limbs, stimulation of the fingers or superficial radial nerve evokes silent period in the thenar muscles and may spread to distal or proximal muscles. In the lower limbs, the silent period can be evoked in the soleus and tibialis posterior upon stimulation of the sural or the plantar nerves [24]. The silent period can also be evoked in the cranial muscles via stimulation of the trigeminal nerve branches. The masseter inhibitory reflex which is discussed later in the chapter is considered an inhibitory reflex and refers to the silent period that interrupts the voluntary activity of the masseter muscle in response to electrical stimulation of the mental nerve [23]. In contrast to the limb cutaneous silent period, the masseter inhibitory reflex consists of two silent periods instead of one.

The silent period can be analyzed qualitatively by visually determining its presence or absence. The duration of the inhibitory period should be at least 10 ms to be classified as cutaneous silent period. Thus, a duration of less than 10 ms is considered absent silent period [25]. The silent period can be quantitively evaluated by measuring its latency and duration. The average latencies and durations are usually used because they vary across individual traces [23].

Abnormal cutaneous silent period has been reported in some patients with Fabry disease and isolated small fiber affection [26]. However, it was insensitive in patients with mild and moderate small fiber neuropathy [27]. Prolonged latency and shortened duration of the lower limb cutaneous silent period were found in diabetic patients with clinical evidence of small fiber neuropathy and normal nerve conventional nerve conduction studies, with a sensitivity of 32.3% and specificity of 96.7% [28].

The silent period is also useful in the assessment of the syringomyelia. Absent silent period in the hand has been found in syringomyelia patients with sensory loss and complete lesion of the posterior horn of the spinal cord [29]. In addition, cutaneous silent period may help in differentiating between radiculopathy and myelopathy and between severe radiculopathy and root avulsion. It is typically normal in radiculopathy due to preservation of the A-delta fibers [30] while it becomes abnormal in myelopathy and in complete nerve root avulsion [31]. Moreover, delayed silent periods with normal duration have been reported in fibromyalgia which may be attributed to central dysfunction or small fiber dysfunction [32, 33].

Of note, despite the reported abnormalities in cutaneous silent period in the previously mentioned disorders, no difference in silent periods was found between patients with or without pain in carpal tunnel syndrome and polyneuropathies [34, 35].

Somatosensory Evoked Potentials

Somatosensory evoked potentials (SEPs) are potentials evoked in response to sensory nerve stimulation. The test is mediated by the dorsal column namely gracile and cuneate tracts. Similar to the nerve conduction studies, somatosensory evoked potentials assess only the non-nociceptive system particularly the large-diameter, myelinated A-beta fibers and the dorsal-leminscal system, but they do not give any clue on the functional status of the spinothalamic system or the small nerve fibers.

The test is performed by direct electrical stimulation of a mixed or purely sensory nerve. The evoked potentials can be recorded from multiple levels along the nervous system including peripheral nerve, spinal cord, and cortex [36]. The ideal theoretical approach is to stimulate purely sensory nerves like the digital nerves, sural, superficial peroneal, saphenous, or lateral femoral cutaneous nerve of the thigh. However, this approach is not practical because it usually does not elicit a satisfactory waveform. Instead, stimulation of mixed nerves including median, ulnar, tibial, or fibular nerves is the commonly used approach in clinical practice. Mixed nerve stimulation activates group Ia muscle afferent as well as cutaneous group II afferents [37]. Recording from the peripheral nerve ensures integrity of the peripheral part of the somatosensory pathway. Spinal cord recordings reflect conduction along the spinal cord, and cortical recordings reflect the projection of the ascending afferent signal to the cortex after it passes the relay nuclie [38]. The value of the SEP test lies in its ability to localize the lesion to a certain level of the nervous system, but it cannot definitely determine a specific diagnosis. Also, a normal SEP study does not exclude presence of an organic disease. The upper limb somatosensory evoked potential is commonly obtained by stimulation of the median nerve at the wrist and recording from the Erb's point, cervical spinous processes, and cortex including parietal and frontal scalp regions [36]. The lower limb somatosensory evoked potential is obtained by tibial or common fibular nerve stimulation and simultaneous recording from the nerve at the popliteal fossa level, lumbar or thoracic spinous processes, and cortex [36]. The evoked waveform varies in configuration according to the studied limb and the recording level. The waveforms are analyzed as regards latency, amplitude, and interpeak intervals. Side-to-side comparison can be helpful especially when absolute parameters are borderline. The latency is the most important and sensitive parameter to analyze while the amplitude of the SEP waveform is not used as a criterion of abnormalities given its high variability [38]. Rather, side-to-side comparison of the amplitude can be more useful to detect axonal lesion. A side-to-side difference in amplitude >50% can be considered abnormal [38].

The SEP abnormalities may take the form of absent response, delayed latency, increased central conduction time, or significant side-to-side difference in amplitude. Delayed latency reflects demyelinating lesion, while absent response or reduced amplitude in the presence of a normal latency reflects axonal lesion.

The clinical diagnostic uses of the somatosensory evoked potentials as recommended by the International Federation of Clinical Neurophysiology (IFCN) include multiple sclerosis, transverse myelitis, and spinal cord injuries [36]. It may also be indicated in brain injury or stroke.

In multiple sclerosis, SEPs can identify clinically silent lesions in patients with vague symptoms or when imaging tools are not available or normal. The most common abnormalities are delayed cortical potentials with leg stimulation and increased central conduction time. Absent cortical potential with normal cervical and lumbar potentials suggests a lesion proximal to the cervical spines [38]. In addition, SEP can be used to monitor disease progression or treatment efficacy. However, several pitfalls exist. A deterioration in SEP over time does not necessarily denote new lesions. Also, SEP may change despite stable clinical status [36]. Given these pitfalls, the IFCN does not recommend the use of SEP to follow up patients with definite multiple sclerosis [36].

In transverse myelitis and spinal cord injuries, SEPs can determine the degree of cord dysfunction and can be used to determine prognosis and to predict recovery (Fig. 12.4). A preserved or an improving response post-injury is indicative of good prognosis [38].

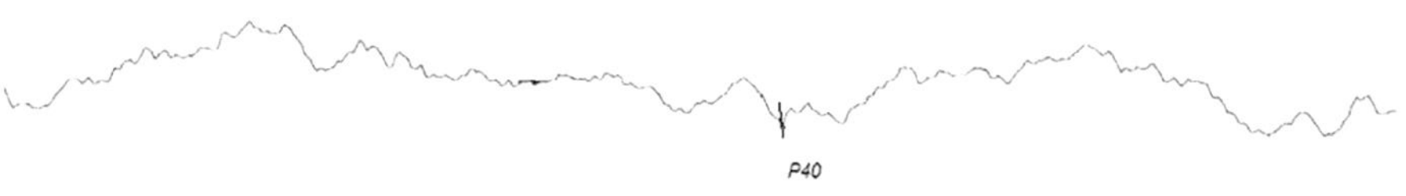

Fig. 12.4 Delayed latency of the tibial nerve somatosensory evoked potential in a patient with partial spinal cord injury.

In peripheral nerve disorders, SEP can be used to assess the proximal segments of the peripheral nerves as in Guillian Barre syndrome or meralgia paresthetica [39]. In meralgia paresthetica, the diagnostic value of dermatomal somatosensory evoked potential was found to be superior to the routine sensory nerve conduction study of the lateral femoral cutaneous nerve of thigh [40].

SEPs have also been used to evaluate brachial plexopathies including the thoracic outlet syndrome, but nerve conduction and electromyography studies are more informative in these disorders. Furthermore, the value of SEPs in radiculopathies is limited. In mono-radiculopathies, mixed nerve SEP is commonly normal because the abnormality of a single root is masked by other healthy roots. Stimulation of pure sensory nerves or specific dermatomes (dermatomal SEP) may be of more help in radiculopathies, but they are difficult to interpret, and their sensitivity and specificity are low [36, 39].

One type of somatosensory evoked potentials is the trigeminal somatosensory evoked potential which evaluates the conduction along the trigeminal pathway from the peripheral to the somatosensory cortex. Tongue somatosensory evoked potential is a variant of trigeminal somatosensory evoked potentials Somatosensory evoked potentials (SEPs) Neurophysiological testssomatosensory evoked potentials (SEPs) Neuropathic painneurophysiological testssomatosensory evoked potentials (SEPs) that was found to be affected in patients with multiple sclerosis and deteriorates with the progression of the disease [41].

Similar to nerve conduction studies, SEP is unable to evaluate the small nerve fibers. The test is also technically demanding which limits its utility in clinical practice.

Laser Evoked Potentials

Laser evoked potentials refer to cortical potentials evoked in response to laser radiant heat pulses. It is considered the most reliable tool to evaluate the nociceptive pathway according to the guidelines of the EFNS [10]. Similarly, the IFCN recommends the laser evoked potential as an assessment tool for neuropathic pain [36]. Laser stimulation delivers radiant-heat pulses that selectively activate A-delta and C fibers. The most commonly used stimulator is CO_2 laser stimulator. The technique involves stimulation of skin areas or dermatomes while recording from the cortex namely the Cz point using silver disc electrodes that are referenced to linked ear lobes. However, the IFCN recommends the use of four recording electrodes [36]. The common stimulation sites include the perioral area in the face, dorsum of the hand, and dorsum of the foot but stimulation of cervical or thoracic territories can be utilized especially in post-heretic neuralgia as it commonly affects the proximal dermatomes. Although laser stimulation activates both A-delta and C fibers, the evoked cortical response entirely represents A-delta fiber activation [42]. Isolated C fiber stimulation requires suppression of the A delta component and modification of the technique. The test is usually well-tolerated by the patients and may cause only minimal redness or skin pigmentation at the stimulation site.

The resultant waveform consists of a negative component followed by a positive component known as N2-P2 complex. The perceptive threshold, latency of each component, and peak-to-peak amplitude of the resultant waveforms are analyzed. The latency of the recorded complex varies according to the stimulation site. Variable reference values of laser evoked potentials have been reported [36, 43]. To use the published reference values in clinical practice, the stimulation technique used in the reference study should be followed and the latency should be adjusted for height. An abnormal test may take the form of an absent waveform, delayed latency, or reduced amplitude. Similar to the somatosensory evoked potentials, absolute values of the amplitude are highly variable among individuals [43]. Therefore, an abnormal amplitude can only be determined through side-to-side comparison.

Laser evoked potentials can be used to evaluate peripheral and central neuropathic pain and can differentiate between neuropathic and non-neuropathic or psychogenic pain [44]. Reduced amplitude or absent waveform have been reported in post-herpetic neuralgia, radiculopathy, diabetic polyneuropathy, and Fabry's disease reflecting axonal lesion [45, 46]. The test can be more sensitive than the SEP and the dermatomal SEPs in post-herpetic neuralgia or radiculopathy because it depends on the stimulation of the thin A-delta fibers that do not overlap to the same extent as the thick myelinated fibers [42–45].

Laser evoked potentials can also be used to evaluate patients with trigeminal neuralgia, trigeminal neuropathy, and Wallenberg syndrome. The potentials can be evoked by supraorbital, upper lip, or lower lip stimulation while recording from the vertex [47]. An abnormal laser evoked potential denotes trigeminal system dysfunction, but a normal test does not exclude trigeminal neuralgia [47]. Of note, the trigeminal laser evoked potentials cannot evaluate the A-beta fibers that are typically damaged by structural lesions like skull base tumors.

Laser evoked potentials not only has a diagnostic role in neuropathic pain, but it allows understanding of pain mechanisms [48] and can also be used to determine the sensory profile of the patients complaining of neuropathic pain [49]. Interestingly, suppression of the laser evoked potentials is observed in cases of ongoing pain, while partial preservation of the potentials is observed in patients with provoked pain including allodynia and hyperalgesia. Thus, laser evoked potentials may have a role in providing optimum treatment by designing the treatment plan according to the sensory profile [49].

The main limitations of the laser evoked potential are its inability to localize the level of the lesion in the nociceptive pathway, and the expensive cost of the laser stimulators.

Contact-heat evoked potentials and pain-related evoked could be of use in neuropathic pain, but their validity and diagnostic accuracy are not yet clear. Additional techniques like direct intraepidermal electrical stimulation to selectively activate A-delta fibers may be helpful in the future [50].

Trigeminal Reflexes

The diagnosis of trigeminal neuralgia is primarily a clinical one. However, several neurophysiological tests can help in the assessment of trigeminal neuralgia especially when secondary causes are suspected including post-herpetic neuralgia, suspected vascular malformations, and cerebellopontine angle tumors. The two most commonly used tests are the blink reflex, the jaw reflex, and the masseter inhibitory reflex.

The blink reflex is a true reflex which has an afferent and efferent. The afferent of the reflex is mediated by the ophthalmic branch of the trigeminal nerve and the efferent is mediated by the facial nerve. The test involves stimulation of the supraorbital branch of the ophthalmic division of the trigeminal nerve while recording from the lower mid-portion of the orbicularis oculi. The resultant responses consist of an early ipsilateral R1, and late ipsilateral R2 and contralateral R2 responses. The responses are analyzed as regards absolute latencies and side-to-side difference in latencies. R1, ipsilateral R2 and contralateral R2 latencies should be less than 13 ms, 41 ms, and 44 ms, respectively [51]. Side-to-side difference in R1, ipsilateral R2, and contralateral R2 latencies should be <1.5 ms, 5 ms, and 7 ms respectively [51]. Peripheral lesion of the trigeminal nerve affects R1 more than R2 latency. In contrast, central medullary lesion affecting the trigeminal sensory system as in multiple sclerosis and cerebellopontine angle tumors usually cause delay in R2 latency with normal R1 latency [51].

The Jaw reflex is another brain stem reflex. Its afferents are mediated by type Ia fibers from the muscle spindles of the masseter muscles. The reflex is elicited by taping the patient's chin with a reflex hammer while simultaneously recording electromyographic activity from the two masseter muscles using surface electrodes or small concentric needle electrode [52]. The latency is the most useful parameter, and it ranges from 5 to 10 ms with a mean of 6.8 ms [53].

The masseter inhibitory reflex refers to reflex inhibition of the jaw closing muscles that typically appears as two electrical silent periods during voluntary contraction of the jaw-closing muscles. Similar to jaw reflex, surface electrodes or needle electrodes are used to record the EMG activity of the masseter muscle. The reflex is elicited by electrical stimulation of the mental nerve while the patient clenches the teeth to produce a full interference pattern. The reflex consists of an early SP1 and late SP2 silent periods interrupting the voluntary electromyographic activity of the masseter muscle. SP1 latency ranges from 10 to 15 ms, and SP2 latency ranges from 40 to 50 ms. A side-to-side difference in SP1 latency >2 ms and in SP2 latency >6 ms is considered abnormal [52].

The R1 blink reflex and the SP1 masseter inhibitory period are the most sensitive parameters in symptomatic trigeminal pain [47]. The trigeminal reflexes are typically normal in patients with idiopathic or classical trigeminal neuralgia. Abnormal reflexes usually implicate structural causes of the neuralgia and may necessitate further investigations to rule out conditions that require surgical interference. In trigeminal neuropathy, blink reflex becomes abnormal if the supraorbital branch or the ophthalmic division is affected while the masseter inhibitory reflex becomes abnormal if the mental branch or the infraorbital branch is affected [52].

Similar to nerve conduction studies and somatosensory evoked potentials, trigeminal reflexes evaluate only the large non-nociceptive afferent fibers.

Microneurography

Microneurography is a test in which individual action potentials are recorded from single fibers allowing quantification of spontaneous activity from nociceptive fibers [54]. It is considered the only tool than can record and quantify positive sensory signs that are either mediated by large-myelinated fibres like tactile paresthesia and dysesthesias or those mediated by small-myelinated and unmyelinated fibres like spontaneous pains [55].

Microneurography is a minimally invasive and safe technique. However, the test is mainly used in research projects rather than in clinical practice because it is technically demanding, time consuming, and requires experienced examiner and cooperative patient.

Microstructure Testing

Tests that evaluate nerve microstructure are valuable tools in the diagnostic workup of neuropathic pain. These tests include skin biopsy and nerve biopsy. Skin biopsy allows the evaluation of epidermal nerve fibers and nerve biopsy allows the microscopic evaluation of a nerve sample. Skin biopsy has gained great attention in the past years and has now become an important integral tool in many centers around the world to diagnose peripheral nerve disorders especially small fiber neuropathy. On the other hand, utility of nerve biopsy has declined throughout the last years because of the increased availability of genetic testing, the increased utility of skin biopsy, and the emergence of non-invasive nerve imaging tools. However, nerve biopsy is still indicated and indispensable in specific situations as will be discussed in the next section.

Skin Biopsy

Skin punch biopsy is currently considered the most specific and sensitive test to diagnose small fiber neuropathy and has now become a standard in the diagnostic workup of small fiber neuropathy based on the recommendations of the European Federation of Neurological Societies and the Peripheral Nerve Society (Level A Recommendation) [56]. Skin biopsy may change the diagnosis and/or the management in about 50 % of the patients suspected of having small fiber neuropathy [57].

Skin biopsy was found to be of higher diagnostic utility than the quantitative sensory testing which is considered a relatively subjective test [56, 58]. Nevertheless, combining more than one diagnostic test may further increase the diagnostic yield of small fiber neuropathy. Combined use of skin biopsy, quantitative sensory testing, laser evoked potential, and electrochemical skin conductance yielded a sensitivity of 90%, a specificity of 87%, a positive predictive value of 90%, and a negative predictive value of 91% [59].

Small fiber neuropathy selectively involves the small, myelinated A-delta and unmyelinated C-fibers with sparing of the large and myelinated fibers. Thus, the motor and sensory nerve conduction studies are typically normal in such disorder. Based on this fact, skin biopsy should be performed for any patient having peripheral sensory symptoms and signs of unknown etiology and normal nerve conduction studies.

Unlike nerve biopsy, skin biopsy is considered a minimally invasive and safe procedure. It can be performed in an outpatient clinic where only topical anaesthesia is required, and does not need suture. The test has several advantages: It can be performed anywhere on the body and can be repeated over time to follow up the disease progression and treatment effect. The adverse effects of the test are minimal. It may cause minimal discomfort, limited local infection or minimal bleeding at the site of punch biopsy [56].

The technique involves obtaining a 3 mm circular punch skin biopsy from either proximal thigh, distal thigh or distal calf which is then processed for immunohistochemical staining with antibodies against protein gene product 9.5. followed by counting the epidermal nerve fibers per linear measurement to determine the density of epidermal nerve fibers. Normal reference values of epidermal nerve fiber density at the distal leg pooled from eight labs are available and valid to be used in clinical practice [60]. Each lab can set its own reference values as well. Decreased density of epidermal nerve fibers compared to the published reference values or the normative data of each lab is diagnostic for small fiber neuropathy. Of note, the reduced epidermal fiber density does not correlate with neuropathic pain intensity [56].

Skin biopsy allows the identification of small fiber involvement in various disorders including metabolic, toxic, immune-mediated, and endocrine disorders [61]. Interestingly, involvement of small fibers diagnosed via skin biopsy has been reported in fibromyalgia [62, 63], a disease which was primarily thought to be caused by dysfunction in central pain processing mechanisms. Abnormal skin biopsy in fibromyalgia patients implicate a peripheral element in its pathogenesis and changes the diagnostic and therapeutic approaches for such challenging disorder [64].

Obtaining the biopsy from the distal leg is the common approach but obtaining the biopsy from both distal and proximal sites and calculating the leg: thigh intraepidermal nerve-fiber density ratio was found to be a useful parameter to discriminate between length-dependent small-fiber neuropathy and small-fiber sensory ganglionopathy [65]. In small fiber neuropathy, the leg: thigh intraepidermal nerve fiber density ratio decreases due to preferential loss of nerve fibers distally, while in sensory ganglionopathy, the nerve fiber loss occurs proximally and distally in a balanced pattern [65].

Intraepidermal nerve fibers can also be quantified from a skin blister sample obtained by applying a suction capsule to the skin [66]. This technique is totally painless and give results comparable to skin biopsy [67], but it does not allow the assessment of dermal and sweat gland nerve fibers [56]. Also, its reliability in small fiber neuropathy has not been established yet.

Parameters other than the intraepidermal fiber density may yield useful information. These include intraepidermal nerve fiber swelling, subdermal nerve plexus density, hair follicles, sweat glands, and microcirculation. Intraepidermal nerve fiber swelling may predict the progression of neuropathy [68, 69]. Subepidermal nerve plexus density was found to be highly sensitive and specific for the diagnosis of painful sensory neuropathies especially if large diameter fibers are involved [70]. Vessel densities and neurovascular densities were reported to be lower in diabetic patients compared to controls [71]. Unlike the routine skin biopsy that requires only 3 mm punch biopsy to calculate the intraepidermal nerve fiber density, evaluation of sweat glands, hair follicles, and arterio-venous anastomosis requires a 6–8 mm skin biopsy [56].

As mentioned earlier, skin biopsy is considered the most specific test for small fiber neuropathy, but the clinicians are advised to use a combination of clinical, electrodiagnostic and structural parameters. Reliable diagnosis of small fiber neuropathy depends on reporting clinical symptoms and signs suggestive of involvement of small nerve fibers, non-involvement of large diameter nerve fibers evidenced by normal nerve conduction studies, and low intraepidermal nerve fiber density in skin biopsy [72, 73]. The interested reader can also refer to the diagnostic criteria of small fiber neuropathy and the grading system in diabetic patients that had been previously proposed [11, 74].

Although skin biopsy is primarily indicated for cases with suspected small fiber neuropathy, it can yield useful information in large-fiber peripheral neuropathies as well. It allows the assessment of the most distal sensory receptors and their myelinated fibers which can be affected early on in length-dependent neuropathies [61] and sheds the light on the morphological and pathological changes that occur in hereditary and acquired polyneuropathies through the analysis of the dermal myelinated fibers and their receptors, and nodal/extranodal architecture [61]. It also allows the detection of small fiber involvement in large-fiber neuropathies. Moreover, the EFNS provided Level B recommendation for the utility of skin biopsy and intraepidermal nerve fiber density in the assessment of the rate of sensory axon regeneration in peripheral neuropathies [58].

The main limitations of the skin biopsy are its inability to determine the exact cause of small fiber neuropathy and low availability in diagnostic centers.

Nerve Biopsy

Most of the patients with neuropathic pain do not require nerve biopsy because they are usually diagnosed via the initial workup that includes electrophysiological, laboratory, and/or genetic testing. Further, the emergence of the less-invasive skin biopsy and the non-invasive magnetic resonance neurography and nerve ultrasound limited the utility of nerve biopsy in recent years. Despite this trend, nerve biopsy is still indicated in certain cases [75]. The most important indications of nerve biopsy include rapidly progressive neuropathy, mononeuritis multiplex, atypical neuropathy like atypical chronic inflammatory demyelinating polyneuropathy, nerve/nerve sheath tumors, suspected vasculitic, pure leprotic, sarcoid, and amyloid neuropathies [76, 77]. The value of nerve biopsy emerges when other diagnostic tests of these disorders are negative. On the other hand, evidence-based review by multiple societies found no evidence supporting the role of nerve biopsy in defining the cause of distal symmetric polyneuropathies [76]. Hence, the decision to perform nerve biopsy should be based on case-by-case discussion. The reader can also refer to the practical flow chart provided by Nathani et al in 2021 which can be helpful to decide the need for nerve biopsy [77].

Since we are in the era of genetic analysis, nerve biopsy is not routinely indicated in suspected hereditary neuropathies as Charcot-Marie Tooth Syndrome because combined data from the family history, clinical examination, electrophysiological studies, and genetic analysis can usually confirm the disease. However, nerve biopsy can be useful in sporadic or familial cases when electrophysiological and genetic tests fail to confirm the diagnosis [78].

Nerve biopsy is usually obtained from the sural nerve, but it can be obtained from the superficial fibular nerve or the superficial radial nerve if the symptoms predominately involve the upper limbs. The obtained biopsy is assessed for inflammatory and vascular changes, amyloid deposition, alterations in axonal density and the Schwann cell-myelin-axon unit [79].

Inflammatory changes are commonly observed in (1) infectious neuropathy like leprotic neuropathy, HIV-induced, and cytomegalovirus-induced neuropathy (2) autoimmune neuropathies like those associated with lupus, rheumatoid arthritis, systemic sclerosis, and sarcoidosis. Vascular changes in the peripheral nerves can be found in different vasculitic disorders including systemic vasculitis, non-systemic vasculitic neuropathy, vasculitis associated with connective tissue diseases, or vasculitis secondary to other causes like malignancy [79]. The clinician can use the guidelines developed by the Peripheral Nerve Society for the diagnosis of non-systemic vasculitic neuropathy [80]. These guidelines include classification of vasculitic neuropathy into pathologically definite and pathologically probable based on nerve biopsy findings, definition of clinically probable vasculitic neuropathy, and the exclusion criteria of non-systemic vasculitic neuropathy. A suggested approach to improve the diagnostic accuracy of vasculitic neuropathy is to include muscle or skin biopsy with the nerve biopsy. Combined superficial peroneal nerve/peroneus brevis biopsy may improve the diagnostic yield of vasculitis [81]. However, the combined sural nerve/vastus lateralis biopsy was not found to be of added value [82]. Adding full thickness skin biopsy to nerve biopsy may also increase the diagnostic yield of vasculitic neuropathy through the identification of perivascular mononuclear inflammation [77].

Nerve biopsy can provide definite diagnosis of pure neuritic leprosy. In lepromatous leprosy, the diagnosis depends In finding acid-fast lepra bacilli within Schwann cells. On the other hand, tuberculoid leprosy is characterized by epithelioid granulomas, endoneurial inflammation with or without necrosis, and low bacillary load [83].

The biopsy findings in hereditary polyneuropathies vary with the polyneuropathy subtype. Axonal loss is seen in axonal hereditary polyneuropathies while demyelinating variants are characterized by onion-bulb formation and segmental demyelination [79]. However, onion-bulb formation can be seen also in other demyelinating non-inherited polyneuropathies like chronic inflammatory demyelinating polyneuropathies. In contrast, hereditary polyneuropathy with liability to pressure palsy is associated with areas of thickened myelin sheath and sausage-like swellings known as tomacula [79].

The main limitations of nerve biopsy are its invasive nature, high cost, and risk of complications like persistent sensory loss, chronic pain, or formation of neuroma [84, 85]. As noted earlier, the emergence of other less invasive and non-invasive diagnostic tools like skin biopsy, nerve ultrasonography, and magnetic resonance neurography has limited the utility of nerve biopsy in recent years.

Neuroimaging

A full overview of every imaging tool that can be used in the diagnostic workup of neuropathic pain is beyond the aim of this chapter because the choice of the imaging tool is case-dependent. So, the following section focuses on the three emerging and promising imaging tools: functional neuroimaging, neuromuscular ultrasound, and magnetic resonance neurography (MR neurography).

The role and the indications of the classical imaging tools like computed tomography (CT) and magnetic resonance imaging (MRI) are well known to the clinicians. Generally speaking, brain CT and MRI are helpful if central causes like multiple sclerosis, post stroke pain, or lateral medullary lesions are suspected. While spinal CT and MRI are useful in suspected spinal cord lesions, disc-related disorders, tumors, or syringomyelia. Brain MRI can also be useful in trigeminal neuralgia. It is mainly indicated when cerebral structural lesions are suspected. However, imaging may be needed even in primary idiopathic cases to detect vascular compression. Magnetic resonance tomographic angiography was found to highly sensitive and specific for the detection of this vascular compression [86].

The aforementioned imaging tools provide excellent anatomical information but depending on them as sole diagnostic tools is not the ideal approach because concomitant functional assessment is usually needed in most of the cases. Moreover, finding a structural lesion does not necessarily mean that it truly caused the neuropathic pain [87, 88].

Functional Neuroimaging

Functional neuroimaging tools include positron emission tomography (PET), single photon emission computed tomography (SPECT), and functional MRI. (fMRI). The value of functional neuroimaging as a diagnostic tool in neuropathic pain is not clearly known. However, the tools can help us understand the pathophysiological brain changes underlying neuropathic pain. These tools allowed the identification of the 'pain matrix' (network of brain areas) involved in pain reception, the exploration of various changes in brain region activity, and the cerebral blood flow in response to pain, and response to treatment [89]. For example, decreased resting cerebral blood flow activity was observed in spontaneous neuropathic pain with improvement of blood flow post treatment [90]. On the other hand, provoked neuropathic pain has been found associated with increased activity in the thalamic, insular, and somatosensory regions [91].

Functional neuroimaging has been used to investigate diabetic neuropathy, complex regional pain syndrome, syringomyelia, spinal cord injury, trigeminal neuropathy, and trigeminal neuralgia [92–97]. Diffusion tensor imaging has been also used to study neuropathic pain. Various changes in diffusivity have been reported in brain ischemia, multiple sclerosis, traumatic nerve injury, and brain tumors [98]. Moreover, several studies have demonstrated the ability of functional neuroimaging to detect brain changes in response to various drug treatment, motor cortex stimulation, and spinal cord stimulation [99–101].

Further validation of these results related to neuroimaging and standardization of the examination protocols in the future will allow confident integration of functional neuroimaging in the diagnostic workup of neuropathic pain.

Neuromuscular Ultrasound

Neuromuscular ultrasound has become a valuable diagnostic tool for the assessment of various neuromuscular disorders and thus can play a crucial role in the diagnostic workup of neuropathic pain. Nerve ultrasonography complements the electrodiagnostic tests and allows structural assessment of nerves and muscles.

The power of ultrasound lies in its integration with electrodiagnosis inside the EMG labs. Such integration facilitates clinical-electrophysiological-sonographic correlation which is mandatory for accurate diagnosis. Nerve ultrasonography is commonly performed after performing the electrodiagnostic tests. However, the clinician may need to perform extra electrodiagnostic tests based on sonographic findings. In other instances, ultrasound may be performed prior to the electrodiagnostic testing as a screening test. Thus, setting the ultrasound machine inside EMG labs, hand-to-hand with the electrodiagnostic machine is the best approach to allow the modification of the diagnostic workup. The low cost of ultrasound, its wide availability, dynamic ability enabled its easy integration in many EMG labs around the world

Ultrasound allows tracing of the entire course of almost all peripheral nerves including nerve branches and small nerves given its high spatial resolution. In the axial view, the healthy nerve appears as an oval or rounded honeycomb structure composed of hypoechoic dots representing nerve fascicles, embedded in a hyperechoic background representing the interfascicular connective tissue. In the longitudinal view, the nerve takes a cable-like appearance consisting of hypoechoic bundles alternating with hyperechoic thin bands.

The sonographic parameters that are usually assessed include nerve size, echotexture, mobility, and vascularity. By far, the most important parameter is the nerve cross-sectional area measured in the transverse view. The sonographic pathological signs include nerve enlargement which could be focal or diffuse, nerve atrophy, echotexture alteration, abnormal mobility, or nerve hypervascularity. It is important to note that these abnormalities are not specific. and they represent reactions to any nerve disorder. Therefore, analysis of the pattern and distribution of these abnormalities is of paramount importance to relate the abnormalities to a specific disorder.

The application domains of nerve ultrasonography are numerous and expands every day. These include but not limited to entrapment neuropathies, traumatic peripheral nerve injuries, and generalized nerve and muscle disorders [102].

Nerve ultrasonography has currently become routine in the diagnostic workup of entrapment neuropathies. Its value has been reported in carpal tunnel syndrome, ulnar neuropathy at the elbow, radial neuropathy, fibular neuropathy, tarsal tunnel syndrome, and even in rare entrapment of small sensory nerves like focal sural, superficial fibular, and superficial radial neuropathies [103–114].

Nerve ultrasound has numerous values in focal mononeuropathies. It contributes significant structural information that impact the diagnosis and management in more than third of the patients presented with mononeuropathy [115]. Nerve ultrasonography can diagnose entrapment neuropathies when the electrodiagnostic tests are non-localizing [116–118] (Fig. 12.5) and can further refine the entrapment site in cases confirmed by electrodiagnosis. For instance, ultrasound can determine the exact site of nerve entrapment in ulnar neuropathy at the elbow and whether it occurs at the cubital tunnel proper, ulnar groove, or at the supracondylar level. Additionally, ultrasound may reveal structural causes of neuropathic pain like ganglion, tenosynovitis, tendinitis, or soft tissue masses [119–121]. Further, it can detect anatomic variants that may predispose the patient to entrapment neuropathies or may itself cause neuropathic pain [122–125] (Fig. 12.6). Ultrasound may also diagnose causes of postoperative neuropathic pain like nerve encasement by scar tissue or iatrogenic injuries post nerve release (Figs. 12.7 and 12.8). Moreover, muscle ultrasound complements nerve ultrasound the same way needle electromyography complements nerve conduction studies. It detects muscle atrophy and hyperechogenicity secondary to muscle denervation and can indirectly localize the lesion to specific nerves or nerve branches by observing selective muscle involvement.

The hallmark sonographic feature of local nerve entrapment is increased nerve cross-sectional area proximal to the entrapment site with nerve flattening at the compression site (notch sign). Other features may include hypoechogenicity, loss of the fascicular pattern, hyper vascularity, and/or abnormal mobility.

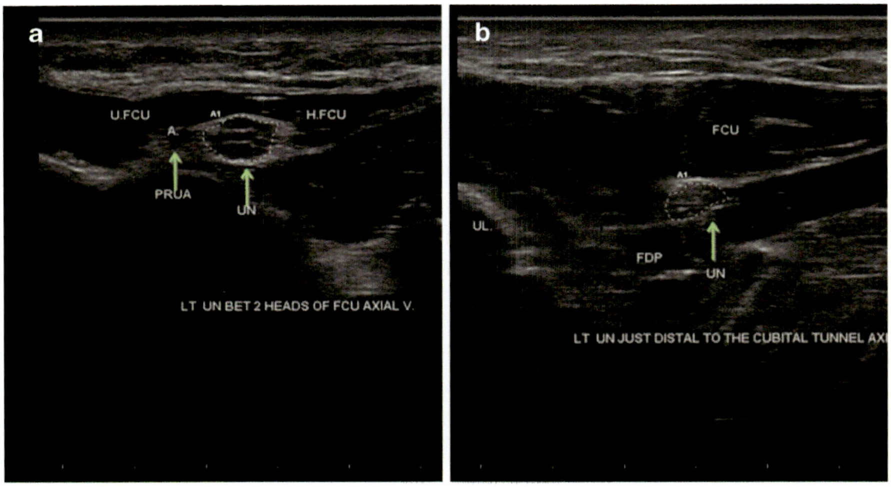

Fig. 12.5 B-mode axial views of the left ulnar nerve at the cubital tunnel proper level (**a**), and distal to it (**b**) in a patient presented with weakness of distal ulnar-innervated muscles and neuropathic pain along the little and ring fingers. Electrodiagnostic tests showed severe diffuse axonal lesion but failed to localize the lesion. In (**a**), the nerve abruptly enlarged at the cubital tunnel level with a cross-sectional area of 13 mm^2, compared to (**b**) in which nerve cross-sectional area measured 7 mm^2. Ultrasound allowed accurate localization of ulnar nerve entrapment and confirmed nerve entrapment

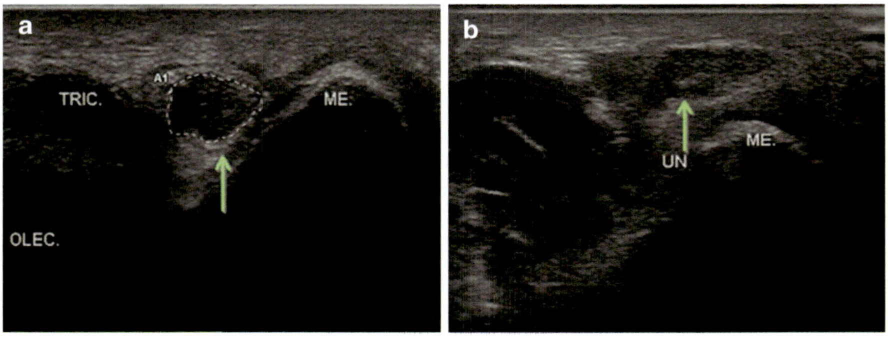

Fig. 12.6 B-mode axial image of the left ulnar nerve in a patient with ulnar neuropathy at the elbow showing ulnar nerve subluxation (**a**) shows ulnar nerve enlarged and lying behind the medial epicondyle during elbow extension. (**b**) shows nerve subluxation (arrow) during full elbow flexion (the nerve jumps on top of the medial epicondyle)

When it comes to traumatic nerve injuries, ultrasound can play a crucial role. Neuromuscular ultrasound was found to modify the diagnostic and the therapeutic approaches in 58% of the traumatic nerve injury cases [126]. It allows the assessment of nerve continuity and can differentiate between neurotemesis and axonotemesis when electrodiagnostic tests cannot in the first several weeks of the

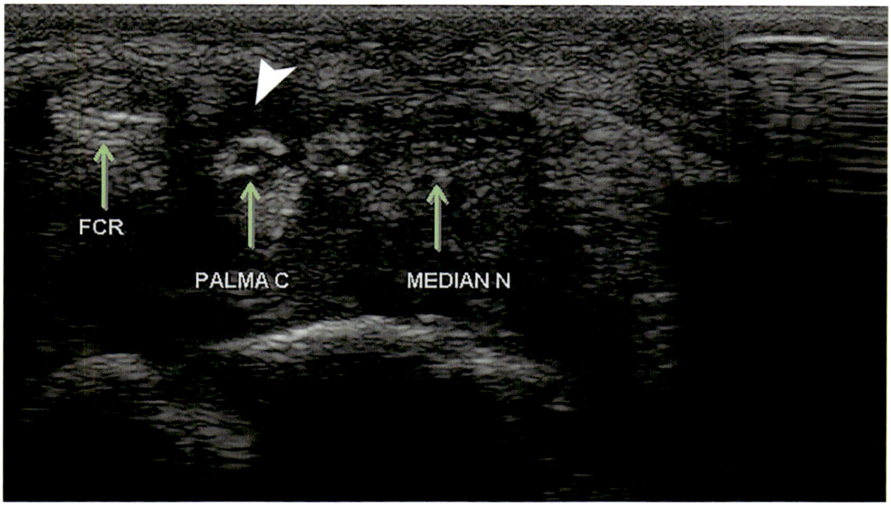

Fig. 12.7 B-mode axial image of the palmar cutaneous branch of the median nerve (Palma C in the figure) in a patient complained of neuropathic pain along the palm post-carpal tunnel release. The nerve appears encased by scar tissue (arrowhead) and its outer border is hyperechoic and thickened

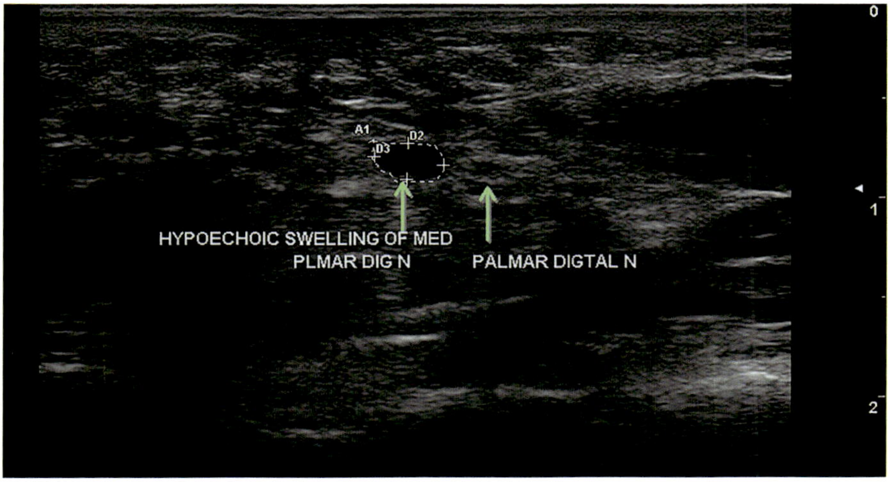

Fig. 12.8 B-mode axial image of one of the common palmar digital branches of the median nerve in a patient complaining of intense neuropathic pain and tingling along the fingers post-carpal tunnel release showing hypoechoic swelling of the medial common palmar digital nerve with positive ultrasound Tinel's sign suggestive of neuroma

trauma (Fig. 12.9). In cases of nerve discontinuity, ultraosund can determine the length of nerve gap, the position of the proximal and distal nerve stumps, and can identify stump neuroma. Such information allows optimum preoperative planning.

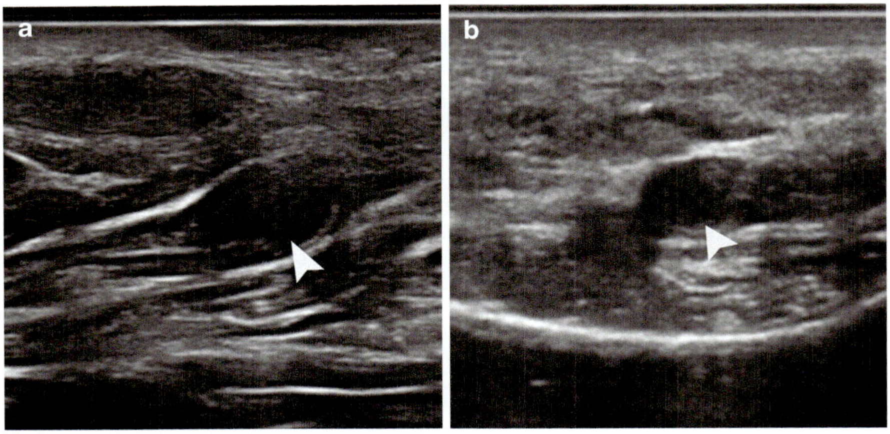

Fig. 12.9 B-mode longitudinal views of the ulnar nerve in a patient with traumatic nerve injury. Electrodiagnosis could not differentiate between axonotemesis and neurotemesis, but ultrasound revealed nerve discontinuity. (**a**) shows the proximal nerve stump and (**b**) shows the distal nerve stump (arrowheads). Nerve gap measured 4 cm

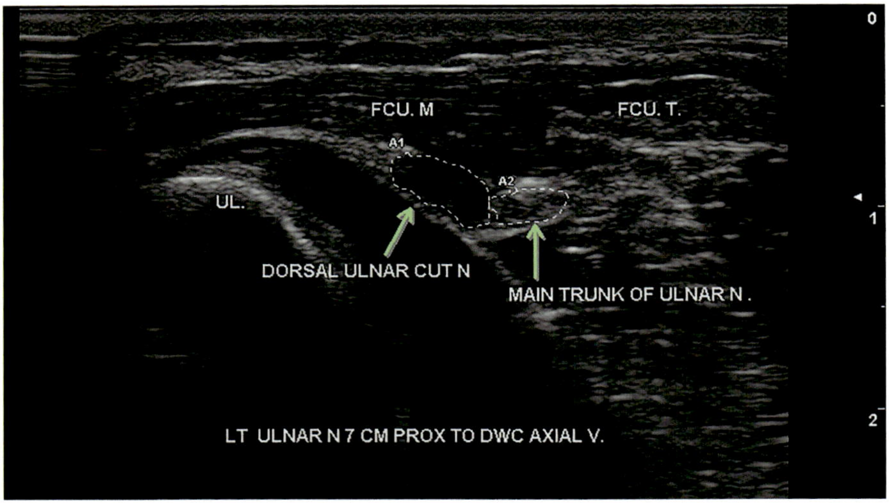

Fig. 12.10 B-mode axial image of the ulnar nerve in a patient with traumatic left ulnar nerve injury and severe neuropathic pain along the ulnar side of the palm showing abrupt enlargement and hypoechogenicity of the dorsal ulnar cutaneous branch of the ulnar nerve suggestive of neuroma. Notice the normal echotexture and size of the main trunk of the ulnar nerve

Moreover, ultrasound can accurately detect structural factors that can interfere with the reinnervation of traumatized continuous nerves like neuroma-in-continuity or scar tissue encasing the nerves (Fig. 12.10). Postoperatively, ultrasound can help determine the outcome depending on finding favorable or unfavorable sonographic findings [127].

Although brachial plexus imaging can be challenging, ultrasound can readily visualize the brachial plexus especially its supraclavicular portion, detects trunk or root enlargements, and identify structural compressive factors and traumatic neuroma or transection [128, 129]. Additionally, ultrasound can help diagnose thoracic outlet syndrome via its ability to detect compressing fibrous band and its dynamic capability which allows the detection of dynamic compression of the trunks or cords by the surrounding muscles [130, 131]. Ultrasound has proven to be of great value in brachial neuritis. It can detect nerve constriction, nerve torsion, or fascicular entwinement [132, 133]. Nerve torsion is a characteristic structural feature of brachial neuritis that necessitates surgical interference. Thus, ultrasound should be routinely performed in every case suspected of having brachial neuritis to avoid missing important anatomical information that cannot be detected via electrodiagnosis.

In addition to its value in focal mononeuropathies, nerve ultrasonography can also be used to assess patients complaining of neuropathic pain secondary to polyneuropathies. It can be used as a screening test to guide electrodiagnostic workup or other workups through pattern analysis of the sonographic abnormalities. Almost all polyneuropathies manifest as nerve enlargement, but the pattern and distribution of nerve enlargements may provide a clue to a specific type of polyneuropathy. For example, leprotic neuropathy is associated with nerve enlargements, nerve hypervascularity, and epineural thickening of the ulnar nerve [134], while diffuse and homogenous enlargements of the peripheral nerves, brachial plexus, and nerve roots have been observed in amyloidosis [135]. In vasculitic neuropathies, ultrasound may reveal focal nerve enlargements of lower limb peripheral nerves or peripheral nerves of the arm proximal to the usual entrapment sites with sparing of the brachial plexus. Thus, ultrasound may help in the differentiation between vasculitic neuropathies and axonal polyneuropathies [136, 137]. Ultrasound can also be used prior to nerve biopsy in vasculitic neuropathy to determine the affected nerve segment appropriate for biopsy [138].

Ultrasound findings in diabetic polyneuropathy are conflicting. Enlargement in nerve cross-sectional areas at entrapment and non-entrapment sites has been reported [139, 140], with normal cross-sectional areas of the peripheral nerve being reported as well [141]. The reason behind these controversial findings is not exactly known but it is generally believed that the degree of nerve enlargement is more evident in demyelinating polyneuropathy in comparison to axonal polyneuropathy [142]. Variation in the results may also be related to different inclusion criteria and clinical status of the patients enrolled in different studies.

In acquired demyelinating polyneuropathy, ultrasound shows peculiar findings. Chronic inflammatory demyelinating polyneuropathy (CIDP) is associated with multifocal peripheral nerve enlargements at non-entrapment sites, fascicular enlargements, and brachial plexus and cervical root enlargements [143–147]. AIDP (AIDP) is associated with enlargement of proximal segments of the peripheral nerves such as sural nerve, and cervical nerve roots appearing early in the course of the disease but gradually decreasing in response to treatment [148–150]. In contrast, the nerve enlargements in the AMSAN variant of AIDP predominantly affect the distal nerve segments [148]. With the development of nerve ultrasound as a diagnostic modality, ultrasound classification and scoring systems have been developed in an effort to distinguish between different nerve disorders. One example is the Bochum Ultrasound Score which can reliably differentiate between AIDP and CIDP with a sensitivity of 90% and a specificity of 94.4% and can differentiate between subacute CIDP and AIDP with a sensitivity of 80% and a specificity of 100% [151]. Such scores may facilitate future development of diagnostic criteria of different nerve disorders based on sonographic findings.

Unlike the acquired demyelinating polyneuropathies, hereditary polyneuropathy like Charcot-Marrie Tooth syndrome is characterized by diffuse symmetrical nerve enlargements and striking fascicular enlargements [152, 153]. However, hereditary polyneuropathy with liability to pressure palsies is associated with multifocal nerve enlargements commonly observed at the common entrapment sites [153–156]. This pattern distinguishes hereditary polyneuropathy with liability to pressure palsy from CIDP in which the multifocal nerve enlargements are typically observed at non-entrapment sites.

With regards to small fiber neuropathy, nerve ultrasound is not expected to have a role because the current ultraosund resolution does not allow visualization of the small nerve fibers in the skin. However, nerve ultrasound has demonstrated increased sural nerve cross-sectional area in patients with small fiber neuropathy [157]. The implication of such finding on the diagnostic approach of small fiber neuropathy is unknown and needs further investigation.

The improvement in ultrasound technology and the emergence of ultra-high frequency probes may allow detailed assessment of fascicles count, fascicle cross-sectional area, and nerve echogenicity. Interestingly, sural nerve hyperechogenicity was found to be correlated with inflammatory infiltrates on sural nerve biopsy [158]. This advancement can provide a non-invasive insight onto nerve pathology in the future.

In addition to the previously reviewed applications of nerve ultrasonography, we can benefit from ultrasound to facilitate other diagnostic tests. For instance, ultrasound can be used to guide nerve conduction studies of small nerves via pre-study nerve mapping to ensure accurate positioning of the stimulator and the recording electrodes [159]. It can also guide near-nerve stimulation of difficult nerves, or guide core needle nerve biopsy in patients with suspected peripheral nerve sheath tumors [160].

As any other diagnostic tool, nerve ultrasonography has its own limitations. Its ability to visualize deep nerves is low due to decreased resolution with increasing depth. It also cannot visualize structures deep to the bone. Moreover, ultrasound scanning of small sensory nerves can be challenging. However, it can reliably capture abnormalities of tiny sensory nerves such as lateral cutaneous nerve of the thigh, digital sensory nerves, superficial sensory ulnar branch, and superficial radial nerve even when electrodiagnostic studies are negative or technically difficult (Fig. 12.11). Other limitations of ultrasound include its dependence on the sonographer's skill, and long learning curve.

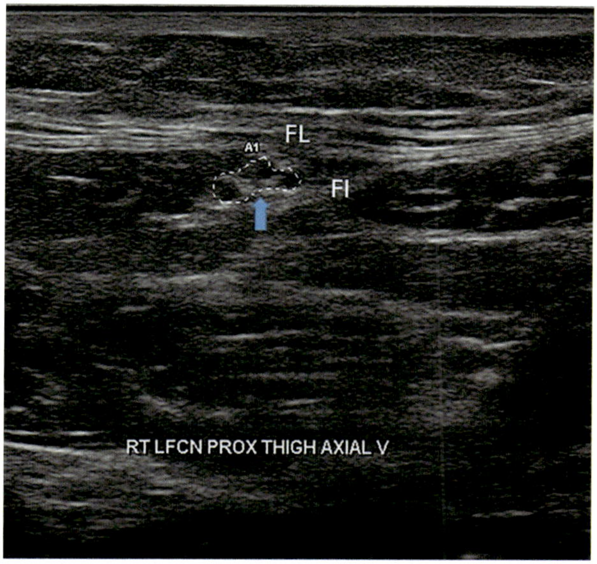

Fig. 12.11 B-mode axial image of the lateral femoral cutaneous nerve of the thigh in patient with suspected meralgia paresthetica. Nerve conduction study failed to elicit a sensory response due to obesity. Ultrasound revealed an enlargement of the nerve cross-sectional area (measured 8 mm^2 vs. 4 mm^2 on the healthy side)

Magnetic Resonance Neurography

Magnetic resonance neurography (MR neurography) simply refers to magnetic resonance imaging of the peripheral nerves. It is quite similar to the traditional MRI but depends on thin, high resolution sequences to allow visualization of the nerve signal, fascicular pattern, and perineural fat.

Similar to nerve ultrasound, MR neurography allows structural assessment of the peripheral nerves and the plexus. It can be utilized to image any nerve in the body, but it is most commonly used to assess brachial plexus, lumbosacral plexus, nerve roots, and the sciatic nerve. Although ultrasound allows visualization of the brachial plexus and the sciatic nerve, MR neurography can provide better imaging window for these structures especially the infraclavicular part of the brachial plexus and the sciatic nerve at the piriformis level because of their deep positions.

The main indications of MR neurography are brachial plexopathies, thoracic outlet syndrome, lumbosacral plexopathies, radiculopathy, piriformis syndrome, and pudendal neuropathy.

Normally, the nerve appears isointense to the muscle with uniform regular arrangement of the fascicles, straight nerve course without angulation, minimal intraepineural fat, and clear halo of perineural fat [161]. The abnormality mainly takes the form of hyperintense nerve signal and/or nerve thickening [162]. The nerve hyperintensity can be graded as mild, moderate, or severe [161]. Mild hyperintensity cannot be considered pathological because it can be seen in some nerves at certain levels along their courses due to friction or traction during activities of daily livening. Thus, it is recommended to consider only the moderate and the severe hyperintensity as pathological signs [161].

Other MR neurography signs of neuropathies include focal deviation of the nerve course, irregular nerve shape, fascicular enlargements/disruption, epineural thickening, and muscle denervation [161]. Nerve enhancement can be also abnormal and should drive the attention towards an inflammatory neuropathy, infectious neuropathy, or nerve tumor [161]. During MR neurography, the muscles can be assessed to detect muscle atrophy and/or denervation signs. MR neurography can determine the phase of muscle denervation. In acute muscle denervation, the muscle appears hyperintense [163]. In the subacute phase, the muscle signal intensity decreases and replacement of muscle fibers by fat starts. In the chronic phase, the muscle appears atrophic and may be completely replaced by fat or fibrous tissue [163]. Muscles distal to the nerve lesion are typically involved and denervation signs involving muscles innervated by a specific nerve are signs of neuropathy of that nerve [161].

The distribution of nerve abnormalities seen in MR neurography vary in different disorders. Therefore, determining the pattern of abnormalities is important. In Parsonage-Turner syndrome, the increased nerve signal and nerve thickening involve mainly the roots especially the C5 root, and it is associated with edema, fatty infiltration, and atrophy of the innervated muscles [164]. Despite these observed abnormalities, the reported sensitivity of MR neurography in brachial neuritis is relatively low ranging from 41% to 71% [165]. Thus, MR neurography can confirm the diagnosis but a normal study does not exclude brachial neuritis.

To assess the generalized nerve disorders, whole body MR based on diffusion weighted whole-body imaging with background body signal suppression is recommended. In chronic inflammatory demyelinating polyneuropathy, increased volumes of the brachial plexus, lumbar plexus, and nerve roots were observed and acquired a symmetrical pattern [166–168]. In contrast, nerve hypertrophy in multifocal acquired demyelinating sensory and motor neuropathy is multifocal and asymmetric [163]. Charcot-Marie Tooth disease is characterized by diffuse symmetrical enlargements of peripheral nerves, brachial and lumbosacral brachial plexus [163].

Moreover, MR neurography proved to be useful in the assessment of mononeuropathies like radial neuropathy, sciatic neuropathy, and fibular neuropathy allowing the detection of nerve morphological changes, injury site, and structural factors compressing the nerve [169–172].

Given the good ability of MR neurography to visualize nerve roots and plexus, it can be used to map and quantitatively evaluate compressed nerve roots or traumatized plexus prior to surgical intervention [173–175]. Further, it can determine the type of the brachial plexus lesion (pre-ganglionic versus postganglionic, root avulsion versus root continuity), and the level of the lesion (involving roots, trunk, or cords) [175]. These information helps the surgeon plan the appropriate surgical approach. Moreover, MRI neurography is superior to ultrasound in the diagnosis of neurogenic thoracic outlet syndrome. It can also reliably identify radiation-induced plexopathy and neoplastic infiltration of the plexus [176, 177].

As to the diagnostic sensitivity of MR neurography and nerve ultrasonography, the investigators reported different results. Zaidman et al found ultrasound to be of higher sensitivity than MRI in identifying abnormalities of upper limb peripheral nerve lesions (93.5% vs. 67% respectively) with ultrasound proven superiority in identifying multifocal lesions [178]. On the other hand, Aggarwal et al found MR neurography to be more sensitive than ultrasound (95.31% vs. 81.25% respectively) [179]. MR neurography was more sensitive in the detection of nerve continuity and change in nerve size, but both MR neurography and ultrasound were equally sensitive in the detection of neuroma [179]. These variation in the reported sensitivities should not hinder the utility of any of the two tools because the sensitivity of each tool is good enough to justify its use. Additionally, each tool has its own advantages and limitations. MR neurography has higher contrast resolution, allows better visualization of deeply situated nerves, plexus, and nerve roots. However, it is expensive, and is not readily available in all medical centers, time consuming, and lacks the dynamic ability. In contrast, ultrasound has higher spatial resolution allowing better visualization of nerve branches and small nerves. Ultrasound has also the advantage of being widely available, affordable, real-time, and dynamic bed side tool. The characteristic dynamic ability of ultrasound allows tracing of the nerves and assessment of nerve mobility, nerve gliding, and muscle movements. Nonetheless, ultrasound is not effective at imaging structures hidden by bone. Also beam attenuation with increased depth may impair visualization of deep nerves. Given these facts, MR neurography and nerve ultrasonography should be looked at as complementary tools, each has its own power and area of application. MR neurography is best suited for the assessment of brachial and lumbosacral plexus, nerve roots, and deeply situated nerves, while nerve ultrasonography is best suited for the superficial peripheral nerves, nerve branches, and small nerves.

The advancement in MRI techniques led to the development of functional MR neurography. Functional MR neurography is based on diffusion-weighted imaging and diffusion tensor imaging sequences. In contrast to the conventional MR neurography which only provides information about nerve morphology, functional MR neurography allows quantitative functional assessment of peripheral nerves and plexus. Functional MR neurography is promising because it provides valuable information about fiber organization, axonal flow, and myelin integrity which can help determine the degree of nerve injury [180]. Functional MR neurography have been investigated in various nerve disorders including radiculopathy, entrapment neuropathies, post carpal tunnel release, diabetic polyneuropathy, ulnar neuropathy, nerve tumors, and brachial plexopathy [181–187]. It could also be useful in the pre- and post-operative assessment of traumatic peripheral nerve and brachial plexus injuries through determining treatment, predicting the outcome, and follow up the recovery process [180, 188]. As a general rule, successful integration of the peripheral nerve imaging depends on clinical-electrophysiological-structural correlations.

In addition to the previously mentioned applications of MR neurography and functional MR neurography in adults, these tools have a diagnostic potential in children as well [189]. Further validation of these techniques in the future will help integrating them on a wide scale in adults and pediatrics.

Laboratory and Genetic Testing

The laboratory tests do not provide objective evidence of somatosensory dysfunction, but they can help identify specific causes. There is no specific laboratory panel for neuropathic pain. As a result, the laboratory tests are requested based on the clinical judgment. The list of the laboratory tests is endless. Examples of the most commonly requested tests are briefly mentioned here.

Complete blood picture, erythrocyte sedimentation rate, and C-reactive protein are considered general screening tests. Blood sugar tests and glucose tolerance tests are indicated in distal sensorimotor polyneuropathies. Thyroid function tests are helpful if thyroid diseases are suspected as the cause of polyneuropathy. Vitamin B 12 serum level is also important to exclude vitamin deficiency. Autoimmune screening may be indicated in suspected autoimmune polyneuropathies. Cerebrospinal fluid analysis is very helpful in suspected Guillian-Barre syndrome and paraneoplastic sensory ganglionopathy. In an evidence-based review, the American Association of Electrodiagnostic and Neuromuscular Medicine (AAENM) recommended the performance of screening laboratory tests for all patients with distal symmetric polyneuropathy (level C Recommendation) [190]. The same evidence-based review revealed that the tests with the highest yield of abnormalities in distal symmetric polyneuropathy include blood glucose level, serum vitamin B12 level with its metabolites, and serum protein immunofixation electrophoresis [190].

Genetic testing in clinical practice remains mainly indicated in cases of suspected hereditary polyneuropathies. However, genetics of neuropathic pain in non-hereditary neuropathies has drawn the attention of researchers in recent years. Sodium channel gene mutation has been reported in painful peripheral neuropathy [191, 192]. Moreover, recent studies have investigated the effect of genetic variants and genetic manipulation in somatosensory function and neuropathic pain [193, 194]. Further studies in this field may open the door for gene therapies for neuropathic pain.

Other Tests

Tests that assess the sudomotor function like the sympathetic skin response and quantitative sudomotor axon reflex can be utilized with the previously discussed tests if neuropathic pain is associated with autonomic symptoms as in diabetic polyneuropathy and small fiber neuropathy. Corneal confocal microscopy is another evolving test that could be of value in early diagnosis of diabetic sensorimotor polyneuropathy. These three tests are briefly highlighted in the next section.

Quantitative Sudomotor Axon Reflex Test

Quantitative sudomotor axon reflex is a quantitative test of sudomotor function. The test depends on delivery of acetylcholine to the skin of the forearm, arm, or lower limbs via iontophoresis and subsequent measurement of sweat volume. The reflex is mediated by postganglionic sympathetic C fibers that innervates the sweat glands. Reduced sweat volume denotes postganglionic sympathetic sudomotor axonal dysfunction or autonomic neuropathy [195].

Incorporating the sudomotor axon reflex test in the diagnostic workup of small fiber neuropathy may increase the diagnostic yield [196]. Also, combined used of this test and the cutaneous silent period increased its sensitivity to diagnose small fiber neuropathy in diabetic or pre-diabetic patients [197]. The test is easy to perform, safe, and well tolerated, but is not readily available everywhere.

Sympathetic Skin Response

Sympathetic skin response is a test that assesses the sympathetic cholinergic pathway allowing evaluation of sudomotor function. It refers to a potential generated by sweat glands in response to various stimuli. The test can be easily conducted using any standard EMG machine. A common technique is to electrically stimulate the median nerve at the wrist while recording from the palmar surface of the hand. Several trials are usually recorded, and the resultant potential is evaluated as regards the latency and amplitude. Lost response, delayed latency, or reduced amplitude are considered abnormal.

An abnormal response can be seen in any central or peripheral nerve disorder that can cause sudomotor dysfunction including polyneuropathies, multiple sclerosis, and spinal cord lesions [198].

Despite the easy technique of the test, it is subjected to habituation and is affected by temperature and humidity. Moreover, its high interindividual variations and lack of reference values for latency and amplitude limit its diagnostic ability in individual patients [199]. As a result, the sympathetic skin response should be utilized in conjunction with other sudomotor tests and its results in patients suspected of having polyneuropathies should be interpreted in the light of clinical and electrophysiological data [200, 201].

Corneal Confocal Microscopy

Corneal focal microscopy is a non-invasive in vivo microscopic imaging of the corneal sub-basal nerve plexus. The test involves quantification of several parameters including corneal nerve fiber density, corneal nerve fiber length, corneal nerve branch density, and corneal nerve fiber tortuosity [202].

Corneal focal microscopy has been recently used to evaluate diabetic sensorimotor polyneuropathy. The test may allow early identification of nerve fiber loss in diabetic polyneuropathy even in recently diagnosed cases or before the development of clinical neuropathic symptoms [203, 204]. It can also be used to assess the severity of nerve fiber pathology and detection of early nerve fiber regeneration post-treatment [205, 206].

Despite its non-invasive nature and its easy technique, the utility of corneal confocal microscopy is limited due to its high cost and limited availability in medical centers.

Conclusion

The definite diagnosis of neuropathic pain requires objective evidence of somatosensory system dysfunction. The toolbox that the clinicians can use to reach this definite diagnosis include several diagnostic tests as discussed throughout the chapter. The optimum diagnostic approach depends on the wise choice of the diagnostic tests that are tailored to each patient according to the clinical status, and the provisional diagnosis. In peripheral neuropathic pain, it is also important to clinically define the type of fibers that are mostly involved to request the most appropriate test as shown in the provided flowchart (Fig. 12.12). The advances in the neuroimaging field will definitely open the door to their full routine integration in the diagnostic workup of neuropathic pain.

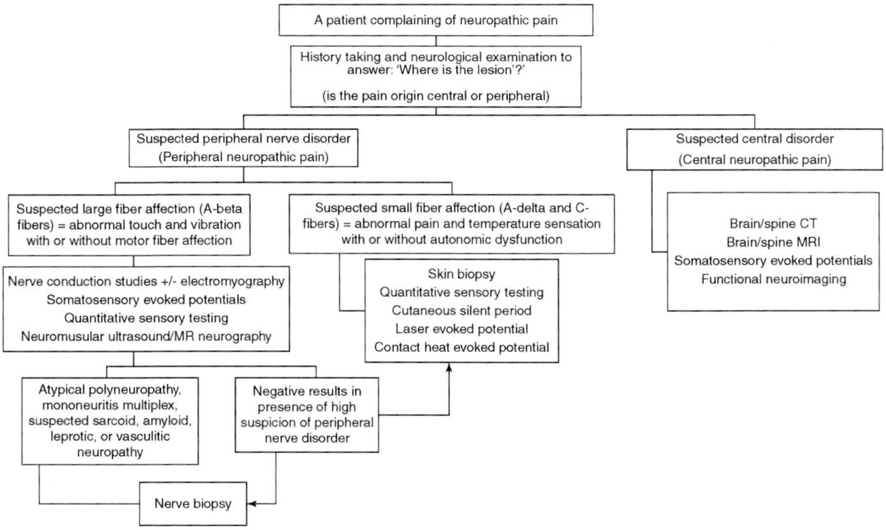

Fig. 12.12 Flow chart showing a general diagnostic approach to neuropathic pain and which tests to choose

References

1. Treede RD, Jensen TS, Campbell JN, Cruccu G, Dostrovsky JO, Griffin JW, Hansson P, Hughes R, Nurmikko T, Serra J. Neuropathic pain: redefinition and a grading system for clinical and research purposes. Neurology. 2008;70(18):1630–5.
2. Jensen TS, Baron R, Haanpää M, Kalso E, Loeser JD, Rice AS, Treede RD. A new definition of neuropathic pain. Pain. 2011;152(10):2204–5.
3. Krumova EK, Geber C, Westermann A, Maier C. Neuropathic pain: is quantitative sensory testing helpful? Curr Diab Rep. 2012;12(4):393–402.
4. Zaslansky R, Yarnitsky D. Clinical applications of quantitative sensory testing (QST). J Neurol Sci. 1998;153(2):215–38.
5. Kelly KG, Cook T, Backonja MM. Pain ratings at the thresholds are necessary for interpretation of quantitative sensory testing. Muscle Nerve. 2005;32(2):179–84.
6. Haanpää M, Attal N, Backonja M, Baron R, Bennett M, Bouhassira D, Cruccu G, Hansson P, Haythornthwaite JA, Iannetti GD, Jensen TS, Kauppila T, Nurmikko TJ, Rice ASC, Rowbotham M, Serra J, Sommer C, Smith BH, Treede RD. NeuPSIG guidelines on neuropathic pain assessment. Pain. 2011;152(1):14–27.
7. La Cesa S, Tamburin S, Tugnoli V, Sandrini G, Paolucci S, Lacerenza M, Marchettini P, Cruccu G, Truini A. How to diagnose neuropathic pain? The contribution from clinical examination, pain questionnaires and diagnostic tests. Neurol Sci. 2015;36(12):2169–75.
8. Cruccu G, Sommer C, Anand P, Attal N, Baron R, Garcia-Larrea L, Haanpaa M, Jensen TS, Serra J, Treede RD. EFNS guidelines on neuropathic pain assessment: revised 2009. Eur J Neurol. 2010;17(8):1010–8.
9. Gwilym SE, Keltner JR, Warnaby CE, Carr AJ, Chizh B, Chessell I, Tracey I. Psychophysical and functional imaging evidence supporting the presence of central sensitization in a cohort of osteoarthritis patients. Arthritis Rheum. 2009;61(9):1226–34.
10. Cruccu G, Anand P, Attal N, Garcia-Larrea L, Haanpää M, Jørum E, Serra J, Jensen TS. EFNS guidelines on neuropathic pain assessment. Eur J Neurol. 2004;11(3):153–62.
11. Devigili G, Tugnoli V, Penza P, Camozzi F, Lombardi R, Melli G, Broglio L, Granieri E, Lauria G. The diagnostic criteria for small fibre neuropathy: from symptoms to neuropathology. Brain. 2008;131(Pt 7):1912–25.
12. Themistocleous AC, Ramirez JD, Serra J, Bennett DL. The clinical approach to small fibre neuropathy and painful channelopathy. Pract Neurol. 2014;14(6):368–79.
13. Preston DC, Shapiro BE. Polyneuropathy. In: Preston DC, Shapiro BE, editors. Electromyography and neuromuscular disorders: clinical-electrophysiologic-ultrasound correlations. 4th ed. Philadelphia: Elsevier Butterworth Heinemann; 2021. p. 491–524.
14. Tankisi H, Pugdahl K, Beniczky S, Andersen H, Fuglsang-Frederiksen A. Evidence-based recommendations for examination and diagnostic strategies of polyneuropathy electrodiagnosis. Clin Neurophysiol Pract. 2019;4:214–22.
15. Albers JW, Kelly JJ Jr. Acquired inflammatory demyelinating polyneuropathies: clinical and electrodiagnostic features. Muscle Nerve. 1989;12(6):435–51.
16. Gordon PH, Wilbourn AJ. Early electrodiagnostic findings in Guillain-Barré syndrome. Arch Neurol. 2001;58(6):913–7.
17. Jin J, Hu F, Qin X, Liu X, Li M, Dang Y, Dang J. Very early neurophysiological study in Guillain-Barre syndrome. Eur Neurol. 2018;80(1-2):100–5.
18. Umapathi T, Lim CSJ, Ng BCJ, Goh EJH, Ohnmar O. A simplified, graded, electrodiagnostic criterion for Guillain-Barré syndrome that incorporates sensory nerve conduction studies. Sci Rep. 2019;9(1):7724.
19. Uncini A, Kuwabara S. Electrodiagnostic criteria for Guillain-Barrè syndrome: a critical revision and the need for an update. Clin Neurophysiol. 2012;123(8):1487–95.
20. Kuntzer T, Antoine JC, Steck AJ. Clinical features and pathophysiological basis of sensory neuronopathies (ganglionopathies). Muscle Nerve. 2004;30(3):255–68.

21. Sghirlanzoni A, Pareyson D, Lauria G. Sensory neuron diseases. Lancet Neurol. 2005;4(6):349–61.
22. Gwathmey KG. Sensory neuronopathies. Muscle Nerve. 2016;53(1):8–19.
23. Floeter MK. Cutaneous silent periods. Muscle Nerve. 2003;28(4):391–401.
24. Shahani BT, Young RR. Studies of the normal human silent period. In: Desmedt JE, editor. New developments in electromyography and clinical neurophysiology. Basel: Karger; 1973.
25. Kofler M, Leis AA, Valls-Solé J. Cutaneous silent periods - part 1: update on physiological mechanisms. Clin Neurophysiol. 2019;130(4):588–603.
26. Syed NA, Sandbrink F, Luciano CA, Altarescu G, Weibel T, Schiffmann R, Floeter MK. Cutaneous silent periods in patients with Fabry disease. Muscle Nerve. 2000;23(8):1179–86.
27. Luciano CA, Russell JW, Banerjee TK, Quirk JM, Scott LJ, Dambrosia JM, Barton NW, Schiffmann R. Physiological characterization of neuropathy in Fabry's disease. Muscle Nerve. 2002;26(5):622–9.
28. Koytak PK, Isak B, Borucu D, Uluc K, Tanridag T, Us O. Assessment of symptomatic diabetic patients with normal nerve conduction studies: utility of cutaneous silent periods and autonomic tests. Muscle Nerve. 2011;43(3):317–23.
29. Kaneko K, Kawai S, Fuchigami Y, Morita H, Ofuji A. Cutaneous silent period in syringomyelia. Muscle Nerve. 1997;20(7):884–6.
30. Leis AA, Kofler M, Šte˘tkár˘ová I, Stokic' DS. The cutaneous silent period is preserved in cervical radiculopathy: significance for the diagnosis of cervical myelopathy. Eur Spine J. 2011;20(2):236–9.
31. Leis AA, Kofler M. Silent period. In: Aminoff MJ, Daroff RB, editors. Encyclopedia of the neurological sciences. 2nd ed. Oxford: Academic; 2014. p. 164–8.
32. Sahin O, Yildiz S, Yildiz N. Cutaneous silent period in fibromyalgia. Neurol Res. 2011;33(4):339–43.
33. Umay E, Ulas U, Unlu E, Akgün H, Cakci A, Odabasi Z. Importance of cutaneous silent period in fibromyalgia and its relationship with disease characteristics, psychological disorders and quality of life of patients. Rev Bras Reumatol. 2013;53(3):288–95.
34. Truini A, Galeotti F, Biasiotta A, Gabriele M, Inghilleri M, Petrucci MT, Cruccu G. Dissociation between cutaneous silent period and laser evoked potentials in assessing neuropathic pain. Muscle Nerve. 2009a;39(3):369–73.
35. Yaman M, Uludüz D, Solak O, Pay G, Kiziltan ME. The cutaneous silent period in carpal tunnel syndrome. Electromyogr Clin Neurophysiol. 2007a;47(4-5):215–20.
36. Cruccu G, Aminoff MJ, Curio G, Guerit JM, Kakigi R, Mauguiere F, Rossini PM, Treede RD, Garcia-Larrea L. Recommendations for the clinical use of somatosensory-evoked potentials. Clin Neurophysiol. 2008;119(8):1705–19.
37. Halonen JP, Jones S, Shawkat F. Contribution of cutaneous and muscle afferent fibres to cortical SEPs following median and radial nerve stimulation in man. Electroencephalogr Clin Neurophysiol. 1988;71(5):331–5.
38. Misulis KE, Fakhoury T. Somatosensory evoked potentials. In: Misulis KE, Fakhoury, editors. Spehlmann's evoked potential primer. 3rd ed. Woburn: Butterworth Heinemann; 2001. p. 83–186.
39. Aminoff MJ, Eisen AA. AAEM minimonograph 19: somatosensory evoked potentials. Muscle Nerve. 1998;21(3):277–90.
40. el-Tantawi GA. Reliability of sensory nerve-conduction and somatosensory evoked potentials for diagnosis of meralgia paraesthetica. Clin Neurophysiol. 2009;120(7):1346–51.
41. Gabelić T, Skorić MK, Adamec I, Mayer D, Habek M. Tongue somatosensory-evoked potentials: evaluation of the afferent trigeminal pathway in patients with early multiple sclerosis. Clin EEG Neurosci. 2013;44(4):286–90.
42. Valeriani M, Pazzaglia C, Cruccu G, Truini A. Clinical usefulness of laser evoked potentials. Neurophysiol Clin. 2012;42(5):345–53.

43. Truini A, Galeotti F, Romaniello A, Virtuoso M, Iannetti GD, Cruccu G. Laser-evoked potentials: normative values. Clin Neurophysiol. 2005;116(4):821–6.
44. Treede RD, Lorenz J, Baumgrtner U. Clinical usefulness of laser-evoked potentials. Neurophysiol Clin. 2003;33(6):303–14.
45. Truini A, Haanpää M, Zucchi R, Galeotti F, Iannetti GD, Romaniello A, Cruccu G. Laser-evoked potentials in post-herpetic neuralgia. Clin Neurophysiol. 2003;114(4):702–9.
46. Valeriani M, Mariotti P, Le Pera D, Restuccia D, De Armas L, Maiese T, Vigevano F, Antuzzi D, Zampino G, Ricci R, Tonali P. Functional assessment of A delta and C fibers in patients with Fabry's disease. Muscle Nerve. 2004;30(6):708–13.
47. Cruccu G, Galeotti F, Iannetti GD, Romaniello A, Truini A, Manfredi M. Trigeminal neuralgia: update on reflex and evoked potential studies. Mov Disord. 2002;17(Suppl 2):S37–40.
48. Garcia-Larrea L, Convers P, Magnin M, André-Obadia N, Peyron R, Laurent B, Mauguière F. Laser-evoked potential abnormalities in central pain patients: the influence of spontaneous and provoked pain. Brain. 2002;125:2766–81.
49. Cruccu G, Truini A. Sensory profiles: a new strategy for selecting patients in treatment trials for neuropathic pain. Pain. 2009;146(1-2):5–6.
50. Garcia-Larrea L, Hagiwara K. Electrophysiology in diagnosis and management of neuropathic pain. Rev Neurol (Paris). 2019;175(1-2):26–37.
51. Preston DC, Shapiro BE. Blink reflex. In: Preston DC, Shapiro BE, editors. Electromyography and neuromuscular disorders: clinical-electrophysiologic-ultrasound correlations. 4th ed. Philadelphia: Elsevier Butterworth Heinemann; 2021. p. 52–6.
52. Aramideh M, Ongerboer de Visser BW. Brainstem reflexes: electrodiagnostic techniques, physiology, normative data, and clinical applications. Muscle Nerve. 2002;26(1):14–30.
53. Cruccu G, Ongerboer de Visser BW. The jaw reflexes. In: Deuschi G, Eisen A, editors. Recommendations for the practice of clinical neurophysiology: guidelines of the international federation of clinical physiology (EEG Suppl. 52). Elsevier; 1999. Available at: Guidelines of the IFCN (2nd Ed, published 1999) - View for Free – Elsevier.
54. Jørum E, Schmelz M. Chapter 29 Microneurography in the assessment of neuropathic pain. Handb Clin Neurol. 2006;81:427–38.
55. Serra J. The role of neurophysiology. J Peripher Nerv Syst. 2014;19(Suppl 2):S22–4.
56. Lauria G, Hsieh ST, Johansson O, Kennedy WR, Leger JM, Mellgren SI, Nolano M, Merkies IS, Polydefkis M, Smith AG, Sommer C, Valls-Solé J. European Federation of Neurological Societies; Peripheral Nerve Society. European Federation of Neurological Societies/Peripheral Nerve Society Guideline on the use of skin biopsy in the diagnosis of small fiber neuropathy. Report of a joint task force of the European Federation of Neurological Societies and the Peripheral Nerve Society. Eur J Neurol. 2010;17(7):903–12.
57. Boruchow SA, Gibbons CH. Utility of skin biopsy in management of small fiber neuropathy. Muscle Nerve. 2013;48(6):877–82.
58. Lauria G, Cornblath DR, Johansson O, McArthur JC, Mellgren SI, Nolano M, Rosenberg N, Sommer C, European Federation of Neurological Societies. EFNS guidelines on the use of skin biopsy in the diagnosis of peripheral neuropathy. Eur J Neurol. 2005;12(10):747–58.
59. Fabry V, Gerdelat A, Acket B, Cintas P, Rousseau V, Uro-Coste E, Evrard SM, Pavy-Le TA. Which method for diagnosing small fiber neuropathy? Front Neurol. 2020;11:342.
60. Lauria G, Bakkers M, Schmitz C, Lombardi R, Penza P, Devigili G, Smith AG, Hsieh ST, Mellgren SI, Umapathi T, Ziegler D, Faber CG, Merkies IS. Intraepidermal nerve fiber density at the distal leg: a worldwide normative reference study. J Peripher Nerv Syst. 2010;15(3):202–7.
61. Nolano M, Tozza S, Caporaso G, Provitera V. Contribution of skin biopsy in peripheral neuropathies. Brain Sci. 2020;10(12):989.
62. Levine TD, Saperstein DS. Routine use of punch biopsy to diagnose small fiber neuropathy in fibromyalgia patients. Clin Rheumatol. 2015;34(3):413–7.
63. Giannoccaro MP, Donadio V, Incensi A, Avoni P, Liguori R. Small nerve fiber involvement in patients referred for fibromyalgia. Muscle Nerve. 2014;49(5):757–9.

64. Grayston R, Czanner G, Elhadd K, Goebel A, Frank B, Üçeyler N, Malik RA, Alam U. A systematic review and meta-analysis of the prevalence of small fiber pathology in fibromyalgia: implications for a new paradigm in fibromyalgia etiopathogenesis. Semin Arthritis Rheum. 2019;48(5):933–40.
65. Provitera V, Gibbons CH, Wendelschafer-Crabb G, Donadio V, Vitale DF, Loavenbruck A, Stancanelli A, Caporaso G, Liguori R, Wang N, Santoro L, Kennedy WR, Nolano M. The role of skin biopsy in differentiating small-fiber neuropathy from ganglionopathy. Eur J Neurol. 2018;25(6):848–53.
66. Kennedy WR, Nolano M, Wendelschafer-Crabb G, Johnson TL, Tamura E. A skin blister method to study epidermal nerves in peripheral nerve disease. Muscle Nerve. 1999;22(3):360–71.
67. Panoutsopoulou IG, Wendelschafer-Crabb G, Hodges JS, Kennedy WR. Skin blister and skin biopsy to quantify epidermal nerves: a comparative study. Neurology. 2009;72(14):1205–10.
68. Lauria G, Morbin M, Lombardi R, et al. Axonal swellings predict the degeneration of epidermal nerve fibers in painful neuropathies. Neurology. 2003;61(5):631–6.
69. Herrmann DN, McDermott MP, Henderson D, Chen L, Akowuah K, Schifitto G, The North East Aids Dementia (Nead) Consortium. Epidermal nerve fiber density, axonal swellings and QST as predictors of HIV distal sensory neuropathy. Muscle Nerve. 2004;29(3):420–7.
70. Vlcková-Moravcová E, Bednarík J, Dusek L, Toyka KV, Sommer C. Diagnostic validity of epidermal nerve fiber densities in painful sensory neuropathies. Muscle Nerve. 2008;37(1):50–60.
71. Sohn E, Suh BC, Wang N, Freeman R, Gibbons CH. A novel method to quantify cutaneous vascular innervation. Muscle Nerve. 2020;62(4):492–501.
72. England JD, Gronseth GS, Franklin G, Miller RG, Asbury AK, Carter GT, Cohen JA, Fisher MA, Howard JF, Kinsella LJ, Latov N, Lewis RA, Low PA, Sumner AJ. Distal symmetric polyneuropathy: a definition for clinical research: report of the American Academy of Neurology, the American Association of Electrodiagnostic Medicine, and the American Academy of physical medicine and rehabilitation. Neurology. 2005;64(2):199–207.
73. Haroutounian S, Todorovic MS, Leinders M, Campagnolo M, Gewandter JS, Dworkin RH, Freeman R. Diagnostic criteria for idiopathic small fiber neuropathy: a systematic review. Muscle Nerve. 2021;63(2):170–7.
74. Tesfaye S, Boulton AJ, Dyck PJ, Freeman R, Horowitz M, Kempler P, Lauria G, Malik RA, Spallone V, Vinik A, Bernardi L, Valensi P, Toronto Diabetic Neuropathy Expert Group. Diabetic neuropathies: update on definitions, diagnostic criteria, estimation of severity, and treatments. Diabetes Care. 2010;33(10):2285–93.
75. Berini SE, Dyck PJB. The utility of nerve biopsy in carefully selected patients in modern neuromuscular practice. Muscle Nerve. 2019;59(6):635–7.
76. England JD, Gronseth GS, Franklin G, Carter GT, Kinsella LJ, Cohen JA, Asbury AK, Szigeti K, Lupski JR, Latov N, Lewis RA, Low PA, Fisher MA, Herrmann D, Howard JF, Lauria G, Miller RG, Polydefkis M, Sumner AJ, American Academy of Neurology, American Association of Neuromuscular and Electrodiagnostic Medicine, American Academy of Physical Medicine and Rehabilitation. Practice parameter: the evaluation of distal symmetric polyneuropathy: the role of autonomic testing, nerve biopsy, and skin biopsy (an evidence-based review). Report of the American Academy of Neurology, the American Association of Neuromuscular and Electrodiagnostic Medicine, and the American Academy of Physical Medicine and Rehabilitation. PM R. 2009;1(1):14–22.
77. Nathani D, Spies J, Barnett MH, Pollard J, Wang MX, Sommer C, Kiernan MC. Nerve biopsy: current indications and decision tools. Muscle Nerve. 2021. https://doi.org/10.1002/mus.27201.
78. Duchesne M, Mathis S, Richard L, Magdelaine C, Corcia P, Nouioua S, Tazir M, Magy L, Vallat JM. Nerve biopsy is still useful in some inherited neuropathies. J Neuropathol Exp Neurol. 2018;77(2):88–99.

79. Chkheidze R, Pytel P. What every neuropathologist needs to know: peripheral nerve biopsy. J Neuropathol Exp Neurol. 2020;79(4):355–64.
80. Collins MP, Dyck PJ, Gronseth GS, Guillevin L, Hadden RD, Heuss D, Léger JM, Notermans NC, Pollard JD, Said G, Sobue G, Vrancken AF, Kissel JT, Peripheral Nerve Society. Peripheral nerve society guideline on the classification, diagnosis, investigation, and immunosuppressive therapy of non-systemic vasculitic neuropathy: executive summary. J Peripher Nerv Syst. 2010;15(3):176–84.
81. Vrancken AF, Gathier CS, Cats EA, Notermans NC, Collins MP. The additional yield of combined nerve/muscle biopsy in vasculitic neuropathy. Eur J Neurol. 2011;18(1):49–58.
82. Bennett DL, Groves M, Blake J, Holton JL, King RH, Orrell RW, Ginsberg L, Reilly MM. The use of nerve and muscle biopsy in the diagnosis of vasculitis: a 5 year retrospective study. J Neurol Neurosurg Psychiatry. 2008;79(12):1376–81.
83. Hui M, Uppin MS, Challa S, Meena AK, Kaul S. Pure neuritic leprosy: resolving diagnostic issues in acid fast bacilli (AFB)-negative nerve biopsies: a single centre experience from South India. Ann Indian Acad Neurol. 2015;18(3):292–7.
84. Dyck PJ, Dyck PJB, Engelstad JK. Pathologic alterations of nerves. In: Dyck PJ, Thomas PK, editors. Peripheral neuropathy. Elsevier; 2005. p. 733–829.
85. Ruth A, Schulmeyer FJ, Roesch M, Woertgen C, Brawanski A. Diagnostic and therapeutic value due to suspected diagnosis, long-term complications, and indication for sural nerve biopsy. Clin Neurol Neurosurg. 2005;107(3):214–7.
86. Meaney JF, Eldridge PR, Dunn LT, Nixon TE, Whitehouse GH, Miles JB. Demonstration of neurovascular compression in trigeminal neuralgia with magnetic resonance imaging. Comparison with surgical findings in 52 consecutive operative cases. J Neurosurg. 1995;83(5):799–805.
87. Macgowan DJL, Janal MN, Clark MC, Wharton RN, Lazar RM, Sacco RL, Mohr JP. Central poststroke pain and Wallenberg's lateral medullary infarction: frequency, character, and determinants in 63 patients. Neurology. 1997;49(1):120–5.
88. Rudick RA, Miller AE. Multiple sclerosis or multiple possibilities. The continuing problem of misdiagnosis. Neurology. 2012;78(24):1904–6.
89. Alomar S, Bakhaidar M. Neuroimaging of neuropathic pain: review of current status and future directions. Neurosurg Rev. 2018;41(3):771–7.
90. Iadarola MJ, Max MB, Berman KF, Byas-Smith MG, Coghill RC, Gracely RH, Bennett GJ. Unilateral decrease in thalamic activity observed with positron emission tomography in patients with chronic neuropathic pain. Pain. 1995;63(1):55–64.
91. Peyron R, Laurent B, García-Larrea L. Functional imaging of brain responses to pain. A review and meta-analysis (2000). Neurophysiol Clin. 2000;30(5):263–88.
92. Cauda F, Sacco K, D'Agata F, Duca S, Cocito D, Geminiani G, Migliorati F, Isoardo G. Low-frequency BOLD fluctuations demonstrate altered thalamocortical connectivity in diabetic neuropathic pain. BMC Neurosci. 2009;10:138.
93. Geha PY, Baliki MN, Harden RN, Bauer WR, Parrish TB, Apkarian AV. The brain in chronic CRPS pain: abnormal gray-white matter interactions in emotional and autonomic regions. Neuron. 2008;60(4):570–81.
94. Ducreux D, Attal N, Parker F, Bouhassira D. Mechanisms of central neuropathic pain: a combined psychophysical and fMRI study in syringomyelia. Brain. 2006;(Pt 4):963–76.
95. Gustin SM, Wrigley PJ, Siddall PJ, Henderson LA. Brain anatomy changes associated with persistent neuropathic pain following spinal cord injury. Cereb Cortex. 2010;20(6):1409–19.
96. DaSilva AF, Becerra L, Pendse G, Chizh B, Tully S, Borsook D. Colocalized structural and functional changes in the cortex of patients with trigeminal neuropathic pain. PLoS One. 2008;3(10):e3396.
97. Abarca-Olivas J, Feliu-Rey E, Sempere AP, Sanchez-Payá J, Baño-Ruiz E, Caminero-Canas MA, Nieto-Navarro J, Botella-Asunción C. Volumetric measurement of the posterior fossa and its components using magnetic resonance imaging in idiopathic trigeminal neuralgia. Rev Neurol. 2010;51(9):520–4.

98. Sundgren PC, Dong Q, Gómez-Hassan D, Mukherji SK, Maly P, Welsh R. Diffusion tensor imaging of the brain: review of clinical applications. Neuroradiology. 2004;46(5):339–50.
99. Kong J, Loggia ML, Zyloney C, Tu P, LaViolette P, Gollub RL. Exploring the brain in pain: activations, deactivations and their relation. Pain. 2010;148(2):257–67.
100. Maarrawi J, Peyron R, Mertens P, Costes N, Magnin M, Sindou M, Laurent B, Garcia-Larrea L. Brain opioid receptor density predicts motor cortex stimulation efficacy for chronic pain. Pain. 2013;154(11):2563–8.
101. Moens M, Sunaert S, Mariën P, Brouns R, De Smedt A, Droogmans S, Van Schuerbeek P, Peeters R, Poelaert J, Nuttin B. Spinal cord stimulation modulates cerebral function: an fMRI study. Neuroradiology. 2012;54(12):1399–407.
102. Walker FO, Cartwright MS, Alter KE, Visser LH, Hobson-Webb LD, Padua L, Strakowski JA, Preston DC, Boon AJ, Axer H, van Alfen N, Tawfik EA, Wilder-Smith E, Yoon JS, Kim BJ, Breiner A, Bland JDP, Grimm A, Zaidman CM. Indications for neuromuscular ultrasound: expert opinion and review of the literature. Clin Neurophysiol. 2018;129(12):2658–79.
103. Cartwright MS, Walker FO. Neuromuscular ultrasound in common entrapment neuropathies. Muscle Nerve. 2013;48(5):696–704.
104. Cartwright MS, Hobson-Webb LD, Boon AJ, Alter KE, Hunt CH, Flores VH, Werner RA, Shook SJ, Thomas TD, Primack SJ, Walker FO, American Association of Neuromuscular and Electrodiagnostic Medicine. Evidence-based guideline: neuromuscular ultrasound for the diagnosis of carpal tunnel syndrome. Muscle Nerve. 2012;46(2):287–93.
105. Park GY, Kwon DR, Seok JI, Park DS, Cho HK. Usefulness of ultrasound assessment of median nerve mobility in carpal tunnel syndrome. Acta Radiol. 2018;59(12):1494–9.
106. Wiesler ER, Chloros GD, Cartwright MS, Shin HW, Walker FO. Ultrasound in the diagnosis of ulnar neuropathy at the cubital tunnel. J Hand Surg Am. 2006;31(7):1088–93.
107. Ellegaard HR, Fuglsang-Frederiksen A, Hess A, Johnsen B, Qerama E. High-resolution ultrasound in ulnar neuropathy at the elbow: a prospective study. Muscle Nerve. 2015;52(5):759–66.
108. Lo YL, Fook-Chong S, Leoh TH, Dan YF, Tan YE, Lee MP, Gan HY, Chan LL. Rapid ultrasonographic diagnosis of radial entrapment neuropathy at the spiral groove. J Neurol Sci. 2008;271(1-2):75–9.
109. Martinoli C, Bianchi S, Pugliese F, Bacigalupo L, Gauglio C, Valle M, Derchi LE. Sonography of entrapment neuropathies in the upper limb (wrist excluded). J Clin Ultrasound. 2004;32(9):438–50.
110. Visser LH, Hens V, Soethout M, De Deugd-Maria V, Pijnenburg J, Brekelmans GJ. Diagnostic value of high-resolution sonography in common fibular neuropathy at the fibular head. Muscle Nerve. 2013;48(2):171–8.
111. Bignotti B, Cadoni A, Assini A, Martinoli C, Tagliafico A. Fascicular involvement in common fibular neuropathy: evaluation with ultrasound. Muscle Nerve. 2016;53(4):532–7.
112. Fantino O. Role of ultrasound in posteromedial tarsal tunnel syndrome: 81 cases. J Ultrasound. 2014;17(2):99–112.
113. Samarawickrama D, Therimadasamy AK, Chan YC, Vijayan J, Wilder-Smith EP. Nerve ultrasound in electrophysiologically verified tarsal tunnel syndrome. Muscle Nerve. 2016;53(6):906–12.
114. Kim Y, Kim DH, Kim NH, Kim BH, Park BK. Dorsal sural neuropathy: electrophysiological, ultrasonographic, and magnetic resonance imaging findings. Muscle Nerve. 2012;46(4):597–600.
115. Pelosi L, Leadbetter R, Mulroy E. Utility of neuromuscular ultrasound in the investigation of common mononeuropathies in everyday neurophysiology practice. Muscle Nerve. 2021;63(4):467–71.
116. Aseem F, Williams JW, Walker FO, Cartwright MS. Neuromuscular ultrasound in patients with carpal tunnel syndrome and normal nerve conduction studies. Muscle Nerve. 2017;55(6):913–5.
117. Alrajeh M, Preston DC. Neuromuscular ultrasound in electrically non-localizable ulnar neuropathy. Muscle Nerve. 2018;58(5):655–9.

118. Aktürk S, Büyükavcı R, Ersoy Y. Median nerve ultrasound in carpal tunnel syndrome with normal electrodiagnostic tests. Acta Neurol Belg. 2020;120(1):43–7.
119. Visser LH. High-resolution sonography of the common peroneal nerve: detection of intraneural ganglia. Neurology. 2006;67(8):1473–5.
120. Yalcin E, Akyuz M, Onder B. Early radial digital neuropathy of the thumb due to flexor pollicis longus tendinitis: value of ultrasound in an uncommon mild neuropathy. Muscle Nerve. 2013;47(5):772–5.
121. Chari B, McNally E. Nerve entrapment in ankle and foot: ultrasound imaging. Semin Musculoskelet Radiol. 2018;22(3):354–63.
122. De Franco P, Erra C, Granata G, Coraci D, Padua R, Padua L. Sonographic diagnosis of anatomical variations associated with carpal tunnel syndrome. J Clin Ultrasound. 2014;42(6):371–4.
123. Cammarata MJ, Hill JB, Sharma S. Ulnar nerve compression due to anconeus epitrochlearis: a case report and review of the literature. JBJS Case Connect. 2019;9(2):e0189.
124. Cushman DM, Walker SE. Symptomatic accessory branch of the superficial peroneal nerve identified by ultrasound. Muscle Nerve. 2020;62:E46–7.
125. Pisapia JM, Ali ZS, Hudgins ED, Khoury V, Heuer GG, Zager EL. Ultrasonography detects ulnar nerve dislocation despite normal electrophysiology and magnetic resonance imaging. World Neurosurg. 2017;99:809.
126. Padua L, Di Pasquale A, Liotta G, Granata G, Pazzaglia C, Erra C, Briani C, Coraci D, De Franco P, Antonini G, Martinoli C. Ultrasound as a useful tool in the diagnosis and management of traumatic nerve lesions. Clin Neurophysiol. 2013;124(6):1237–43.
127. Peer S, Bodner G, Meirer R, Willeit J, Piza-Katzer H. Examination of postoperative peripheral nerve lesions with high-resolution sonography. AJR Am J Roentgenol. 2001;177(2):415–9.
128. Nwawka OK, Casaletto E, Wolfe SW, Feinberg JH. Ultrasound imaging of brachial plexus trauma in gunshot injury. Muscle Nerve. 2019;59(6):707–11.
129. Jakobsen RL, Fuglsang-Frederiksen A, Hellfritzsch MB, Qerama E. A prospective study of high resolution ultrasound in brachial plexopathies - correlation with electrophysiological measurements. Clin Neurophysiol. 2019;130(7):1144–50.
130. Arányi Z, Csillik A, Böhm J, Schelle T. Ultrasonographic identification of fibromuscular bands associated with neurogenic thoracic outlet syndrome: the "wedge-sickle" sign. Ultrasound Med Biol. 2016;42(10):2357–66.
131. Sucher BM. Thoracic outlet syndrome-postural type: ultrasound imaging of pectoralis minor and brachial plexus abnormalities. PM R. 2012;4(1):65–72.
132. Arányi Z, Csillik A, Dévay K, Rosero M, Barsi P, Böhm J, Schelle T. Ultrasonographic identification of nerve pathology in neuralgic amyotrophy: enlargement, constriction, fascicular entwinement, and torsion. Muscle Nerve. 2015;52(4):503–11.
133. ArÁnyi Z, Csillik A, DéVay K, Rosero M, Barsi P, Böhm J, Schelle T. Ultrasonography in neuralgic amyotrophy: sensitivity, spectrum of findings, and clinical correlations. Muscle Nerve. 2017;56(6):1054–62.
134. Visser LH, Jain S, Lokesh B, Suneetha S, Subbanna J. Morphological changes of the epineurium in leprosy: a new finding detected by high-resolution sonography. Muscle Nerve. 2012;46(1):38–41.
135. Rasenack M, Proebstel AK, Athanasopoulou IM, Décard BF, Grimm A. Nerve hypertrophy in primary amyloidosis. Muscle Nerve. 2016;54(3):510–2.
136. Grimm A, Décard BF, Bischof A, Axer H. Ultrasound of the peripheral nerves in systemic vasculitic neuropathies. J Neurol Sci. 2014;347(1-2):44–9.
137. Goedee HS, van der Pol WL, van Asseldonk JH, Vrancken AFJE, Notermans NC, Visser LH, van den Berg LH. Nerve sonography to detect peripheral nerve involvement in vasculitis syndromes. Neurol Clin Pract. 2016;6(4):293–303.
138. Chipman JN, Mott RT, Stanton CA, Cartwright MS. Ultrasonographic Tinel sign. Muscle Nerve. 2009;40(6):1033–5.

139. Pitarokoili K, Kerasnoudis A, Behrendt V, Labedi A, Ayzenberg I, Gold R, Yoon MS. Facing the diagnostic challenge: nerve ultrasound in diabetic patients with neuropathic symptoms. Muscle Nerve. 2016;54(1):18–24.
140. Breiner A, Qrimli M, Ebadi H, Alabdali M, Lovblom LE, Abraham A, Albulahi H, Perkins BA, Bril V. Peripheral nerve high-resolution ultrasound in diabetes. Muscle Nerve. 2017;55(2):171–8.
141. Zaidman CM, Al-Lozi M, Pestronk A. Peripheral nerve size in normals and patients with polyneuropathy: an ultrasound study. Muscle Nerve. 2009;40(6):960–6.
142. Hobson-Webb LD, Massey JM, Juel VC. Nerve ultrasound in diabetic polyneuropathy: correlation with clinical characteristics and electrodiagnostic testing. Muscle Nerve. 2013;47(3):379–84.
143. Di Pasquale A, Morino S, Loreti S, Bucci E, Vanacore N, Antonini G. Peripheral nerve ultrasound changes in CIDP and correlations with nerve conduction velocity. Neurology. 2015;84(8):803–9.
144. Jang JH, Cho CS, Yang KS, Seok HY, Kim BJ. Pattern analysis of nerve enlargement using ultrasonography in chronic inflammatory demyelinating polyneuropathy. Clin Neurophysiol. 2014;125(9):1893–9.
145. Goedee HS, van der Pol WL, van Asseldonk JH, Franssen H, Notermans NC, Vrancken AJ, van Es MA, Nikolakopoulos S, Visser LH, van den Berg LH. Diagnostic value of sonography in treatment-naïve chronic inflammatory neuropathies. Neurology. 2017;88(2):143–51.
146. Matsuoka N, Kohriyama T, Ochi K, Nishitani M, Sueda Y, Mimori Y, Nakamura S, Matsumoto M. Detection of cervical nerve root hypertrophy by ultrasonography in chronic inflammatory demyelinating polyradiculoneuropathy. J Neurol Sci. 2004;219(1-2):15–21.
147. Zaidman CM, Pestronk A. Nerve size in chronic inflammatory demyelinating neuropathy varies with disease activity and therapy response over time: a retrospective ultrasound study. Muscle Nerve. 2014;50(5):733–8.
148. Mori A, Nodera H, Takamatsu N, Maruyama-Saladini K, Osaki Y, Shimatani Y, Kaji R. Sonographic evaluation of peripheral nerves in subtypes of Guillain-Barré syndrome. J Neurol Sci. 2016;364:154–9.
149. Gallardo E, Sedano MJ, Orizaola P, Sánchez-Juan P, González-Suárez A, García A, Terán-Villagrá N, Ruiz-Soto M, Álvaro RL, Berciano MT, Lafarga M, Berciano J. Spinal nerve involvement in early Guillain-Barré syndrome: a clinico-electrophysiological, ultrasonographic and pathological study. Clin Neurophysiol. 2015;126(4):810–9.
150. Razali SNO, Arumugam T, Yuki N, Rozalli FI, Goh KJ, Shahrizaila N. Serial peripheral nerve ultrasound in Guillain-Barré syndrome. Clin Neurophysiol. 2016;127(2):1652–6.
151. Kerasnoudis A, Pitarokoili K, Behrendt V, Gold R, Yoon MS. Nerve ultrasound score in distinguishing chronic from acute inflammatory demyelinating polyneuropathy. Clin Neurophysiol. 2014;125(3):635–41.
152. Martinoli C, Schenone A, Bianchi S, Mandich P, Caponetto C, Abbruzzese M, Derchi LE. Sonography of the median nerve in Charcot-Marie-tooth disease. AJR Am J Roentgenol. 2002;178(6):1553–6.
153. Padua L, Coraci D, Lucchetta M, Paolasso I, Pazzaglia C, Granata G, Cacciavillani M, Luigetti M, Manganelli F, Pisciotta C, Piscosquito G, Pareyson D, Briani C. Different nerve ultrasound patterns in charcot-marie-tooth types and hereditary neuropathy with liability to pressure palsies. Muscle Nerve. 2018;57(1):E18–23.
154. Hooper DR, Lawson W, Smith L, Baker SK. Sonographic features in hereditary neuropathy with liability to pressure palsies. Muscle Nerve. 2011;44(6):862–7.
155. Ginanneschi F, Filippou G, Giannini F, Carluccio MA, Adinolfi A, Frediani B, Dotti MT, Rossi A. Sonographic and electrodiagnostic features of hereditary neuropathy with liability to pressure palsies. J Peripher Nerv Syst. 2012;17(4):391–8.
156. Bayrak AO, Bayrak IK, Battaloglu E, Ozes B, Yildiz O, Onar MK. Ultrasonographic findings in hereditary neuropathy with liability to pressure palsies. Neurol Res. 2015;37(2):106–11.

157. Ebadi H, Siddiqui H, Ebadi S, Ngo M, Breiner A, Bril V. Peripheral nerve ultrasound in small Fiber polyneuropathy. Ultrasound Med Biol. 2015;41(11):2820–6.
158. Puma A, Grecu N, Villa L, Butori C, Besson T, Cambieri C, Cavalli M, Azulay N, Sacconi S, Raffaelli C. Ultra-high-frequency ultrasound imaging of sural nerve: a comparative study with nerve biopsy in progressive neuropathies. Muscle Nerve. 2021;63(1):46–51.
159. Wei KC, Chiu YH, Wu CH, Liang HW, Wang TG. Ultrasound guidance may have advantages over landmark-based guidance for some nerve conduction studies. Muscle Nerve. 2021;63(4):472–6.
160. Tøttrup M, Eriksen JD, Hellfritzsch MB, Sørensen FB, Baad-Hansen T. Diagnostic accuracy of ultrasound-guided core biopsy of peripheral nerve sheath tumors. J Clin Ultrasound. 2020;48(3):134–8.
161. Chhabra A. Magnetic resonance neurography-simple guide to performance and interpretation. Semin Roentgenol. 2013;48(2):111–25.
162. Martín Noguerol T, Barousse R. Update in the evaluation of peripheral nerves by MRI, from morphological to functional neurography. Radiologia. 2020;62(2):90–101.
163. Gasparotti R, Padua L, Briani C, Lauria G. New technologies for the assessment of neuropathies. Nat Rev Neurol. 2017;13(4):203–16.
164. Upadhyaya V, Upadhyaya DN, Bansal R, Pandey T, Pandey AK. MR neurography in parsonage-turner syndrome. Indian J Radiol Imaging. 2019;29(3):264–70.
165. Crim J, Ingalls K. Accuracy of MR neurography in the diagnosis of brachial plexopathy. Eur J Radiol. 2017;95:24–7.
166. Ishikawa T, Asakura K, Mizutani Y, Ueda A, Murate KI, Hikichi C, Shima S, Kizawa M, Komori M, Murayama K, Toyama H, Ito S, Mutoh T. MR neurography for the evaluation of CIDP. Muscle Nerve. 2017;55(4):483–9.
167. Hiwatashi A, Togao O, Yamashita K, Kikuchi K, Momosaka D, Nakatake H, Yamasaki R, Ogata H, Yoneyama M, Kira JI, Honda H. Simultaneous MR neurography and apparent T2 mapping in brachial plexus: evaluation of patients with chronic inflammatory demyelinating polyradiculoneuropathy. Magn Reson Imaging. 2019;55:112–7.
168. Wu F, Wang W, Zhao Y, Liu B, Wang Y, Yang Y, Ren Y, Liu H. MR neurography of lumbosacral nerve roots: diagnostic value in chronic inflammatory demyelinating polyradiculoneuropathy and correlation with electrophysiological parameters. Eur J Radiol. 2020;124:108816.
169. Faridian-Aragh N, Chalian M, Soldatos T, Thawait GK, Deune EG, Belzberg AJ, Carrino JA, Chhabra A. High-resolution 3T MR neurography of radial neuropathy. J Neuroradiol. 2011;38(5):265–74.
170. Polesello GC, Queiroz MC, Linhares JPT, Amaral DT, Ono NK. Anatomical variation of piriformis muscle as a cause of deep gluteal pain: diagnosis using MR neurography and treatment. Rev Bras Ortop. 2013;48(1):114–7.
171. Cejas C, Aguilar M, Falcón L, Caneo N, Acuña MC. Neurografía por resonancia magnética de alta resolución (3 Tesla) del nervio ciático [High resolution (3 T) magnetic resonance neurography of the sciatic nerve]. Radiologia. 2013;55(3):195–202.
172. Pineda D, Barroso F, Cháves H, Cejas C. High resolution 3T magnetic resonance neurography of the peroneal nerve. Radiologia. 2014;56(2):107–17.
173. Eguchi Y, Enomoto K, Sato T, Watanabe A, Sakai T, Norimoto M, Yoneyama M, Aoki Y, Suzuki M, Yamanaka H, Tamai H, Kobayashi T, Orita S, Suzuki M, Inage K, Shiga Y, Hirosawa N, Inoue M, Koda M, Furuya T, Nakamura J, Hagiwara S, Akazawa T, Takahashi H, Takahashi K, Ohtori S. Simultaneous MR neurography and apparent T2 mapping of cervical nerve roots before microendoscopic surgery to treat patient with radiculopathy due to cervical disc herniation: Preliminary results. J Clin Neurosci. 2020;74:213–9.
174. Sato T, Eguchi Y, Norimoto M, Inoue M, Enomoto K, Watanabe A, Sakai T, Yoneyama M, Aoki Y, Orita S, Narita M, Inage K, Shiga Y, Umimura T, Sato M, Suzuki M, Takaoka H, Mizuki N, Kim G, Hozumi T, Hirosawa N, Furuya T, Maki S, Nakamura J, Hagiwara S, Koda M, Akazawa T, Takahashi H, Takahashi K, Ohtori S. Diagnosis of lumbar radiculopathy using simultaneous MR neurography and apparent T2 mapping. J Clin Neurosci. 2020;78:339–46.

175. Upadhyaya V, Upadhyaya DN, Kumar A, Gujral RB. MR neurography in traumatic brachial plexopathy. Eur J Radiol. 2015;84(5):927–32.
176. Cai Z, Li Y, Hu Z, Fu R, Rong X, Wu R, Cheng J, Huang X, Luo J, Tang Y. Radiation-induced brachial plexopathy in patients with nasopharyngeal carcinoma: a retrospective study. Oncotarget. 2016;7(14):18887–95.
177. Qayyum A, MacVicar AD, Padhani AR, Revell P, Husband JE. Symptomatic brachial plexopathy following treatment for breast cancer: utility of MR imaging with surface-coil techniques. Radiology. 2000;214(3):837–42.
178. Zaidman CM, Seelig MJ, Baker JC, Mackinnon SE, Pestronk A. Detection of peripheral nerve pathology: comparison of ultrasound and MRI. Neurology. 2013;80(18):1634–40.
179. Aggarwal A, Srivastava DN, Jana M, Sharma R, Gamanagatti S, Kumar A, Kumar V, Malhotra R, Goyal V, Garg K. Comparison of different sequences of magnetic resonance imaging and ultrasonography with nerve conduction studies in peripheral neuropathies. World Neurosurg. 2017;108:185–200.
180. Martín Noguerol T, Barousse R, Gómez Cabrera M, Socolovsky M, Bencardino JT, Luna A. Functional MR neurography in evaluation of peripheral nerve trauma and postsurgical assessment. Radiographics. 2019;39(2):427–46.
181. Eguchi Y, Ohtori S, Yamashita M, Yamauchi K, Suzuki M, Orita S, Kamoda H, Arai G, Ishikawa T, Miyagi M, Ochiai N, Kishida S, Inoue G, Masuda Y, Ochi S, Kikawa T, Toyone T, Takaso M, Aoki Y, Takahashi K. Diffusion-weighted magnetic resonance imaging of symptomatic nerve root of patients with lumbar disk herniation. Neuroradiology. 2011;53(9):633–41.
182. Guggenberger R, Markovic D, Eppenberger P, Chhabra A, Schiller A, Nanz D, Prüssmann K, Andreisek G. Assessment of median nerve with MR neurography by using diffusion-tensor imaging: normative and pathologic diffusion values. Radiology. 2012;265(1):194–203.
183. Naraghi A, da Gama LL, Menezes R, Khanna M, Sussman M, Anastakis D, White LM. Diffusion tensor imaging of the median nerve before and after carpal tunnel release in patients with carpal tunnel syndrome: feasibility study. Skelet Radiol. 2013;42(10):1403–12.
184. Vaeggemose M, Haakma W, Pham M, Ringgaard S, Tankisi H, Ejskjaer N, Heiland S, Poulsen PL, Andersen H. Diffusion tensor imaging MR neurography detects polyneuropathy in type 2 diabetes. J Diabetes Complicat. 2020;34(2):107439.
185. Bäumer P, Pham M, Ruetters M, Heiland S, Heckel A, Radbruch A, Bendszus M, Weiler M. Peripheral neuropathy: detection with diffusion-tensor imaging. Radiology. 2014;273(1):185–93.
186. Chhabra A, Thakkar RS, Andreisek G, Chalian M, Belzberg AJ, Blakeley J, Hoke A, Thawait GK, Eng J, Carrino JA. Anatomic MR imaging and functional diffusion tensor imaging of peripheral nerve tumors and tumorlike conditions. AJNR Am J Neuroradiol. 2013;34(4):802–7.
187. Wang X, Harrison C, Mariappan YK, Gopalakrishnan K, Chhabra A, Lenkinski RE, Madhuranthakam AJ. MR Neurography of brachial plexus at 3.0 T with robust fat and blood suppression. Radiology. 2017;283(2):538–46.
188. Martín Noguerol T, Barousse R, Socolovsky M, Luna A. Quantitative magnetic resonance (MR) neurography for evaluation of peripheral nerves and plexus injuries. Quant Imaging Med Surg. 2017;7(4):398–421.
189. Merlini L, Vargas MI, Anooshiravani M, Viallon M, Fluss J, Hanquinet S. Look for the nerves! MR neurography adds essential diagnostic value to routine MRI in pediatric practice: a pictorial overview. J Neuroradiol. 2011;38(3):141–7.
190. England JD, Gronseth GS, Franklin G, Carter GT, Kinsella LJ, Cohen JA, Asbury AK, Szigeti K, Lupski JR, Latov N, Lewis RA, Low PA, Fisher MA, Herrmann DN, Howard JF, Lauria G, Miller RG, Polydefkis M, Sumner AJ, American Academy of Neurology; American Association of Neuromuscular and Electrodiagnostic Medicine; American Academy of Physical Medicine and Rehabilitation. Practice parameter: the evaluation of distal symmetric polyneuropathy: the role of laboratory and genetic testing (an evidence-based review).

Report of the American Academy of Neurology, the American Association of Neuromuscular and Electrodiagnostic Medicine, and the American Academy of Physical Medicine and Rehabilitation. PM R. 2009;1(1):5–13.
191. Waxman SG, Merkies ISJ, Gerrits MM, Dib-Hajj SD, Lauria G, Cox JJ, Wood JN, Woods CG, Drenth JPH, Faber CG. Sodium channel genes in pain-related disorders: phenotype-genotype associations and recommendations for clinical use. Lancet Neurol. 2014;13(11):1152–60.
192. Hoeijmakers JG, Faber CG, Merkies IS, Waxman SG. Painful peripheral neuropathy and sodium channel mutations. Neurosci Lett. 2015;596:51–9.
193. Sachau J, Bruckmueller H, Gierthmühlen J, Magerl W, Kaehler M, Haenisch S, Binder A, Caliebe A, Maier C, Treede RD, Tölle T, Cascorbi I, Baron R. SIGMA-1 receptor gene variants affect the somatosensory phenotype in neuropathic pain patients. J Pain. 2019;20(2):201–14.
194. Shiers S, Mwirigi J, Pradhan G, Kume M, Black B, Barragan-Iglesias P, Moy JK, Dussor G, Pancrazio JJ, Kroener S, Price TJ. Reversal of peripheral nerve injury-induced neuropathic pain and cognitive dysfunction via genetic and tomivosertib targeting of MNK. Neuropsychopharmacology. 2020;45(3):524–33.
195. Low PA. Quantitative sudomotor axon reflex test (QSART). In: Encyclopedia of the neurological sciences. Elsevier; 2014. p. 1023–4. https://doi.org/10.1016/B978-0-12-385157-4.00510-8.
196. Thaisetthawatkul P, Fernandes Filho JA, Herrmann DN. Contribution of QSART to the diagnosis of small fiber neuropathy. Muscle Nerve. 2013;48(6):883–8.
197. Kamel JT, Vogrin SJ, Knight-Sadler RJ, Willems NK, Seiderer L, Cook MJ, MacIsaac RJ, Roberts LJ. Combining cutaneous silent periods with quantitative sudomotor axon reflex testing in the assessment of diabetic small fiber neuropathy. Clin Neurophysiol. 2015;126(5):1047–53.
198. Vetrugno R, Liguori R, Cortelli P, Montagna P. Sympathetic skin response: basic mechanisms and clinical applications. Clin Auton Res. 2003;13(4):256–70.
199. Gibbons C, Freeman R. The evaluation of small fiber function-autonomic and quantitative sensory testing. Neurol Clin. 2004;22(3):683–702.
200. Loavenbruck AJ, Hodges JS, Provitera V, Nolano M, Wendelshafer-Crabb G, Kennedy WR. A device to measure secretion of individual sweat glands for diagnosis of peripheral neuropathy. J Peripher Nerv Syst. 2017;22(2):139–48.
201. Buchmann SJ, Penzlin AI, Kubasch ML, Illigens BM, Siepmann T. Assessment of sudomotor function. Clin Auton Res. 2019;29(1):41–53.
202. Papanas N, Ziegler D. Corneal confocal microscopy: recent progress in the evaluation of diabetic neuropathy. J Diabetes Investig. 2015;6(4):381–9.
203. Jiang MS, Yuan Y, Gu ZX, Zhuang SL. Corneal confocal microscopy for assessment of diabetic peripheral neuropathy: a meta-analysis. Br J Ophthalmol. 2016;100(1):9–14.
204. Azmi S, Ferdousi M, Petropoulos IN, Ponirakis G, Alam U, Fadavi H, Asghar O, Marshall A, Atkinson AJ, Jones W, Boulton AJ, Tavakoli M, Jeziorska M, Malik RA. Corneal confocal microscopy identifies small-fiber neuropathy in subjects with impaired glucose tolerance who develop type 2 diabetes. Diabetes Care. 2015;38(8):1502–8.
205. Tavakoli M, Kallinikos P, Iqbal A, Herbert A, Fadavi H, Efron N, Boulton AJ, Malik A, R. Corneal confocal microscopy detects improvement in corneal nerve morphology with an improvement in risk factors for diabetic neuropathy. Diabet Med. 2011;28(10):1261–7.
206. Dahan A, Dunne A, Swartjes M, Proto PL, Heij L, Vogels O, van Velzen M, Sarton E, Niesters M, Tannemaat MR, Cerami A, Brines M. ARA 290 improves symptoms in patients with sarcoidosis-associated small nerve fiber loss and increases corneal nerve fiber density. Mol Med. 2013;19(1):334–45.

Chapter 13
Outcome Measures for Chronic Pain

Natalie Winter

Assessment of chronic pain is very complex and challenging due to the subjective and individually varying perception of pain and the numerous factors influencing it. Nevertheless, in the field of research and clinical routine, standardized methods for recording pain-related parameters are mandatory to enable a more profound evaluation of therapy success and the comparability of different therapy strategies. Various questionnaires and rating scales, also called instruments, have therefore been established for the assessment and outcome measures of pain.

In chronic pain, objective parameters like blood-pressure or certain serum parameters have not been described yet, or are insufficiently informative because they do not correlate with individual suffering or complex constructs such as depression or quality of life [1]. In recent years, therefore, the focus has increasingly been set on the patient's perspective in the assessment of therapeutic success, in the field of clinical research and in the evaluation of health care services [2]. To further operationalize patient's reports, the terms 'patient-reported outcomes' (PRO), 'patient-reported outcome measures' (PROM) and patient-reported experience measures (PREM) were established. PROs are any reports coming directly from patients about how they feel in relation to a health condition and its therapy, without interpretation of the patient's responses by a clinician, or anyone else [2, 3]. They include any treatment or outcome evaluation obtained directly from patients through interviews, diaries or other data collection tools such as hand-held devices and web-based forms [3]. The corresponding PROM is the instrument used to measure PROs. They mostly contain standardized, validated questionnaires that are completed by patients to ascertain perceptions of their health status, perceived level of

N. Winter (✉)
Department of Neurology and Epileptology, Hertie Institute for Clinical Brain Research, University of Tuebingen, Tuebingen, Germany
e-mail: natalie.winter@med.uni-tuebingen.de

© The Author(s), under exclusive license to Springer Nature Switzerland AG 2022

J. de Castro, Y. El Miedany (eds.), *Advances in Chronic and Neuropathic Pain*, Contemporary Rheumatology, https://doi.org/10.1007/978-3-031-10687-3_13

impairment, disability, and health-related quality of life [4]. The focus of PROMs might be generic (designed for the use in populations with different medical conditions), disease-specific or condition-specific (designed for the use in a particular disease state, condition, intervention or treatment of interest) [1, 4].

PREMs are tools that gather information on patients' views of their experience whilst receiving care. They are an indicator of the quality of patient care, although they do not measure it directly. Questionnaires are most common forms for PREMs. In contrast to PROMs, PREMs focus on the impact of the process of the care on the patient's experience e.g. communication and timeliness of assistance [4].

When developing and using PROMs and PREMs, the following psychometric properties should be considered:

- Validity—the instrument measures what it is supposed to measure [1, 5]
- Content validity—describes the extent to which the measurements of a construct fully capture its content in all its aspects [5]
- Reliability—the instrument assesses the feature of interest reliably and consistently over time
- Sensitivity to change—the instrument detects treatment-induced changes

The authors of IMMPACT (Initiative on Methods, Measurement and Pain Assessment in Clinical Trials) also recommend that the parameters appropriateness, interpretability and availability should be taken into account when developing and applying PROMs [6]. Although PROs and PROMs are increasingly used, verification and validation of test procedures is not performed on a regular basis. In addition, many limitations result from the heterogeneity of the instruments used [1]. One approach to address this problem is to establish core outcome sets (COS) —defined as a minimum set of most critical outcome domains and corresponding instruments [1, 6, 7]. These sets represent the minimum that should be measured and reported in all clinical trials of a specific condition, but COS are also suitable for use in routine care, clinical audit and research other than randomized trials [8–10]. A register for COS for all diseases as well as instructions for creating COS can be found at https://comet-initiative.org/. In the field of chronic pain research, various expert consortia have already developed recommendations for COS depending on disease, interventions and outcome definitions (Table 13.1). As chronic pain has multiple effects on patients, COS should cover several domains depending on the context of question [5–7]:

- Pain Intensity
- Pain Interference and Physical functioning
- Emotional functioning
- Patient reported global rating

For each domain, there are different instruments, each with different application specifications. In the following, the most frequently used tests will be presented.

Table 13.1 Examples of existing core outcome set recommendations in chronic pain conditions (modified from Pogatzki et al. [1])

Core outcome sets—domains	IMMPACT [6, 7]-chronic pain	PedIMMPACT [32]–(acute and) chronic pain	Low back pain [33, 34]-Low back Pain	COMPACT [35]–CRPS
Pain	– NRS – Usage of rescue medicine – VRS if NRS might be problematic	– 3–4 years: Poker Chip Tool – 4–12 years: Faces Pain Scale-Revised – ≥8 years: VAS – Pain diary	– NRS – 1-week interval – RMDQ – Oswestry Disability Index 2.1	*Intensity*: – NRS – PROMIS-29 Profile 2 *Neuropathic Components*: – SF-MPQ2
Physical functioning	– Multidimensional Pain Inventory Interference Scale *or* – Brief Pain Inventory Interference items	– Functional Disability Inventory [36] – <7 years PedsQL	– Oswestry Disability Index 2.1 – RMDQ	+ social participation: – PROMIS-29 profile 2 – EQ-5D-5L
Emotional functioning	– BDI *or* – Profile of mood states	– Children's Depression Inventory – Revised Child Anxiety and Depression Scale (RCADS) –<7 years PedsQL	–	– PROMIS-29 Profile 2 – PROMIS suicidal ideation question *Self-Efficacy*: – Pain Self-efficacy Questionnaire
Symptoms and adverse events	Passive Capture	Active Capture *(further research needed)*	Number of deaths	*Disease Severity*: – CRPS Severity Score – CRPS symptoms question
Patient's global impression/ ratings of change	Patient Global Impression of Change	–	–	Patient Global Impression of Change

(continued)

Table 13.1 (continued)

Core outcome sets—domains	IMMPACT [6, 7]-chronic pain	PedIMMPACT [32]–(acute and) chronic pain	Low back pain [33, 34]-Low back Pain	COMPACT [35]–CRPS
Other domains	*Patient's disposition and acquisition data*: CONSORT guidelines [37]	*Role Functioning*: – School attendance – PedMIDAS (persistent headache) [38] – PedsQL *Sleep*: – Sleep Habits Questionnaire *(further research needed)* *Economic Factors*: Instruments in progress	*Health-related quality of life*: – Short form health survey 12 – 10-item PROMIS Global Health	*Catastrophizing*: Pain Catastrophizing Scale

COMPACT: Core Outcome Measurement for CRPS Clinical Studies; CONSORT: Consolidated Standards of Reporting Trials; CRPS: complex regional pain syndrome; IMMPACT: Initiative on Methods, Measurement and Pain Assessment in Clinical Trials; NRS: Numeric Rating Scale; PedMIDAS: Pediatric Migraine Disability Assessment; PedsQL: Pediatric Quality of Life Inventory; PROMIS: Patient-reported Outcomes Measurement Information System; RMDQ: The Roland & Morris Disability Questionnaire; SF-MPQ2: short form McGill Questionnaire 2; VAS: Visual Analogue Scale; VRS: Verbal Rating Scale

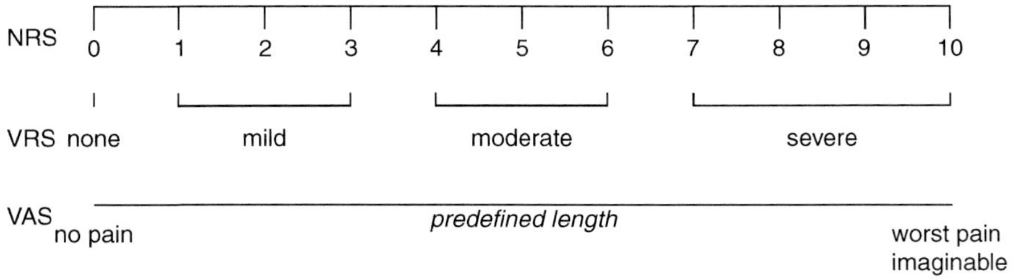

Fig. 13.1 Comparison of Numeric Rating Scale (NRS) , Verbal Rating Scale (VRS) and Visual Analogue Scale (VAS)

Pain Intensity

The most commonly used scales for measuring acute and chronic pain intensity are the **Numeric Rating Scale** (NRS) , **Verbal Rating Scale** (VRS) and **Visual Analogue Scale** (VAS) [11]. The NRS is a unidimensional 11-point scale ranging from 0 points = no pain to 10 points = worst pain (Fig. 13.1). It shows very good correlation with the VAS (correlation ranges from 0.86 to 0.95), in which the patient is asked to mark the pain intensity on a line with a defined length (Fig. 13.1). In terms of sensitivity to changes, both scales are superior to the VRS, which only consists of four terms describing pain intensity: 'none', 'mild, 'moderate' and 'severe'. In some versions of VRS a fifth category, 'very severe pain', is added. A computerized simulation study of simultaneous recorded data of VAS, NRS and VRS observations documented that the power to detect a difference in pain intensity was higher with the NRS and the VAS data in comparison to the VRS data. Furthermore, the power to detect a difference increases with the magnitude of the difference in pain intensities before and after pain treatment [11, 12]. The IMMPACT authors recommend using VRS as an additional tool to increase comparability between studies [6]. The VRS is also easier to understand, especially for older participants, and quickly completed, so that dropout rates can be reduced if the NRS or VAS are inadequately completed. The VRS and NRS are more suitable for telephone interviews.

The test-retest reliability is very high for NRS for both literate and illiterate people ($r = 0.96$ and 0.95 respectively, studied on patients with rheumatoid arthritis) and VAS (literate $r = 0.94$, illiterate $r = 0.71$, studied on patients with rheumatoid arthritis) [5]. All three scales are freely available.

The **short form McGill Questionnaire 2** (SF-MPQ2) is the specifically extended version of the McGill Questionnaire to include evaluation of neuropathic pain in the assessment of chronic pain. The SF-MPQ2 contains 22 pain descriptors (scored 0–10 using the anchors "none" to "worst possible") on four subscales representing (1) continuous, (2) intermittent, (3) neuropathic, and (4) affective features [13]. For complex regional pain syndrome (CRPS) Dworkin et al. reported good internal consistency for each subscale (ranging from 0.73 to 0.87 across several investigations in large samples). Discriminant validity was supported by significant differences in change scores across a clinical trial in those who considered themselves improved compared with those who did not ($P < 0.002$ for all scales) [14]. Other areas of application for SF-MQ2 include low back pain, painful diabetic neuropathy and cancer pain [13].

Pain Interference and Physical Functioning

Pain Interference refers to all pain-related consequences on relevant aspects of a person's life and include the extent to which pain hinders engagement with social, cognitive, emotional, physical, and recreational activities. Most questionnaires in this area include pain intensity and impact on daily function as well as general functional impairment. **The Roland & Morris Disability Questionnaire** (RMDQ) is a widely used health status measure for low back pain and can be used for clinical purposes or research [5]. The RMDQ contains 24 sentences which describe different limitations of movements or functions for which participants tick those that apply to them that day [5]. The total score ranges from 0 points (no sentences applied) to 24 points (all applied). In several studies psychometric properties have been evaluated: the RMDQ has a good validity and reliability with a range of internal consistency between 0.83 and 0.95 [15, 16], and a range of intraclass correlation coefficients between 0.83 and 0.93 with poorer retest reliability in longer intervals [15, 17–19]. The questionnaire is freely available on the website www.rmdq.org and has already been translated into over 50 languages.

The **Oswestry Disability Index** (ODI) 2.1 has become one of the principal condition-specific outcome measures used in the management of low back pain. The questionnaire is very detailed with 10 categories (pain intensity, personal care, lifting, walking, sitting, standing, sleeping, sex life, social life, traveling), each containing six statements with different degrees of restriction, from which the patient selects the most applicable to him or her. Each category is scored from 0 (no difficulty) to 5 points (maximum difficulty), summed and multiplied by the factor two to obtain a score range from 0 to 100. Test-retest reliability has been shown to be high with intraclass correlation coefficients values ranging from 0.83 to 0.99 [19–23]. Similar to the RMDQ, the reliability decreases with increasing interval between tests. For non-commercial use, the test is free of charge.

As complimentary instruments to disease-specific ones, both the **West Haven-Yale Multidimensional Pain Inventory Interference Scale** (WHYMPI/ MPI) and the **Brief Pain Inventory (BPI) Interference Items** are recommended to measure physical functioning [6]. The WHYMPI is a 52-item, 12-scale inventory that is divided into three parts, which addresses the impact of pain on the patients' lives, the responses of others to the patients' communications of pain, and the extent to which patients participate in common daily activities [24]. Especially the last part is designed to assess physical functioning. The initial study showed good psychometric results: The internal reliability coefficients of all WHYMPI scales ranged from 0.7 to 0.9, the test-retest reliabilities of these scales over a 2-week interval ranged from 0.62 to 0.91 [24].

The BPI was initially designed for the assessment of pain in tumor patients. In the meantime, however, its application in chronic pain associated diseases, such as low back pain, musculoskeletal pain and arthritis, has been widely demonstrated [25–27]. In addition to the MPI, the BPI includes an item to asses pain interference with sleep, which is an important part of the evaluation of physical functioning [6]. A validation study by Tan and his colleagues revealed an acceptable internal consistency (Cronbach alpha coefficients were 0.85 for the intensity items and 0.88 for the interference items), a stable 2-factor structure and responsivity to change [25].

The WHYMPI is freely available. The University of Texas M.D. Anderson Cancer Center holds the copyright, but permission to use the tool can be sought by filling out an online form.

Emotional Functioning

Chronic pain is often accompanied by symptoms of psychological distress and psychiatric disorders, including depression, anxiety and anger [6]. The IMMPACT consensus recommends the **Beck Depression Inventory** (BDI) and the **Profile of Mood Status** (POMS) to assess emotional functioning [6]. Both instruments are very well established in clinical trials as well as in clinical areas such as psychiatry, psychology, cardiology, neurology, obstetrics, nephrology, and others. The BDI consist of 21 items, each item scored from 0 to 3 with cut-offs for the total scores: 0 to 13—minimal depression, 14 to 19—mild depression, 20 to 28 moderate depression, 29 to 63 severe depression [5]. The POMS, on the other hand, measures six different dimensions of fluctuating mood swings over a certain period of time: 'Depression or Dejection', 'Confusion or Bewilderment', 'Fatigue or Inertia', 'Tension or Anxiety', 'Anger or Hostility', 'Vigor or Activity'. Each feeling is rated by the respondent on a scale from 1 (not at all) to 5 (extremely) to what extent it is currently applicable. Internal consistency is high for both instruments: POMS ranges from 0.63 to 0.96 (Cronbach alpha coefficient) [28], and BDI around 0.9 (Cronbach alpha coefficient) with a test-retest reliability of 0.73 to 0.96 [5].

Both instruments are copyrighted.

Patient Reported Global Rating

To measure global change from the patient's perspective, the Patient Global Impression of Change Scale (PGIC) has been very useful and is recommended by the IMMPACT [6, 7] and COMPACT consortium (Core Outcome Measurement for CRPS Clinical Studies). The PGIC is a 7-point verbal scale to rate the change before and after or under treatment ranging from 1 = no change to 6 = a great deal better. PGIC has shown to correlate significantly with changes in other measurements like Roland Morris Disability Questionnaire, Oswestry Disability Index, EQ-5D and Pain Rating Scale [29]. Test-retest reliability was high (ICC 0.9).

Other Domains

The term 'catastrophizing' was formally introduced by Albert Ellis and subsequently adapted by Aaron Beck to describe a maladaptive cognitive style employed by patients with anxiety and depressive disorders [30]. The pain-related term 'catastrophizing' is broadly conceived as a set of exaggerated and negative cognitive and emotional schemata brought to bear during actual or anticipated painful stimulation [30]. The Pain Catastrophizing Scale (PCS) consists of 13 statements that the participant is asked to rate from 0 = not at all to 4 = all the time, depending on how much these statements apply to the participant when in pain. Internal consistency ranged from 0.86 to 0.95 (Cronbach alpha coefficient) with good validity [31]. The PSC is free for use, for commercial research a payment is required.

PROMIS, Neuro Qol, ASCQ-Me

PROMIS (Patient-reported Outcomes Measurement Information System) is a National Institutes of Health initiative to develop and make self-reported and parent-reported measures of global, physical, mental, and social health for adults and children in the general population and those living with a chronic condition available. Other measurement batteries for specific diseases are also freely accessible: **Neuro QoL** are self-reported and proxy-reported measures of physical, mental, and social health for adults and children living with a neurological condition and **ASCQ-ME** offers self-reported measures of physical, mental, and social health for adults living with sickle cell disease. Many of these measurements have already been tested with regard to their validity and reliability and are also available in different languages. However, the exact specifications should be checked before application. All three databases can be accessed via the Website www.healthmeasures.net

References

1. Pogatzki-Zahn E, Schnabel K, Kaiser U. Patient-reported outcome measures for acute and chronic pain: current knowledge and future directions. Curr Opin Anaesthesiol. 2019;32(5):616–22.
2. Weldring T, Smith SMS. Article commentary: patient-reported outcomes (PROs) and patient-reported outcome measures (PROMs). Heal Serv Insights. 2013;6:61–8.
3. Higgins JP, Green S. Cochrane handbook for systematic reviews. Vol. Version 5. The Cochrane Collaboration. 2008. Version 5.1.0.
4. Kingsley C, Patel S. Patient-reported outcome measures and patient-reported experience measures. BJA Educ. 2017;17(4):137–44.
5. Baranidharan G, Williams A, Wilson S, Cameron P, Tan T. Outcome measures [internet]. British Pain Society. 2019 [cited 2021 May 2]. Available from: https://www.britishpainsociety.org/static/uploads/resources/files/Outcome_Measures_January_2019.pdf
6. Dworkin RH, Turk DC, Farrar JT, Haythornthwaite JA, Jensen MP, Katz NP, et al. Core outcome measures for chronic pain clinical trials: IMMPACT recommendations. Pain. 2005;113(1–2):9–19.
7. Turk DC, Dworkin RH, Allen RR, Bellamy N, Brandenburg N, Carr DB, et al. Core outcome domains for chronic pain clinical trials: IMMPACT recommendations. Pain. 2003;106:337–45.
8. Kirkham JJ, Gorst S, Altman DG, Blazeby JM, Clarke M, Tunis S, et al. Core outcome set-STAndardised protocol items: the COS-STAP statement. Trials. 2019;20(1):1–7.
9. Kirkham JJ, Gorst S, Altman DG, Blazeby JM, Clarke M, Devane D, et al. Core outcome set–STAndards for reporting: the COS-STAR statement. PLoS Med. 2016;13(10):1–11.
10. Kirkham JJ, Davis K, Altman DG, Blazeby JM, Clarke M, Tunis S, et al. Core outcome set-STAndards for development: the COS-STAD recommendations. PLoS Med. 2017;14(11):1–10.
11. Breivik H, Borchgrevink PC, Allen SM, Rosseland LA, Romundstad L, Breivik Hals EK, et al. Assessment of pain. Br J Anaesth. 2008;101(1):17–24.
12. Breivik Hals EK, Björnsson GA, Skovlund E. A comparison of pain rating scales by sampling from clinical trial data. Clin J Pain. 2000;16:22–8.
13. Packham TL, Bean D, Johnson MH, Macdermid JC, Grieve S, Mccabe CS, et al. Measurement properties of the SF-MPQ-2 neuropathic qualities subscale in persons with CRPS: validity , responsiveness , and Rasch analysis. Pain Med. 2018;0(0):1–11.
14. Dworkin RH, Turk DC, Trudeau JJ, Benson C, David M, Katz NP, et al. Validation of the short-form McGill pain questionnaire-2 (SF-MPQ-2) in acute low Back pain. J Pain. 2015;2:1–29.
15. Stratford PW, Binkley J, Solomon P, Finch E, Gill C, Moreland J. Defining the minimum level of detectable change for the Roland- Morris questionnaire. Phys Ther. 2018;76(4):359–65.
16. Spanjer J, Groothoff JW, Brouwer S. Instruments used to assess functional limitations in workers applying for disability benefit: a systematic review. Disabil Rehabil. 2011;33:2143–50.
17. Brouwer S, Kuijer W, Dijkstra PU. Reliability and stability of the Roland Morris disability questionnaire: intra class correlation and limits of agreement. Disabil Rehabil. 2004;26(3):162–5.
18. Jordan K, Dunn KM, Lewis M, Croft P. A minimal clinically important difference was derived for the Roland-Morris disability questionnaire for low back pain. J Clin Epidemiol. 2006;59:45–52.
19. Davidson M, Keating JL. A comparison of five low back disability questionnaires: reliability. Phys Ther. 2002;82(1):8–24.
20. Roland M, Fairbank J. The Roland – Morris disability questionnaire and the Oswestry disability questionnaire. Spine (Phila Pa 1976). 2000;25(24):3115–24.
21. Fairbank JCT, Pynsent PB. The Oswestry disability index. Spine (Phila Pa 1976). 2000;25(22):2940–53.
22. Grotle M, Garratt AM, Krogstad H, Stuge B. Research report reliability and construct validity of. Phys Ther. 2012;92(1):111–23.
23. Miekisiak G, Kollataj M, Dobrogowski J, Kloc W. Validation and cross-cultural adaptation of the. Spine (Phila Pa 1976). 2013;38(4):237–43.

24. Kerns R. The west Haven-Yale multidimensional pain inventory the west Haven-Yale multidimensional inventory (WHYMPI). Pain. 1986;23:345–56.
25. Tan G, Jensen MP, Thornby JI, Shanti BF. Validation of the brief pain inventory for chronic nonmalignant pain. J Pain. 2004;5(2):133–7.
26. Keller S, Bann CM, Dodd SL, Schein J, Mendoza TR, Cleeland CS. Validity of the brief pain inventory for use in documenting the outcomes of patients with noncancer pain. Clin J Pain. 2004;20(5):309–18.
27. Celik E, Yalcinkaya E, Atamaz F, Karatas M, Ones K. Validity and reliability of a Turkish brief pain inventory short form when used to evaluate musculoskeletal pain. J Back Musculoskelet Rehabil. 2016;1:1–5.
28. Curran SL, Andrykowski MA, Studts JL. Short form of the profile of mood states (POMS-SF): psychometric information. Psychol Assess. 1995;7(1):80–3.
29. Kamper SJ, Maher CG, Mackay G. Global rating of change scales. J Man Manip Ther. 2009;17(3):163–70.
30. Quartana PJ, M CC, Edwards RR. Pain catastrophizing: a critical review. Expert Rev Neurother. 2009;9(5):745–58.
31. Osman A, Barrios FX, Gutierrez PM, Kopper A, Merrifield T, Grittmann L. The pain catastrophizing scale: further psychometric evaluation with adult samples. J Behav Med. 2000;23(4):351–65.
32. McGrath PJ, Walco GA, Turk DC, Dworkin RH, Brown MT, Davidson K, et al. Core outcome domains and measures for pediatric acute and chronic/recurrent pain clinical trials: PedIMMPACT recommendations. J Pain. 2008;9(9):771–83.
33. Chiarotto A, Boers M, Deyo RA, Al E. Core outcome measurement instruments for clinical trials in non-specific low back pain 1. Pain. 2018;159:481–95.
34. Chiarotto A, Deyo RA, Terwee CB, Boers M, Buchbinder R, Corbin TP, et al. Core outcome domains for clinical trials in non-specific low back pain. Eur Spine J. 2015;24:1127–42.
35. Grieve S, Perez RSGM, Birklein F, Brunner F, Bruehl S, Harden RN, et al. Recommendations for a first core outcome measurement set for complex regional PAin syndrome clinical sTudies (COMPACT). Pain. 2017;158:1083–90.
36. Walker LS, Greene JW. The functional disability inventory: measuring a neglected dimension of child health status. J Pediatr Psychol. 1991;16:39–58.
37. CONSORT [Internet]. [cited 2021 May 2]. Available from: http://www.consort-statement.org/
38. Hershey AD, Powers SW, Vockell AB. Development of a questionnaire to assess disability of. Neurology. 2001;57:2034–9.

Part VI
Management of Chronic and Neuropathic Pains

Chapter 14 Nonpharmacologic Modalities for Chronic Pain

Carl Froilan D. Leochico and Reynaldo R. Rey-Matias

Introduction

Hellen Keller once said, *"Although the world is full of suffering, it is full also of the overcoming of it."* Chronic pain (CP) with or without neuropathic features is considered a major public health problem and among the most common chief complaints encountered in primary care [1, 2]. CP exists beyond the usual tissue healing time for a certain underlying illness [3], and may persist for more than 3–6 months or present intermittently as a recurring symptom [4–7]. Its vast and lingering impact on the physical, neuropsychological, and social aspects of the life of a patient may contribute not just to his/her reduced health-related quality of life, which is among the lowest found for any medical condition [8], but also to the community's economic burden from loss of productivity and increased demand for disability-related compensations [9, 10]. Although there is no universally acceptable standardized or fixed protocol for CP care [11, 12], a lot of treatment options are available, ranging from pharmacologic to nonpharmacologic, and unimodal (a single therapeutic intervention targeting a specific pain mechanism or diagnosis) to multimodal (concurrent use of two or more therapeutic interventions within the realm of one discipline targeting different pain mechanisms), multidisciplinary (multimodal approach by a team composed of different disciplines working separately towards a common

C. F. D. Leochico · R. R. Rey-Matias (✉)
Department of Physical Medicine and Rehabilitation, St. Luke's Medical Center, Global City and Quezon City, Philippines

Department of Rehabilitation Medicine, College of Medicine and Philippine General Hospital, University of the Philippines Manila, Manila, Philippines

School of Medicine, St. Louis University, Baguio City, Philippines
e-mail: rrreymatias@stlukes.com.ph

© The Author(s), under exclusive license to Springer Nature Switzerland AG 2022

J. de Castro, Y. El Miedany (eds.), *Advances in Chronic and Neuropathic Pain*, Contemporary Rheumatology, https://doi.org/10.1007/978-3-031-10687-3_14

goal), and interdisciplinary (multidisciplinary team working in collaboration with the patient and/or family) treatments, which can all be contextualized according to the patient's overall condition, needs, goals, and resources [13].

Treatment Rationale

Previously viewed as being outside the scope of mainstream pain management [14], nonpharmacologic modalities, which are interventions that do not rely on medications to effect analgesia, are now part of the fundamental and holistic care for patients even from the outset of pain to prevent it from "chronification" (progression into persistent pain due to imbalance between pain amplification and inhibition) [11, 15]. While acute pain may be considered a normal, expected, and physiologic response to an underlying tissue injury, CP does not seem to serve a protective function or apparent biological value [15].

In line with Engel's biopsychosocial model [16], CP can result from a complex and dynamic interaction of biological, cognitive, psychological, social, and cultural contexts that may shape the clinical symptoms, severity, duration, functional impact, perceptions, and response to illness experienced by a patient [17]. Given the multifaceted nature of CP, providing at least a multimodal approach to treatment may, therefore, seem rational [17, 18]. Nonetheless, an interdisciplinary approach maximizing the coordinated efforts of healthcare providers from different disciplines (e.g., physicians from relevant specialties and subspecialties, physical therapists, occupational therapists, psychologists, nurses, nutritionists, social workers, and other health professionals) can more comprehensively address the individualized needs of a patient [19], but similar to any other intervention/s its cost-effectiveness has to be considered [17].

The evolution of pain models began with the World Health Organization's three-step ladder (depicting the linear up or down approach to medication use) [20], which eventually gave rise to the four-step ladder (incorporating interventional procedures) [21], and platform model (highlighting both pharmacologic and nonpharmacologic treatments) [22]. The latest model comes in the image of a trolley that advocates dynamic, tailored, and multimodal pain management [12]. The simple and intuitive "analgesic trolley" model consists of several drawers containing pharmacologic options with different mechanisms of action, and nonpharmacologic options whether nonoperative (e.g., therapeutic, educational, or psychological services; complementary and alternative medicine) or operative (e.g., neurolysis; other interventional procedures). It guides a healthcare provider in selecting the most appropriate treatment modalities for his/her patient depending on the following: (1) pain intensity; (2) underlying pathophysiology; (3) complex clinical presentation; (4) comorbid condition/s; and (5) socioenvironmental factors [12].

Nonpharmacologic Modalities

Nonpharmacologic modalities can be used either as stand-alone or in combination with analgesic medications. Their advantages over pharmacologic treatments may include, but are not limited to, their overall safety, tolerability, patient compliance, and potentially long-term benefits [23–25]. Nonpharmacologic modalities may also minimize the dosage of analgesic medications (e.g., opioids) and subsequently their possible side effects [26]. The selection of individual modalities comprising a comprehensive and tailored treatment should consider various clinical factors, such as patient's age, medical history and evaluation, prior interventions, current pain status, safety, preferences, and treatment goals [26]. Nonpharmacologic modalities generally aim to control, rather than eliminate, the pain and its negative impact on the person (e.g., limitations in functional activities and societal roles; anxiety; reduced quality of life) [24, 26]. However, the success of patient-centered nonpharmacologic approach may entail consistent and active participation from the patient and family, who ultimately direct and adhere to the treatment options offered by the healthcare team based on their needs and available resources. Incorporating nonpharmacologic modalities in the treatment armamentarium for a patient suffering from CP encourages "patient self-efficacy, active problem-solving, realistic goal setting, and a functional/rehabilitative outlook" [27].

Turk and Monarch describe a medical condition or "disease" as an objective alteration of the normal or physiological body structure and function, while an "illness" as a subjective experience arising from a "unique interaction among biological, psychological, and social factors" [28]. CP, albeit emerging from underlying peripheral sensory and central sensitization mechanisms [29], can be viewed as an illness that may benefit from rehabilitation and disability management, rather than mere curative approach [30]. In the same way, the biopsychosocial perspective may target the illness more than the disease, taking into account the diverse differences in the pain journey of individual patients [31].

For an organized discussion, this section presents some of the nonpharmacologic modalities according to their intuitively primary or direct benefits as follows: (1) biological or physical; (2) psychological or behavioral; and (3) social or cultural. However, it must be noted that most, if not all, of the nonpharmacologic modalities presented herein may have one or more of these interrelated benefits.

Biological or Physical Treatment Options

Nociception pertains to pain perception as a result of underlying biological or physiological pain mechanisms (e.g., through nerve receptors, specifically free nerve endings for pain; nerve fibers, such as types A-delta or C for acute or chronic pain, respectively) associated with sensory input [31]. The multitude of pain conditions can be categorized into inflammatory, neuropathic, or cancer pain [30]. The mechanism of acute inflammatory pain states involves "stimulation or potentiation of nociceptive transduction at peripheral terminals and central changes contributing to hypersensitivity" [30, 32], which if managed inadequately may lead to CP characterized by central sensitization, an abnormal heightened state of pain perception disproportionate to usual sensory inputs and mechanisms [33]. Neuropathic pain arises from "a lesion or disease of the somatosensory system" [34], spanning from the peripheral nerves to the spinal cord and other areas in the central nervous system. Meanwhile, cancer-related pain can result from tumor infiltration or mechanical compression of adjacent neurologic structures, neuroendocrine substances released by tumors, or effects of treatment [30]. CP can typically accompany neuropathic and cancer-related types of pain [35, 36].

Given the biological mechanisms of CP, various nonpharmacologic modalities have been developed to alleviate primarily the physical aspect of this pain condition.

Thermotherapy

Thermotherapy refers to any therapeutic modality that can either increase (heat therapy) or decrease (cryotherapy) the cutaneous, intraarticular, and/or core temperature of soft tissues with the goal of relieving pain and spasm [37, 38]. Thermoreceptors, localized in the dermal ends of primary somatosensory nerve fibers [39], may alter the neurotransmission of nociceptive or pain impulses [38]. Aside from 'shutting the pain gate,' heat therapy works by vasodilation resulting in enhanced local blood flow, metabolic rate, and tissue extensibility of the treatment area, while cryotherapy facilitates vasoconstriction that initially decreases and then increases local blood flow with the net result of reduction in tissue metabolism, neuronal excitability and conduction, and inflammation [37, 40]. In general, cryotherapy is used during the inflammatory phase of healing to help control swelling [41], whereas heat therapy can be instituted either alone or alternately with cryotherapy (i.e., contrast bath) during the proliferative and remodeling phases. The choice between cryotherapy and heat therapy depends on the patient's medical history, treatment goals, and preference, along with the healthcare provider's experience and judgment [42].

Topical modalities that employ heat therapy can be categorized into superficial and deep heating agents. Superficial heating agents (e.g., hot packs; heating pads; infrared radiation; dry heat in the form of fluidotherapy; paraffin wax bath) achieve a maximum tissue temperature in the skin and subcutaneous tissue and allow heat dissipation to deeper tissues through vasodilation and the insulating properties of fat [43]. Deep heating agents (e.g., therapeutic ultrasound; shortwave diathermy; microwave diathermy) penetrate the skin and subcutaneous tissue and produce a maximum temperature increase (up to therapeutic levels of 40–45° C or 104–113° F) in the underlying tissues, without heating up or damaging the more superficial ones [43, 44]. Therapeutic heat can benefit various painful conditions, such as sprains, strains, fibrositis, muscle injury, arthritis, contractures, chronic pelvic inflammatory disease, etc [44].

The modalities that provide cryotherapy are all superficial cooling agents. Examples include cold packs, ice massage, cold water immersion, and cryotherapy-compression units that employ conduction as their main form of energy transfer. On the other hand, vapocoolant sprays and whirlpool baths transfer energy through evaporation and convection, respectively [43]. A recent systematic review found supportive evidence for the use of either local or nonlocal (whole body) cryotherapy for CP of degenerative or rheumatic origins [40]. Promising results were observed for adhesive capsulitis, myofascial pain syndrome, chronic low back pain, fibromyalgia, rheumatoid arthritis, ankylosing spondylitis, and osteoarthritis. However, insufficient evidence was found for chronic venous disease and multiple sclerosis.

Thermotherapy is a generally safe nonpharmacologic modality, but it is not without known adverse effects inherent to either heat or cold application. Hence, a thorough review of the patient's medical contraindications and precautions, along with adequate knowledge of the mechanism and risks of any available specific modalitiy, should be considered before incorporating thermotherapy in the treatment regimen.

Electrotherapy

Electrotherapy in the form of transcutaneous electrical nerve stimulation (TENS) , which can come in a small, low-cost, battery-powered device delivering alternating current through electrodes applied on or near the painful area, is used widely for CP [45]. TENS works at both peripheral and central levels. It activates large diameter afferent fibers and subsequently the descending inhibitory systems to reduce pain perception [45, 46]. The high-frequency TENS (25–50 Hertz) in particular reduces neuronal excitation and sensitization in the spinal cord through the reduction of glutamate [45, 47]. The effectiveness of TENS is associated with its pulse frequency and intensity that can be increased until levels perceived by the patient as pain-free, although tolerance may develop especially with frequent application using the same parameters [45].

Earlier systematic reviews suggested emerging evidence of TENS for CP such as in osteoarthritis and fibromyalgia, and neuropathic pain such as in diabetes mellitus and spinal cord injury [45]. However, a recent review of prior Cochrane reviews was unable to reach a solid conclusion regarding the effectiveness of TENS for adults with CP due to the very low-quality evidence found in the literature [48]. For the same reason, the 2019 guideline of the American College of Rheumatology/Arthritis Foundation does not recommend TENS for knee and/or hip osteoarthritis [49].

Manual Therapy

Manual therapy refers to passive techniques applied by trained practitioners (e.g., physicians, physiotherapists, chiropractors, osteopaths) to joint, muscle, connective, and/or neurovascular tissues [50]. It comes in different forms, such as oscillatory techniques, high-velocity, low-amplitude thrust techniques, sustained stretching, muscle energy techniques, and massage, depending on the patient's needs, clinician's expertise, treatment goals, and even cultural beliefs [51, 52]. It can provide several physiological, biomechanical or physical, and psychological therapeutic benefits. It reduces pain by activating the gate control theory and descending inhibitory tracts, and inhibits muscles spasm by reducing the pressure or tension of intraarticular or periarticular structures [53]. To improve joint range of motion and quality, 'mobilization' or 'manipulation' can be performed within or beyond an available active range of motion, respectively [54]. Through repetitive movements, manual therapy can produce alterations in tissue extensibility and joint fluid dynamics to facilitate repair and remodeling of injured structures [54, 55]. Employing direct physical contact, it can foster patient-clinician interaction via the "laying of hands," possibly alleviating stress or anxiety [50, 54, 56].

The incidence of major adverse events with manual therapy in general is low, and no catastrophic event like death or stroke has been reported [57]. It may, however, present with minor adverse events like short-term muscle soreness, stiffness, and headache in about 50% of patients [58, 59]. Especially for spinal manipulation, several contraindications should be considered such as the following: joint hypermobility (e.g., syndromes presenting with ligamentous laxity) or instability (e.g., spondylolisthesis); bone disease (e.g., malignancy, infection, fracture, osteoporosis); neurovascular compromise (e.g., spinal cord compression, moderate to severe nerve root compression); rheumatologic disease (e.g., rheumatoid arthritis, ankylosing spondylitis, polymyalgia rheumatica) ; and vascular disorders (e.g., aortic aneurysm, severe blood dyscrasias, vertebrobasilar insufficiency, spinal ischemia) [60].

Prior systematic reviews, including a Cochrane review, showed that spinal manipulative therapy may be as effective and safe as other common interventions like standard medical treatment, physiotherapy, or exercises, in reducing pain and improving function among patients with chronic low back pain [61, 62]. However, due to a high risk of bias found in the included studies, further research, including economic evaluations to determine cost-effectiveness, was recommended. Meanwhile, a more recent randomized controlled trial (RCT) compared the effects of manual therapy (3 sessions at one per week employing high thoracic manipulation, cervical articular mobilization, and suboccipital muscle inhibition), therapeutic exercises for cervical flexors and extensors daily for 3 weeks, and placebo on non-specific chronic neck pain [63]. The two experimental groups showed statistically significant improvements in pain and disability in the short and medium terms. Nonetheless, the authors recognized the need for further studies particularly on the effects of multimodal treatment (e.g., combined manual therapy, therapeutic exercise, and pain education), which might provide more optimal outcomes.

Therapeutic Exercises

Therapeutic exercise refers to a planned, structured, and repetitive "performance of bodily movements, postures, or physical activities" aimed towards the prevention or rehabilitation of impairments, control of health-related risk factors, and maintenance or improvement of function, fitness, and overall well-being [64, 65]. It refers to a wide range of exercise modalities (e.g., land- or water-based range-of-motion, resistance, and/or aerobic exercises; tai chi; balance training; motor control exercise; Pilates method) that can target one or more of the following interrelated components of function: mobility/flexibility, muscle performance (strength, power, muscular endurance), posture, stability, balance, neuromuscular control/coordination, and cardiopulmonary fitness/endurance [64, 65]. It is a fundamental component of any rehabilitation program that can benefit a variety of conditions, including those presenting with CP. Studies show that exercise, especially when done repeatedly, can increase one's level of endogenous opioids resulting in anti-nociception, promote self-efficacy and ability to self-manage pain, and improve health-related quality of life [64, 66].

Different guidelines such as from the National Institute for Health & Care Excellence (NICE) and the American College of Sports Medicine (ACSM) recommend physical activity to help manage chronic primary pain (e.g., fibromyalgia; chronic neck pain; others in which no underlying condition can adequately account for the pain or its impact) [67, 68]. There is evidence of various short- and long-term benefits across different exercise modalities, depending on the type of pain [64, 69]. In general, therapeutic exercises are found to be cost-effective and free from negative outcomes, except for potential problems with patient adherence, which seems to improve when exercise programs are sustainable and suited to one's lifestyle, preferences, abilities, needs, and resources [67].

Psychological or Behavioral Treatment Options

CP can negatively impact sleep, mood, interpersonal relationships, functional and work-related activities, and quality of life [19, 30]. It may result in the development of maladaptive behaviors and ineffective coping strategies, which logically can be managed by incorporating psychological interventions as part of a comprehensive treatment plan [19]. A careful psychological assessment and management can control the vicious cycle of nociception, distress, and disability perpetuated by the emotional and cognitive components of the CP experience [30].

A holistic assessment of the person should look beyond objective physical and ancillary findings in order to address even the unseen, possibly neglected, consequences of CP [29]. The essential psychosocial elements that the healthcare provider needs to evaluate include, but are not limited to, the following: patient's perception of and attitude towards CP; positive and negative coping strategies, including drug dependence and substance use (if any); past medical and family history of psychiatric conditions; and social support [29, 70, 71]. In general, psychological or behavioral interventions aim to reduce the suffering caused by the entire pain experience through patient education, empowerment, and self-efficacy techniques [29].

Cognitive-Behavioral Therapy

Cognitive-behavioral therapy (CBT) is the first-line psychosocial treatment for a wide range of CP conditions, such as headache, low back pain, arthritis, fibromyalgia, orofacial pain, and cancer or its treatment [72]. There is no single standardized protocol for conducting CBT, varying in content (specific techniques), format (group versus one-on-one; in-person versus online), and dose (duration; number of sessions; frequency). Examples of CBT techniques include relaxation training (which can be combined with physiologic techniques like slow diaphragmatic breathing and progressive muscle relaxation exercises), activity pacing, problem solving, cognitive restructuring, behavioral activation, and mindfulness meditation [72–74]. Regardless of the technique, whether administered alone or as adjunct to pharmacologic or other nonpharmacologic interventions, CBT targets negative appraisals, fear avoidance, catastrophizing, and other maladaptive cognitions [75, 76]. A recently updated Cochrane review of psychological therapies for CP, excluding headache, found sufficient evidence supporting the efficacy of CBT, albeit small or very small benefits, on pain, disability, and distress based on 59 studies with over 5000 participants [77]. The review, however, found insufficient evidence to evaluate the adverse events associated with CBT. Nonetheless, the efficacy of CBT is relatively well-established in the literature compared with other psychological interventions that need more research like the following: Acceptance and Commitment Therapy (ACT) (promoting psychological flexibility as alternative to experiential avoidance); guided imagery (incorporating words and music to bring to mind calming images and positive scenarios); hypnosis and suggestion (inducing a state of balance between relaxation and focus), and biofeedback (learning to self-regulate bodily processes through physiologic feedback information, such as from electromyography, heart rate variability, and respiratory, mirror visual, or postural biofeedback) [72, 74, 77–79].

Social or Cultural Treatment Options

Waddell (1987) emphasized that in order to have a complete understanding of a patient's pain experience, his/her sociocultural context needs to be evaluated and considered in the treatment planning and implementation [80]. Missing any of the components of the biopsychosocial approach may result in an inadequate intervention [30]. In Gatchel's conceptual model depicting the biopsychosocial interactive processes involved in health and illness, the social component involves consideration of the following: activities of daily living, environmental stressors, interpersonal relationships, family environment, social support/isolation, social expectations, cultural factors, medicolegal/insurance issues, previous treatment experiences, and work history [30, 81]. Recognized among the important contributors to the multidimensional pain experience, social factors can help individualize patient care by also considering job security, financial status, access to preventative care, past history of physical or sexual abuse, ethnocultural background, external locus of control, and family events like loss of a family member and marital conflicts [29, 82].

The psychological and social aspects of treatment for CP are generally intertwined and ideally involve working with an interdisciplinary team of healthcare professionals (e.g., primary care provider, pain clinician, psychiatrist, psychologist, rehabilitation specialist, physical or occupational therapist, counselor, social worker) [83]. A meta-analysis of 25 interventions (e.g., coping skills training; cognitive restructuring; coaching; patient education about analgesic use; one-on-one counselling; support groups) emphasized the potential utility of various psychosocial modalities as adjunct to medical treatment for cancer-related pain [84]. Few of its included studies, however, were limited by their small sample size, inadequate subject description, and/or lack of randomization among others. Nevertheless, healthcare professionals can select from a variety of psychosocial treatment options based on sound clinical judgment, existing body of knowledge, and patient acceptance [84].

Since social isolation is commonly associated with CP, gradual reintegration to premorbid functioning at home, work/school, and/or community is necessary, wherever and whenever applicable [74]. Lifestyle modifications (e.g., changes in diet and eating behavior; avoidance of vices like smoking or substance use; regular physical activity; stress management; sleep hygiene) may help improve one's self-esteem associated with improvements in pain perception and social participation [74, 82]. In addition, vocational rehabilitation involving strategies initiated towards the later stages of a comprehensive rehabilitation program aims to facilitate early and successful return to work [85]. Examples of components unique to vocational rehabilitation include career exploration, job matching, job-seeking skills training, work placement, supported employment, and social development [86]. These can be accompanied by occupational medicine and rehabilitation components like functional capacity evaluation, job demands analysis, on-the-job support, assistive technology and accommodations, and ergonomics [86].

Future Directions

The potential benefits of various nonpharmacologic modalities for CP may be maximized through shared decision-making involving the patient and healthcare provider/s working collaboratively to ensure that all aspects of the treatment program are acceptable to all parties [87]. Unlike the traditional and often authoritative clinical decision-making process wherein the healthcare provider dictates and the patient is expected to agree with the prescribed intervention, shared decision-making is consistent with the patient-centered approach [88]. However, its effectiveness has yet to be studied [88].

The current body of literature regarding the combination of individual treatment approaches for CP generally remains inconclusive, emphasizing the need for healthcare providers to conduct more methodologically sound research [29, 74]. Nonetheless, it remains prudent to incorporate multimodal interventions for patients based on clinical experience, sound judgment, and practice-based evidence [29].

In certain healthcare settings, in-person access to nonpharmacologic modalities for CP may not be available [74]. In addition, there may be challenges to the coordination of specialized care across disciplines, treatment facilities, and geographic locations of patients and healthcare providers [74, 89]. Hence, if applicable, telehealth using information and communication technologies to remotely deliver healthcare services and overcome the barriers of distance, time, and costs among others can be leveraged either as an adjunct or alternative to in-person pain management [90]. Further research is recommended to determine the characteristics of patients who can significantly benefit from telehealth versus those who need to be seen in person. Amid the ongoing and future technological advancements in healthcare, telehealth for CP may have to explore the cost-effectiveness of various frontiers (e.g., virtual reality, contactless ultrasonic haptic technology) for screening, monitoring, and treatment processes [90].

With the shift from being mere passive recipients of care to taking a more active role in the pain journey, patients can potentially engage in long-term preventive and restorative strategies. A call to action, however, is imperative to ensure adequate knowledge dissemination regarding available treatment options, professional and public education, and proper and inclusive reimbursement schemes [74].

Summary

Nonpharmacologic modalities comprise a fundamental component of the treatment armamentarium to combat the chronic pain epidemic. Patients and healthcare providers alike need to recognize the multidimensional nature of chronic pain in order to arrive at a mutually acceptable treatment program, which results from a careful selection of nonpharmacologic modalities as standalone or adjunct to pharmacologic therapy. Although the body of evidence is still evolving, there are undeniably a lot of generally safe and low-cost physiologic, psychological, and social treatment options available for chronic pain. Keeping in mind the biopsychosocial model in evaluation and treatment of chronic pain, the interventions can be optimized by employing an individualized, patient-centered, interdisciplinary approach. Proper selection and implementation of therapeutic modalities based on sound clinical reasoning are important drivers of a successful outcome. The cost-effectiveness of individual or combined nonpharmacologic modalities, however, can be derived from relevant methodologically sound studies in the future.

References

1. Elliott AM, Smith BH, Penny KI, Cairns Smith W, Alastair Chambers W. The epidemiology of chronic pain in the community. Lancet. 1999;354:1248–52.
2. Duenas M, Ojeda B, Salazar A, Mico JA, Failde I. A review of chronic pain impact on patients, their social environment and the health care system. J Pain Res. 2016;9:457–67.
3. Fishman SM, Rathmell JP, Ballantyne JC. Bonica's management of pain. Wolters Kluwer/ Lippincott Williams & Wilkins; 2009.
4. Russo CM, Brose WG. Chronic pain. Annu Rev Med. 1998;49:123–33.
5. International Association for the Study of Pain (Subcommittee on Taxonomy). Classification of chronic pain: descriptions of chronic pain syndromes and definitions of pain terms. Pain Suppl. 1986;3:S1–226.
6. American Society of Anesthesiologists (Task Force on Pain Management Chronic Pain Section). Practice guidelines for chronic pain management. Anesthesiology. 1997;86:995–1004.
7. Gatchel RJ. Early development of physical and mental deconditioning in painful spinal disorders. In: Mayer T, Mooney V, Gatchel R, editors. Contemporary conservative care for painful spinal disorders. Lea & Febiger; 1991. p. 278–89.
8. Becker N, et al. Pain epidemiology and health related quality of life in chronic non-malignant pain patients referred to a Danish multidisciplinary pain center. Pain. 1997;73:393–400.
9. Langley P, Pérez Hernández C, Margarit Ferri C, Ruiz Hidalgo D, Lubián López M. Pain, health related quality of life and healthcare resource utilization in Spain. J Med Econ. 2011;14:628–38.
10. Dansie EJ, Turk DC. Assessment of patients with chronic pain. Br J Anaesth. 2013;111:19–25.
11. Cascella M. Introductory chapter: the rationale for a multimodal approach to pain treatment. In: From conventional to innovative approaches for pain treatment. IntechOpen; 2019. https://doi.org/10.5772/intechopen.85864.
12. Cuomo A, Bimonte S, Forte CA, Botti G, Cascella M. Multimodal approaches and tailored therapies for pain management: the trolley analgesic model. J Pain Res. 2019;12:711–4.
13. International Association for the Study of Pain. Task force on multimodal pain treatment defines terms for chronic pain care. 2017. Available at: https://www.iasp-pain.org/PublicationsNews/NewsDetail.aspx?ItemNumber=6981. Accessed: 24th July 2021.
14. Mathews M. Multimodal treatment of pain. Neurosurg Clin N Am. 2014;25:803–8.
15. Morlion B, et al. Pain chronification: what should a non-pain medicine specialist know? Curr Med Res Opin. 2018;34:1169–78.
16. Engel G. The need for a new medical model: a challenge for biomedicine. Science (80-). 1977;196:129–36.
17. Ospina, M. & Harstall, C. Multidisciplinary pain programs for chronic pain: evidence from systematic reviews. (2003).
18. Guzman J. Multidisciplinary rehabilitation for chronic low back pain: systematic review. BMJ. 2001;322:1511–6.
19. Dale R, Stacey B. Multimodal treatment of chronic pain. Med Clin North Am. 2016;100:55–64.
20. Ventafridda V, Saita L, Ripamonti C, De Conno F. WHO guidelines for the use of analgesics in cancer pain. Int J Tissue React. 1985;7:93–6.
21. Vargas-Schaffer G. Is the WHO analgesic ladder still valid? Can Fam Physician. 56:514–7.
22. Leung L. From ladder to platform: a new concept for pain management. J Prim Health Care. 2012;4:254.
23. Houzé B, El-Khatib H, Arbour C. Efficacy, tolerability, and safety of non-pharmacological therapies for chronic pain: an umbrella review on various CAM approaches. Prog Neuro-Psychopharmacology Biol Psychiatry. 2017;79:192–205.
24. Anthony YL. Appraisal of nonpharmacological chronic pain management. Walden University; 2017.
25. Chang K-L, Fillingim R, Hurley RW, Schmidt S. Chronic pain management: nonpharmacological therapies for chronic pain. FP Essent. 2015;432:21–6.

26. El Geziry A, Toble Y, Al Kadhi F, Mohammad P, Al Nobani M. Non-pharmacological pain management. In: Pain Management in Special Circumstances. IntechOpen; 2018. https://doi.org/10.5772/intechopen.79689.
27. Becker WC, et al. Barriers and facilitators to use of non-pharmacological treatments in chronic pain. BMC Fam Pract. 2017;18:41.
28. Turk, D. C. & Monarch, E. S. Biopsychosocial perspective on chronic pain. in Psychological approaches to pain management: a practitioner's handbook (eds. Turk, D. C. & Gatchel, R. J.) 3–24 (The Guilford Press, New York 2018).
29. Argoff CE, Albrecht P, Irving G, Rice F. Multimodal analgesia for chronic pain: rationale and future directions. Pain Med. 2009;10:S53–66.
30. Gatchel RJ, Peng YB, Peters ML, Fuchs PN, Turk DC. The biopsychosocial approach to chronic pain: scientific advances and future directions. Psychol Bull. 2007;133:581–624.
31. Gatchel RJ, Howard KJ. The biopsychosocial approach. Available at: https://www.practicalpainmanagement.com/treatments/psychological/biopsychosocial-approach. Accessed: 27th July 2021.
32. Levine, J. Reichling, D. Peripheral mechanisms of inflammatory pain. in Textbook of pain (eds. Wall, P. Melzack, R.) 59–84 (Churchill Livingstone, Edinburgh 1999).
33. Latremoliere A, Woolf CJ. Central sensitization: a generator of pain hypersensitivity by central neural plasticity. J Pain. 2009;10:895–926.
34. International Association for the Study of Pain. IASP terminology. Available at: https://www.iasp-pain.org/Education/Content.aspx?ItemNumber=1698. Accessed: 26th July 2021.
35. Colloca L, et al. Neuropathic pain. Nat Rev Dis Prim. 2017;3:17002.
36. Nersesyan H, Slavin KV. Current aproach to cancer pain management: availability and implications of different treatment options. Ther Clin Risk Manag. 2007;3:381–400.
37. Hurley MV, Bearne LM. Non-exercise physical therapies for musculoskeletal conditions. Best Pract Res Clin Rheumatol. 2008;22:419–33.
38. Nadler SF, Weingand K, Kruse RJ. The physiologic basis and clinical applications of cryotherapy and thermotherapy for the pain practitioner. Pain Physician. 2004;7:395–9.
39. Nakamura K. Afferent pathways for autonomic and shivering thermoeffectors; 2018. p. 263–79. https://doi.org/10.1016/B978-0-444-63912-7.00016-3.
40. Garcia C, Karri J, Zacharias NA, Abd-Elsayed A. Use of cryotherapy for managing chronic pain: an evidence-based narrative. Pain Ther. 2021;10:81–100.
41. Kuo C-C, Lin C-C, Lee W-J, Huang W-T. Comparing the antiswelling and analgesic effects of three different ice pack therapy durations. J Nurs Res. 2013;21:186–93.
42. Sluka KA, Christy MR, Peterson WL, Rudd SL, Troy SM. Reduction of pain-related behaviors with either cold or heat treatment in an animal model of acute arthritis. Arch Phys Med Rehabil. 1999;80:313–7.
43. Weber, D. C. & Hoppe, K. M. Physical agent modalities. in Braddom's physical medicine and rehabilitation (ed. Braddom, R. L.) 449–467 (Elsevier, Philadelphia, PA 2011).
44. Guy AW, Lehmann JF, Stonebridge JB. Therapeutic applications of electromagnetic power. Proc IEEE. 1974;62:55–75.
45. Vance CG, Dailey DL, Rakel BA, Sluka KA. Using TENS for pain control: the state of the evidence. Pain Manag. 2014;4:197–209.
46. Levin MF, Hui-Chan CWY. Conventional and acupuncture-like transcutaneous electrical nerve stimulation excite similar afferent fibers. Arch Phys Med Rehabil. 1993;74:54–60.
47. Ma Y-T, Sluka KA. Reduction in inflammation-induced sensitization of dorsal horn neurons by transcutaneous electrical nerve stimulation in anesthetized rats. Exp Brain Res. 2001;137:94–102.
48. Gibson W, Wand BM, Meads C, Catley MJ, O'Connell NE. Transcutaneous electrical nerve stimulation (TENS) for chronic pain–an overview of Cochrane reviews. Cochrane Database Syst Rev. 2019; https://doi.org/10.1002/14651858.CD011890.pub3.

49. Kolasinski SL, et al. 2019 American College of Rheumatology/Arthritis Foundation guideline for the management of osteoarthritis of the hand, hip, and knee. Arthritis Rheumatol. 2020;72:220–33.
50. Bishop MD, et al. What effect can manual therapy have on a patient's pain experience? Pain Manag. 2015;5:455–64.
51. Bialosky JE, Bishop MD, Cleland JA. Individual expectation: an overlooked, but pertinent, factor in the treatment of individuals experiencing musculoskeletal pain. Phys Ther. 2010;90:1345–55.
52. Bialosky JE, Simon CB, Bishop MD, George SZ. Basis for spinal manipulative therapy: a physical therapist perspective. J Electromyogr Kinesiol. 2012;22:643–7.
53. Zusman M. Spinal manipulative therapy: review of some proposed mechanisms, and a new hypothesis. Aust J Physiother. 1986;32:89–99.
54. Bearne LM, Hurley MV. Physical therapies. In: Rheumatology. Elsevier; 2010. p. 111–22. https://doi.org/10.1016/B978-0-443-06934-5.00008-5.
55. Jayson MI, Dixon AS. Intra-articular pressure in rheumatoid arthritis of the knee: pressure changes during joint use. Ann Rheum Dis. 1970;29:401–8.
56. Hertzman YM. The role of touch in manual therapy - an integrative literature review. Satakunta University of Applied Sciences; 2016.
57. Carnes D, Mars TS, Mullinger B, Froud R, Underwood M. Adverse events and manual therapy: a systematic review. Man Ther. 2010;15:355–63.
58. Carnes D, Mullinger B, Underwood M. Defining adverse events in manual therapies: a modified Delphi consensus study. Man Ther. 2010;15:2–6.
59. Carnes, D., Mars, T., Mullinger, B. & Underwood, M. Adverse events in manual therapy: a systematic review. (2009).
60. World Health Organization (WHO). WHO guidelines on basic training and safety in chiropractic. (2015).
61. Rubinstein SM, et al. Benefits and harms of spinal manipulative therapy for the treatment of chronic low back pain: systematic review and meta-analysis of randomised controlled trials. BMJ l689. 2019; https://doi.org/10.1136/bmj.l689.
62. Rubinstein SM, van Middelkoop M, Assendelft WJ, de Boer MR, van Tulder MW. Spinal manipulative therapy for chronic low-back pain. Cochrane Database Syst Rev. 2011; https://doi.org/10.1002/14651858.CD008112.pub2.
63. Bernal-Utrera C, Gonzalez-Gerez JJ, Anarte-Lazo E, Rodriguez-Blanco C. Manual therapy versus therapeutic exercise in non-specific chronic neck pain: a randomized controlled trial. Trials. 2020;21:682.
64. Geneen LJ, et al. Physical activity and exercise for chronic pain in adults: an overview of Cochrane reviews. Cochrane Database Syst Rev. 2017; https://doi.org/10.1002/14651858.CD011279.pub3.
65. Kisner C, Colby L. Therapeutic exercise: foundational concepts. In: Therapeutic exercise: foundations and techniques. F.A. Davis; 2012.
66. Stagg NJ, et al. Regular exercise reverses sensory hypersensitivity in a rat neuropathic pain model. Anesthesiology. 2011;114:940–8.
67. National Institute for Health and Care Excellence (NICE). Chronic pain (primary and secondary) in over 16s: assessment of all chronic pain and management of chronic primary pain. NICE guideline [NG193] (2021). Available at: https://www.nice.org.uk/guidance/ng193/chapter/Recommendations#assessing-all-types-of-chronic-pain-chronic-primary-pain-chronic-secondary-pain-or-both. Accessed: 31st July 2021.
68. Riebe D, Ehrman JK, Liguori G, Magal M, American College of Sports Medicine. Benefits and risks associated with physical activity. In: ACSM's guidelines for exercise testing and prescription. Wolters Kluwer Health; 2018. p. 1–21.
69. Scottish Intercollegiate Guidelines Network (SIGN). Management of chronic pain. (2013).
70. Hainline B. Chronic pain: physiological, diagnostic, and management considerations. Psychiatr Clin North Am. 2005;28:713–35.

71. Webster LR, Webster RM. Predicting aberrant behaviors in opioid-treated patients: preliminary validation of the opioid risk tool. Pain Med. 2005;6:432–42.
72. Ehde DM, Dillworth TM, Turner JA. Cognitive-behavioral therapy for individuals with chronic pain: efficacy, innovations, and directions for research. Am Psychol. 2014;69:153–66.
73. Turner JA, Romano JM. Cognitive-behavioral therapy for chronic pain. In: Loeser JD, Bonica JJ, editors. *Bonica's management of pain*. Lippincott Williams & Wilkins; 2001. p. 1751–8.
74. Tick H, et al. Evidence-based nonpharmacologic strategies for comprehensive pain care. EXPLORE. 2018;14:177–211.
75. Hofmann SG, Asnaani A, Vonk IJJ, Sawyer AT, Fang A. The efficacy of cognitive behavioral therapy: a review of meta-analyses. Cognit Ther Res. 2012;36:427–40.
76. Lim J-A, et al. Cognitive-behavioral therapy for patients with chronic pain. Medicine (Baltimore). 2018;97:e10867.
77. de Williams AC, Fisher E, Hearn L, Eccleston C. Psychological therapies for the management of chronic pain (excluding headache) in adults. Cochrane Database Syst Rev. 2020;2021
78. Hayes SC, Luoma JB, Bond FW, Masuda A, Lillis J. Acceptance and commitment therapy: model, processes and outcomes. Behav Res Ther. 2006;44:1–25.
79. Sielski R, Rief W, Glombiewski JA. Efficacy of biofeedback in chronic back pain: a meta-analysis. Int J Behav Med. 2017;24:25–41.
80. Waddell G. A new clinical model for the treatment of low-back pain. Spine (Phila. Pa. 1976). 1987;12:632–44.
81. Gatchel RJ. Comorbidity of chronic mental and physical health conditions: the biopsychosocial perspective. Am Psychol. 2004;59:792–805.
82. van Hecke O, Torrance N, Smith BH. Chronic pain epidemiology–where do lifestyle factors fit in? Br J Pain. 2013;7:209–17.
83. Sanders SH, Harden RN, Vicente PJ. Evidence-based clinical practice guidelines for interdisciplinary rehabilitation of chronic nonmalignant pain syndrome patients. Pain Pract. 2005;5:303–15.
84. Devine EC. Meta-analysis of the effect of psychoeducational interventions on pain in adults with cancer. Oncol Nurs Forum. 2003;30:75–89.
85. Institute of Medicine (US). Rehabilitation approaches and issues in chronic pain. In: Osterweis M, Kleinman A, Mechanic D, editors. Pain and disability: clinical, behavioral, and public policy perspectives. (National Academies Press (US); 1987.
86. McAnaney D, Wynne R. The context for vocational rehabilitation. In: National Disability Authority, editor. International good practice in vocational rehabilitation: lessons for Ireland; 2016. p. 8–29.
87. Coronado RA, Bialosky JE. Manual physical therapy for chronic pain: the complex whole is greater than the sum of its parts. J Man Manip Ther. 2017;25:115–7.
88. Tousignant-Laflamme Y, et al. Does shared decision making results in better health related outcomes for individuals with painful musculoskeletal disorders? A systematic review. J Man Manip Ther. 2017;25:144–50.
89. Leochico C, Espiritu A, Ignacio S, Mojica J. Challenges to the emergence of telerehabilitation in a developing country: a systematic review. Front Neurol. 2020; https://doi.org/10.3389/fneur.2020.01007.
90. Perez J, Niburski K, Stoopler M, Ingelmo P. Telehealth and chronic pain management from rapid adaptation to long-term implementation in pain medicine: a narrative review. PAIN Reports. 2021;6:e912.

Chapter 15
Pharmacological Management of Neuropathic Pain

Kunal Targe and Sadiq Bhayani

Neuropathic Pain Introduction and Epidemiology

According to the NeuPSIG (Special Interest Group on Neuropathic Pain) Neuropathic pain is defined as **"pain arising as a direct consequence of a lesion or disease affecting the somatosensory system"** [1].

The exact prevalence of neuropathic pain is not known. Two population-based studies from Europe reported the prevalence of pain of predominantly neuropathic origin [2] or pain with neuropathic characteristics [3] to be 8% and 7%, respectively.

Neuropathic pain is typically divided into central and peripheral, depending on whether the anatomic location of the nerve lesion or disease affects the central or the peripheral nervous system, respectively.

Classic examples of peripheral Neuropathic pain include polyneuropathies such as painful diabetic peripheral neuropathy (DPN) , chemotherapy-induced peripheral neuropathy (CIPN) , and human immunodeficiency virus (HIV) –induced sensory neuropathy as well as focal neuropathies such as in post-herpetic neuralgia (PHN), post-traumatic nerve injury, post-amputation pain, and entrapment neuropathies (Table 15.1). Up to 34% of persons with diabetes mellitus suffer from painful diabetic peripheral neuropathy [4].

Central Neuropathic conditions include, but are not limited to, pain after spinal cord injury (SCI), central post-stroke pain (CPSP), and multiple sclerosis (MS) pain.

The presence of a neuropathic pain component does not preclude the simultaneous presence of a nociceptive component (e.g., in diabetes mellitus: a patient can

K. Targe
Consultant in Pain Medicine, Ashford & St Peter's NHS Foundation Trust, London, UK

S. Bhayani (✉)
Consultant in Pain Medicine, Clevecland Clinic Abu Dhabi, Abu Dhabi, UAE

© The Author(s), under exclusive license to Springer Nature Switzerland AG 2022

J. de Castro, Y. El Miedany (eds.), *Advances in Chronic and Neuropathic Pain*, Contemporary Rheumatology, https://doi.org/10.1007/978-3-031-10687-3_15

Table 15.1 Types of neuropathic pain

Examples of neuropathic pain syndromes
• **peripheral neuropathic pain**
– Painful neuropathy (e.g., diabetic, HIV, post herpetic neuralgia, alcoholic, or post-chemotherapeutic)
– Radiculopathy
– Traumatic nerve lesion
– Post-mastectcomy, –thoracotomy, or -herniotomy syndrome (these may also be mixed neuropathic-nociceptive pain syndromes)
• **central neuropathic pain**
– After a stroke
– After a spinal cord injury
– In multiple sclerosis
• **mixed pain**
– Subgroups of patients with chronic back pain
– Complex regional pain syndrome (CRPS, Sudeck's dystrophy)
– Subgroups of patients with cancer-related pain

have nociceptive pain from a foot ulcer and, at the same time, painful diabetic peripheral neuropathy or cancer-related pain).

An estimated 16–25% of patients with back pain (with or without leg pain) have pain of both nociceptive and neuropathic origin. This combination has been termed "mixed pain" (Table 15.1). To date this concept has not been validated by any clinically applicable gold standard.

In any patient who might have either or both types of pain, evidence for neuropathic pain should be sought by meticulous history taking and physical examination, as the proper analgesic treatment will depend on the particular type of pain that is present. Targeted pharmacological management is indicated based on predominant type of pain the patient has. For mixed pain both opioids, non-opioids & anti-neuropathic medications are indicated.

Diagnosis of Neuropathic Pain

Given the challenge that will be encountered with this new definition of neuropathic pain special interest group (NeuPSIG) also proposed a grading system to guide decisions on the level of certainty with which neuropathic pain can be determined in an individual patient.

Three levels of certainty—possible, probable, and definite neuropathic pain—were proposed. As an activity in the Global Year Against Neuropathic Pain NeuPSIG established a committee to (1) critically evaluate the use of the grading system in the 7 years after its publication, (2) assess the usefulness and limitations of the grading system, and (3) update the grading system if required, for improved application in clinical and research settings. The committee consisted of an expert panel of neurologists, clinical neurophysiologists, neuroscientists, anaesthesiologists, pain specialists, primary care physicians, and population health scientists.

The probability of neuropathic can be determined based on the three following criteria:

1. Patient's history of signs, symptoms, and descriptors suggestive of pain related to a neurologic lesion or disease and pain distribution that is consistent with the suspected lesion or disease.
2. Presence of sensory disturbances upon examination in the painful area and with a neuro-anatomically plausible distribution.
3. Diagnostic tests that confirm a lesion or disease of the somatosensory nervous system

The Mechanisms of Neuropathic Pain as Targets for Pharmacotherapy

Nerve damage has been shown to alter the neurophysiological properties of afferent neurons [5]. Spontaneous ectopic activity arises, damaged axons degenerate and regenerate, and there is heightened sensitivity to afferent stimuli. These phenomena manifest themselves clinically as spontaneous pain, thermal hyperalgesia, and pain attacks [5]. Ectopic activity is induced and maintained by several factors, including voltage-gated neuronal sodium channels and transient receptor potential (TRP) channels [5]. These channels can be modulated with drugs such as carbamazepine, lidocaine, and capsaicin, with resulting relief of pain [6].

Nociceptive impulse transmission in the spinal cord is physiologically modulated by a descending system [5]. Inhibition of the reuptake of these neurotransmitters (serotonin & norepinephrine from the synaptic cleft through the action of anti -depressant drugs leads mainly to an intensification of the analgesic effect [6].

The term "central sensitization" refers to neuronal hyperexcitability that is found mainly in the spinal cord [7]. Its clinical manifestations are intensified spontaneous pain, mechanical allodynia, and hyperalgesia. Central sensitization can be modulated with drugs including gabapentin, pregabalin, and opioids, with resulting relief of pain [6].

Evidence and Guidance for Pharmacotherapy of Neuropathic Pain

The most comprehensive and up-to-date meta-analysis on the treatment of chronic neuropathic pain to date appeared in Lancet Neurology in early 2015 and included 229 randomized, double-blind, placebo-controlled trials [6].

It yielded the following conclusions:

- Wide variations in trial methods, size (patient numbers), and quality make it difficult to compare the utility of older and newer drugs.
- The number needed to treat (NNT) of all first-line drugs, i.e., the number of patients who would need to be treated with a given drug so that one of them, on average, would experience a reduction of pain by at least 50%, lies in the range 3.5–7.7. No recommendation can be given for the preferential use of any particular first-line drug over any other [6].
- Treatment recommendations are the same regardless of the etiology of the pain [8].

It should be pointed out, however, that these conclusions are based in part on assumptions of efficacy across pain syndromes that were made only by analogy. This methodological approach may have put some drugs at a disadvantage in the final assessment.

For example, a review of the use of cannabinoids yielded a more positive evaluation than the meta-analysis did, though a need for further trials was mentioned in the review [9]. As for some other drugs, such as carbamazepine, there is agreement that the available evidence does not clearly support a general recommendation for their use [10]. The meta-analysis also included a statistical estimate of the effect of publication bias (i.e., the tendency of trials with negative findings to remain unpublished), according to which the therapeutic benefit of drugs against neuropathic pain is likely to have been overstated by 10%. This small effect does not negate the treatment recommendations derived from the meta-analysis (Table 15.2).

The primary outcome of effectiveness was based on the proportion of responders to active treatment versus responders to placebo. A reduction in pain intensity equal to or greater than 50% was the primary outcome measure, which was used to calculate the numbers needed to treat (NNT) for each intervention.

NNT is the number of patients needed to treat with a drug to achieve a response (i.e., ≥50% reduction in pain intensity) that is not attributable to placebo. The NNT is the inverse of absolute risk reduction. It was calculated based on the following formula: NNT =1/[P (active) − P (placebo)] where P is the proportion of responders. For example, if 50 of 100 subjects in the active arm and 40 of the 100 subjects in the placebo arm report a reduction in pain intensity equal to or greater than 50%, the NNT is calculated as follows: NNT =1/[(50/100) − (40/100)] =1/(0.50–0.4) =10 Subsequently, of every ten patients treated with the drug, one will have an important (≥50%) degree of pain relief not attributable to placebo.

For determining the balance between the benefit and the potential risks of each intervention, the numbers needed to harm (NNH) were calculated for each drug/drug group. NNH is calculated similarly to NNT (but from the ratios of subjects who withdrew from the study owing to side effects) for active drug versus placebo. Contrary to NNT, a larger NNH implies a safer drug i.e., a smaller ratio of patients is harmed.

It is important to note, though, that although NNH provides a measure of tolerability, it does not, by itself, indicate the seriousness of adverse effects. Rare but

Table 15.2 The pharmacotherapy of neuropathic pain: number of trials, number of patients, number needed to treat, evidence levels (GRADE [11]), and common side effects (modified from [6]). Dtsch Arztebl Int 2016; 113: 616–26. https://doi.org/10.3238/arztebl.2016.0616

	Number of trials	Number of patients	Number needed to treat [95% CI]	Evidence level (GRADE)	Examples of common side effects (may vary depending on drug and manufacturer)
Tricyclic antidepressants	15	948	3.6 [3.0; 4.4]	High	Drowsiness, fatigue, dizziness, hypotension, weight gain
Serotonin-norepinephrine reuptake inhibitors	10	2541	6.4 [5.2; 8.4]	High	Nausea, dry mouth, somnolence, headache
Pregabalin	25	5940	7.7 [6.5; 9.4]	High	Drowsiness, somnolence, peripheral edema, weight gain
Gabapentin	14	3503	7.2 [5.9; 9.1]	High	Somnolence, dizziness
Tramadol	6	741	4.7 [3.6; 6.7]	Intermediate	Dizziness, nausea
High-potency opioids	7	838	4.3 [3.4; 5.8]	Intermediate	Sedation, dizziness, headache, constipation, nausea, itch
Capsaicin 8% patch[a]	6	2073	10.6 [7.4; 18.8]	High	Pain or erythema at the site of application

[a]Only peripheral neuropathic pain. CI, confidence interval. Only evidence of high or intermediate quality was considered in the construction of this table

serious risks as well as side effects that develop over long periods of treatment are unlikely to be captured by clinical trials of a few weeks' duration.

To minimize bias in translating evidence into recommendations, the NeuPSIG treatment guidelines committee used the Grading of Recommendations Assessment, Development, and Evaluation (GRADE), which is a systematic, transparent approach to making judgments about quality of evidence and strength of recommendation. (Tables 15.3 and 15.4).

Guidelines on the pharmacological treatment of neuropathic pain have been proposed by several groups in recent years. These guidelines were based on available scientific evidence (and its consistency), degree of efficacy, safety, and clinical experience with the individual drugs. The available guidelines for the treatment of certain forms of painful neuropathy have been adjusted by different organizations in various countries to accommodate drug availability. There are few differences among these various guidelines although local treatment practices were incorporated into these guidelines.

Treatment guidelines for neuropathic pain recommended by the different groups are in the Table 15.5.

A well-respected international guideline has been proposed by NeuPSIG (Special Interest Group on Neuropathic Pain of the IASP). In their guideline, certain antidepressants (including TCAs and Serotonin Norepinephrine Reuptake Inhibitors

Table 15.3 Recommendations for individual drugs/classes based on the GRADE classification and for first-, second-, and third—line drugs for neuropathic pain

Grade classification	Drugs	Daily dosages and dose regime	Recommendations
Strong for	Gapabentin	1200–3600 mg TID	First-line
	Gabapentin ER/ enacarbil	1200–3600 mg BID	First-line
	Pregabalin	300–600 mg BID	First-line
	SNRIs duloxetine/ venlafaxine	60–120 mg QD (duloxetine); 150–225 mg QD (venlafaxine ER)	First-line
	TCAs	25–150 mg qd or BID	First-line [1]
Weak for	Capsaicin 8% patches	1–4 patches to the painful area for 30–60 min every 3 months	Second-line (PNP) [2]
	Lidocaine patches	1–3 patches to the painful area for up to 12 h	Second-line (PNP)
	Tramadol	200–400 mg BID (tramadol ER) or TID	Second-line
	BTX-A (SC)	50–200 units to the painful area every 3 months	Third-line ; specialist use (PNP)
	Strong opioids	Individual titration	Third line[3]
Inconclusive	Combination therapy		
	Capsaicin cream		
	Carbamazepine		
	Clonidine topical		
	Lacosamide		
	Lamotrigine		
	NMDA antagonists Oxcarbazepine		
	SSRI antidepressants Tapentadol		
	Topiramate		
	Zonisamide		
Weak against	Cannabinoids		
	Valproate		
Strong against	Levetiracetam		
	Mexiletine		

Abbreviations: *SNRIs* serotonin noradrenaline reuptake inhibitors, *TCAs* tricyclic antidepressants, *ER* extended release, *BID* twice daily, *OD* once daily, *PNP* peripheral neuropathic pain

[SNRIs]), certain AEDs (more specifically those acting on alpha-2-delta subunit of the Ca2+ channels), and topical lidocaine are proposed as potential first-line treatment options.

Opioids and tramadol are proposed as general second-line treatment, although these analgesics could also be first-line treatment in some cases. Other drugs belong to third-line treatment although they can be used as second-line treatment in some

Table 15.4 Summary of GRADE recommendations. Drug classes with recommendation for use

	First Line Drugs			Second Line Drugs			Third Line Drugs	
	SNRIs duloxetine venlafaxine	**TCAs**	**Pregabalin Gabapentin Gabapentin ER/ enacarbil**	**Tramadol**	**Capsaicin 8% patches**	**Lidocaine patches[a]**	**Strong opioids**	**BTX-A**
Quality of evidence								
	High	Moderate	High	Moderate	High	Low[a]	Moderate	Low
Balance between desirable and undesirable effects								
Effect size	Moderate	Moderate	Moderate	Moderate	Law	Unknown	Moderate	Moderate
Tolerability and safety[b]	Moderate	Low-Moderate	Moderate-high	Low-moderate	Moderate-high	High	Low-moderate	High
Values and preferences								
	Low-moderate	Low-moderate	Low-moderate	Low-moderate	High	High	Low-moderate	High
Cost and resource allocation								
	Low-moderate	Low	Low-moderate	Low	Moderate-high	Moderate-high	Low-moderate	Moderate-high
Strength of recommendation								
	Strong	Strong	Strong	Weak	Weak	Weak	Weak	Weak
Neuropathic pain conditions	All	All	All	All	Peripheral	Peripheral	All	Peripheral

[a] FDA and EMEA approval for the treatment of postherpetic neuralgia

[b] Common side effects: antidepressants: somnolence, constipation, dry mouth (particularly TCAs), nausea (particularly duloxetine); pregabalin/gabapentin: somnolence, dizziness, weight gain; opioids (including tramadol): constipation, nausea, vomiting, tiredness, somnolence, dizziness, dry mouth, itch; lidocaine patches: local irritation; capsaicin patches: local pain, edema, erythema; botulinum toxin A: local pain

Abbreviation: *SNRIs* serotonin noradrenaline reuptake inhibitors, *TCAs* tricyclic antidepressants, *BTX-A* botulinum toxin type A, *ER* extended release

Table 15.5 Recommended Treatments for Neuropathic Pain Syndromes by the Canadian Pain Society, European Federation of Neurological Sciences (EFNS), and the International Association for the Study of Pain (IASP) Neuropathic Pain Special Interest Group (NeuroPSIG)

Group	First-Line Treatment	Second-Line Treatment	Third-Line Treatment
Canadian Pain Society, CPS[29]	TCAs	SNRIs	Tramadol
	Anticonvulsants	Topical lidocaine	Opioids
EFNS[27]	SNRI	Tramadol	
	Pregabalin	Opioids	
	TCAs		
IASP NeuroPSIG[31]	SNRIs, TCAs	Tramadol	Antidepressants (bupropion, citalopram, paroxetine)
	Gabapentin, Pregabalin	Opioids	Anticonvulsants (carbamazepine, lamotrigine, oxcarbazepine, topiramate, valproic acid)
	Tropical lidocaine		
			Topical low-concentration capsaicin
			Dextromethorphan
			Memantine
			Mexiletine

SNRI serotonin-norepinephrine reuptake inhibitor, *TCA* tricyclic antidepressants

cases. These other drugs include some antidepressants (bupropion, citalopram, paroxetine) and AEDs (Carbamazepine, Lamotrigine, Oxcarbazepine, Topiramate, Valproic acid), Mexiletine, NMDA receptor antagonists including Ketamine, and topical low-concentration Capsaicin.

The absence of a "gold standard" in the treatment of neuropathic pain that is effective in all patients should be considered.

Pharmacology of Drugs Implied to Treat Neuropathic Pain

Antidepressants

Tricyclic Antidepressants

TCAs have been key drugs for the treatment of various neuropathic disorders. TCAs are effective in treating neuropathic due to diabetic neuropathy and PHN irrespective of its antidepressant effect.

Classification

Tricyclic antidepressants can be divided to secondary amines and tertiary amines, depending on the number of methyl (–CH3) groups on the side chain nitrogen.

Secondary amine (Nortriptyline, desipramine) result from the metabolism of tertiary amines (amitriptyline and imipramine, respectively), during which one of the nitrogen methyl groups is lost and replaced by hydrogen (the demethylation process).

Mechanism of Action
TCAs work by blocking serotonin and norepinephrine reuptake pumps increasing their levels within hours with analgesic effects generally by 1 week, but antidepressant effects can take several weeks.

Effect is more likely related to adaptive changes in serotonin and norepinephrine receptor systems over time. Secondary amines have higher affinity to the norepinephrine transporter than the serotonin transporter, while in the reverse is true for tertiary amines. It also has anticholinergic and antihistamine properties which most likely contribute to the sedation in treating insomnia. Secondary amines have lower affinity to muscarinic acetylcholine (mAch) receptors; thus, they have a lower likelihood of anticholinergic side effects, especially at low doses.

There are some differences among tertiary amine TCAs as well. The affinity of imipramine to the blockage of histaminergic H1 receptors, for example, is lower than that of amitriptyline therefore it might be less sedating. Amitriptyline may provide analgesia via other mechanisms including acting as a local anaesthetic (blocking sodium channels).

For neuropathic pain, usually some effect is seen within 4 weeks. For insomnia, anxiety, depression it may be effective immediately, but effects often delayed 2 to 4 weeks.

Pharmacokinetics
TCAs have excellent oral bioavailability and prolonged half-life typically allowing once a day administration. TCAs undergo hepatic metabolism by CYP450 system, especially CYP2D6, 1A2. CYP2D6 inhibitors (duloxetine, paroxetine, fluoxetine, bupropion), cimetidine, and valproic acid can increase drug concentration. Fluvoxamine, a CYP1A2 inhibitor, prevents metabolism to nortriptyline and increased amitriptyline concentrations. Tramadol increases risk of seizures in patients taking TCAs. Phenothiazines may increase tricyclic levels. Enzyme inducers, such as rifamycin, smoking, phenobarbital can lower levels. May reduce absorption and bioavailability of levodopa. TCAs may alter effects of antihypertensive medications and prolongation of QTc, especially problematic in patients taking drugs that induce bradycardia. Use of TCAs within 2 weeks of MAO inhibitors may risk serotonin syndrome.

Side Effects
Side effects of TCAs are due to their anticholinergic and antihistaminic properties. Blockade of alpha-adrenergic-1 receptor may cause orthostasis and sedation. Notable side effects include constipation, dry mouth, blurry vision, increased appetite, nausea, diarrhoea, heartburn, weight gain, urinary retention, sexual dysfunction, sweating, itching, rash, fatigue, weakness, sedation, nervousness, restlessness. Life-threatening or dangerous side effects include orthostatic hypotension

(alpha-adrenergic-1 receptor blockade), tachycardia, QTc prolongation, and rarely death. Other side effects include increased intraocular pressure, paralytic ileus, hyperthermia.

Lowering the dose or switch to another agent can reduce some of the side effects. If tiredness/sedation are bothersome, change to a secondary amine (e.g., nortriptyline). For serious adverse effects lower dose and consider stopping.

Dosing
Most TCAs can be initiated at 10–25 mg once a day at bedtime and titrated in 10- to 25-mg increments every 1–2 weeks to a target dose of about 75 mg/day, which has been the average dose in clinical trials. Doses can be increased further, up to 150 mg/day, based on tolerability; however, some studies question the benefits of doses higher than 100 mg/day. TCA doses are typically titrated to clinical response.

Serotonin: Norepinephrine Reuptake Inhibitors

Duloxetine and venlafaxine are currently the two SNRIs recommended for the treatment of neuropathic pain. Given a pivotal role of serotonin and norepinephrine dual reuptake inhibition for pain control, the binding affinity of SNRIs to serotonin and norepinephrine transporter and reuptake inhibition effect in the synaptic cleft may be crucial in their clinical efficacy. However, differential effect of such medications on serotonin and norepinephrine neurotransmission has been suggested. A recent study has compared the ability between duloxetine and venlafaxine to block serotonin and norepinephrine transporters *in vitro* and *in vivo* [12]. Duloxetine potently inhibits binding to the human serotonin transporters and norepinephrine transporter approximately by 100 times and 300 times greater potency, respectively, comparing with venlafaxine [12]. In addition, duloxetine inhibited serotonin and norepinephrine reuptake with K_i values of 4.6, 16 and 369 nM, respectively, while venlafaxine inhibited reuptake with 17 and 34-fold lower potency, respectively, comparing with duloxetine [12].

Mechanism of Action
Duloxetine was found to be the most potent of the agents tested in blocking the reuptake of serotonin. Venlafaxine, in contrast, selectively bound to the serotonin transporter, but not the norepinephrine transporter.

The net effect of SNRIs results in increment of extracellular 5-HT and NE levels in prefrontal cortex, which is correlated with uptake blockade increasing extracellular levels of the neurotransmitters in the synapse [12]. A number of experimental studies on chronic pain have consistently shown its engagement with prefrontal cortex activity [13, 14]. Cognitive modulations of pain are related to activation of regions of interest in several prefrontal brain areas (dorsolateral prefrontal cortex, ventrolateral prefrontal cortex and anterior cingulated cortex), where eventually modulate the central and peripheral pain pathways in some crucial regions in the CNS and spinal cord (i.e., thalamus, periaqueductal gray and dorsal horn [13, 14]. In fact the dorsolateral prefrontal cortex is directly and indirectly connected to the anterior cingulate cortex and thalamus, and finally to the periaqueductal grey, a critical part of the descending pain modulatory system.

Both duloxetine and venlafaxine have very low affinity to cholinergic, adrenergic, histaminergic, and dopaminergic receptors.

Pharmacokinetics

Duloxetine has oral bioavailability of 30%–80%. Its absorption is slow and takes about 2 h for plasma concentrations to peak. Taking duloxetine with or after meals further delays the absorption but does not seem to affect the peak plasma concentration substantially. Duloxetine is metabolized by the liver CYP450 enzymes, primarily CYP 1A2 and 2D6. The metabolites undergo renal excretion [15].

Venlafaxine is well absorbed orally but undergoes extensive first-pass metabolism, and therefore has only 12%–45% bioavailability depending on the dosage form. Extended-release formulations result in improved bioavailability (Effexor XR product information, Wyeth Pharmaceuticals). Food does not seem to have an effect on bioavailability. Venlafaxine undergoes extensive liver metabolism by the CYP450 2D6 isoenzyme to an active metabolite, N, O-di-desmethylvenlafaxine (Effexor product information, Wyeth Pharmaceuticals).

Dosing

Duloxetine can be started at 60 mg once a day. Effectiveness in clinical studies has been shown with doses of 60 and 120 mg/day. Duloxetine should be used cautiously in patients with renal and hepatic impairment. Most common side effects include nausea, sweating, weight loss, dizziness, drowsiness, and headaches. Hypertension has been reported in 3%–13% of subjects, especially with high doses of 375 mg/day. At doses below 225 mg/day, the average increase in blood pressure was less than 2 mm Hg.

Side Effects

Common side effects include nausea, drowsiness, and dizziness. Gastrointestinal side effects such as constipation, diarrhoea, and dry mouth are often reported. Hypertension and orthostatic hypotension have been reported; fatigue and diaphoresis has been reported at higher rates than with placebo. SNRIs, similarly to SSRIs, may affect the effects of serotonin on platelets and increase the risk of (mainly gastrointestinal) bleeding, particularly in patients on chronic anticoagulant, antiplatelet, NSAID, aspirin, or systemic corticosteroid therapy. The main drug interactions of duloxetine are with other serotonergic drugs (monoamine oxidase inhibitors [MAOIs], SSRIs, tramadol, linezolid, etc.) by increasing the risk of serotonin syndrome, and with drugs affecting coagulation and platelet adhesion by increasing the risk of bleeding. CYP 1A2 inhibitors such as fluvoxamine can cause a substantial increase in duloxetine plasma concentrations.

Palpitation and electrocardiographic abnormalities were reported in 3%–5% of patients. Caution is advised in using high dosages of venlafaxine (>150 mg/day) in patients with cardiac conditions. Abnormal ejaculation/orgasm and erectile dysfunction have been reported with venlafaxine.

Potential drug interaction concerns are with QT-prolonging drugs, serotonergic agents, and drugs that affect coagulation and increase the risk of bleeding. Dosage:

The initial recommended dosage of venlafaxine is 37.5 mg once or twice a day as an immediate-release formulation or 75 mg/day in an extended-release formulation. The doses then can be increased in 37.5- to 75-mg increments every 1–3 weeks to 150 mg/day and, if required, further up to 225 mg/day with appropriate monitoring in cardiac patients. The dosage should be reduced by 25%–50% in patients with mild to moderate renal impairment and by at least 50% in patients with cirrhosis or mild to moderate liver impairment.

Anti-Epileptics

Gabapentanoids

The gabapentinoid drugs gabapentin and pregabalin are antiepileptic drugs that are considered as first-line treatments for the management of neuropathic pain. The mechanisms of action are still unclear despite their widespread use. The gabapentinoids share similar mechanisms of action but differ considerably in their pharmacokinetic and pharmacodynamic characteristics.

Several recommendations on the pharmacological management of neuropathic pain based on a review of randomised controlled trials are available. The Cochrane reviews of evidence for gabapentinoids in neuropathic pain have been recently updated [8, 9]. These reviews show moderate-quality evidence for pregabalin in postherpetic neuralgia, diabetic neuropathy and low-quality evidence for efficacy in post-stroke pain and after spinal cord injury. Pregabalin is not effective in neuropathic pain due to HIV. There is limited evidence for neuropathic back pain, neuropathic cancer pain and other forms of neuropathic pain. Gabapentin is effective to an extent in postherpetic neuralgia and diabetic neuropathy but the evidence in other forms of neuropathic pain is limited.

Clinical practice guidelines have been published by a number of international and regional professional associations, all of which recommend gabapentinoids as first-line therapy.

The National Institute of Clinical Excellence (NICE) guidelines on the management of neuropathic pain recommend gabapentin, pregabalin, amitriptyline or duloxetine as the initial choice of treatment for neuropathic pain with the exception of trigeminal neuralgia [10].

Despite these recommendations, the effects of most analgesics including gabapentinoids in neuropathic pain are modest with meta-analyses indicating that only a minority of patients benefit from pharmacological therapy [6, 16]. The combined number needed to treat (NNT) is 7.7 (6.5–9.4) for pregabalin and 7.2 (5.9–9.2) for gabapentin but this can be as high as 22 in painful diabetic neuropathy. These limited effects can be explained by the modest efficacy of drugs, high placebo response and heterogeneity in diagnostic criteria. The modest efficacy of gabapentinoids is not surprising as elevated levels of $\alpha 2\delta$ are not necessary for the development of neuropathic pain. Pharmacogenomic differences can also explain the inter-individual variability in responses.

Mechanism of Action

Gabapentin and pregabalin do not bind to GABA receptors despite their structural similarity but have a high affinity for the α2δ-1 subunit of voltage-gated calcium channels (VGCCs). α2δ-1 subunits are transported to the dorsal horn from their site of production in DRG (dorsal root ganglion) cell bodies. Elevated levels in the dorsal horn are associated with the development of neuropathic pain [17]. Gabapentinoids inhibit the accumulation of α2δ-1 in the pre-synaptic terminals in the dorsal horn and reduce response to painful stimuli in animal models [17]. α2δ-1 allows enhanced neurotransmitter release at decreased calcium influx. Gabapentinoids can influence nociception by inhibiting the α2δ-1-mediated enhanced neurotransmitter release [18]. Analgesic effects are mediated by the facilitation of descending noradrenergic inhibition, inhibition of descending serotonergic facilitation and by cortical mechanisms affecting the limbic system [19]. It also stimulates the uptake of glutamate by the excitatory amino acid transporters (EAAT) and reduces the brain glutamate levels.

Pharmacokinetics

Pregabalin is rapidly and completely absorbed as compared to gabapentin. Peak plasma concentrations are seen within an hour as compared to 3 h with gabapentin. Oral bioavailability for pregabalin is more than 90% as compared to 30–60% for gabapentin. These differences can be explained by the mechanism of absorption. Although both gabapentinoids are absorbed in the small intestine, pregabalin is also absorbed in the proximal colon. Absorption of gabapentin is solely dependent on Large-neutral Amino Acid Transporter (LAT) that are easily saturable, resulting in dose-dependent pharmacokinetics. As the dose of gabapentin increases, the area under the plasma concentration–time curve (AUC) does not increase proportionally. In contrast, pregabalin has non-saturable absorption with a linear pharmacokinetic profile and less variable bioavailability as it may be transported by carriers in addition to LAT. Food has only a slight effect on the rate and extent of absorption of gabapentin but can substantially delay the absorption of pregabalin without affecting the bioavailability.

Gabapentinoids do not bind to plasma proteins. They are actively transported across the blood–brain barrier by LAT-1. Peak cerebrospinal fluid levels take significantly longer to achieve than peak plasma levels, with a median time of 8 h. They do not influence spinal neurotransmitter concentrations of glutamate, norepinephrine, substance P and calcitonin gene–related peptide. Both are highly water-soluble and the volume of distribution of each is 0.8 and 0.5 L/kg for gabapentin and pregabalin, respectively.

They are not metabolised by the liver and do not affect the cytochrome P450 system, major cytochrome P450 system isoenzymes; however, drug-induced hepatotoxicity has been described in case reports. Elimination is mostly done by the kidney and is proportional to the creatinine clearance. Accumulation can cause renal failure resulting in adverse effects.

Dosing

Gabapentin is initiated at 100–300 mg three times a day and can be increased in 100- to 300- mg increments every 3–7 days to reach target doses. It can be titrated upto

1800–2400 mg/day doses in NeuP, but doses can be increased up to 3600 mg/day. No dose adjustment is required in patients with liver impairment. The dose should be reduced in patients with mild to moderate renal insufficiency, and gabapentin is not recommended in patients with Clcr <30 mL/min. Dose reduction and post dialysis dose supplementation is warranted in patients undergoing haemodialysis.

Pregabalin is initiated at 75 mg twice a day and can be increased in 75 mg-increments every 3–7 days to reach target doses of 300–600 mg/day. Although mostly administered twice a day, several clinical trials have employed thrice daily dosing; this approach may be useful in patients who experience side effects related to high peak plasma concentrations soon after drug intake. Similar to gabapentin, pregabalin is almost entirely excreted renally and does not require dose adjustment in hepatic insufficiency.

Side Effects
Dizziness, somnolescence and gait disturbances are the most common adverse effects. Other common adverse effects affecting the central nervous system (CNS) include impaired concentration, confusion, memory loss, altered mood, movement disorders, sleep disorder, speech impairment and vertigo. Respiratory depression has been described when used in combination with opioids resulting in an increased risk of accidental opioid-related mortality. Weight gain is common with gabapentinoids and can affect up to a quarter of all patients treated with pregabalin, resulting in non-compliance and termination of treatment. Gastrointestinal adverse effects such as abdominal distension, abnormal appetite, constipation, dry mouth, and nausea are common and are dose-related with the exception of constipation. There is increasing awareness of the abuse potential of gabapentinoids, particularly in individuals with a history of opioid abuse. Both gabapentinoids have been reported to stimulate feelings of sociability, euphoria, calm and relaxation and can enhance psychoactive effects of other drugs. The abuse potential of pregabalin is higher as compared to gabapentin due to its pharmacokinetic properties. Withdrawal symptoms are common and appear between 12 h and 7 days after cessation of use, with most cases occurring between 24 and 48 h.

Other Anticonvulsants

Carbamazepine and Oxcarbazepine

Carbamazepine is chemically related to TCAs.

Mechanism of Action
It acts as a use-dependent blocker of voltage-sensitive sodium channels, interacting with the open channel conformation of voltage-sensitive sodium channels reducing hyperactivity in both central and peripheral neurons. It interacts at a specific site of the alpha pore-forming subunit of voltage-sensitive sodium channels. Inhibition of

release of glutamate is also postulated. It also has additional effects on calcium and potassium channels as well as on potentiation of GABAergic inhibition have been proposed, but their clinical relevance is unclear.

Dosing range for Carbamazepine is 400–1200 mg/day. It can be administered as 50 mg four times a day of immediate release or 100 mg twice a day for extended-release formulation. The dose may be titrated in increments of 200 mg/day until target doses of 400–800 mg/day. Dose adjustment is needed in renal and hepatic impairment.

Pharmacokinetics

The bioavailability of carbamazepine is in the range of 75–85% of an ingested Carbamazepine is largely metabolized in the liver. CYP3A4 hepatic enzyme is the major enzyme that metabolizes carbamazepine to its active metabolite, carbamazepine-10,11-epoxide, which is further metabolized to its transdiol form by the enzyme epoxide hydrolase. Other hepatic cytochrome enzymes that contribute to the metabolism of carbamazepine are CYP2C8, CYP3A5, and CYP2B6. Carbamazepine also undergoes hepatic glucuronidation by UGT2B7 enzyme and several other metabolic reactions occur, resulting in the formation of minor hydroxy metabolites and quinone metabolites. Interestingly, carbamazepine induces its own metabolism. This leads to enhanced clearance, reduced half-life, and a reduction in serum levels of carbamazepine Oxcarbazepine is structurally like carbamazepine and has a similar effectiveness profile in epilepsy and neuropathic pain. Although both drugs are eventually metabolized to dihydroxy-carbamazepine, one of the main differences is that oxcarbazepine metabolism does not involve the formation of carbamazepine 10,11-epoxide, an important contributor to carbamazepine toxicity and CYP450 enzyme induction.

The NNT for carbamazepine/oxcarbazepine in NeuP was 5.7 (3.4–18), along with an NNH of 5.5 (4.3–7.9).

Dosing

Oxcarbazepine 300 mg twice a day; this can be increased in increments of 300 mg every 1–2 weeks up to the therapeutic dose of 1800–2400 mg/day. Oxcarbazepine is renally excreted. Elimination half-life of active metabolite MHD is increased therefore initial dose should be reduced by 50%; may need to use slower titration Hepatic Impairment. No dose adjustment recommended for mild to moderate hepatic impairment.

Side Effects

Sedation, dizziness, headache, ataxia, nystagmus, abnormal gait, confusion, nervousness, fatigue, Nausea, vomiting, abdominal pain, dyspepsia, Diplopia, vertigo, abnormal vision.

Most common side effects of carbamazepine and oxcarbazepine are sedation, dizziness, headache, ataxia, nystagmus, abnormal gait, confusion, nervousness, fatigue, nausea, vomiting, abdominal pain, dyspepsia, diplopia, vertigo, abnormal vision. Rare but serious side effects include activation of suicidal ideation, rare blood dyscrasias: leukopenia, thrombocytopenia. Dermatologic reactions are uncommon and rarely severe which include erythema multiforme, toxic epidermal necrolysis, and Stevens–Johnson syndrome. Hyponatremia/SIADH (syndrome of inappropriate antidiuretic hormone secretion) can occur.

Lamotrigine

The primary mechanism of action of lamotrigine is thought to be mediated via inhibition of glutamate release by blocking neuronal voltage-gated sodium channels, although the exact mechanism has not been elucidated. 54 Three positive trials have been published (in CPSP, DPN, and HIV sensory neuropathy), but virtually all large trials in NeuP have been negative. Lamotrigine may cause serious, sometimes life-threatening skin rashes. Dose titration should be performed slowly, by starting at 25 mg/day, with slow increases at 2-week intervals to 50, 100, and then 200 mg/day (up to a maximum 400 mg/day). More rapid dose titration increases the risk of serious skin reactions. It is important to note that the titration schedule is different in patients who are taking other drugs (primary anticonvulsants) that can inhibit or induce the hepatic metabolism of lamotrigine.

Topiramate

The drug appears to have several mechanisms of action, including activation of GABAA receptors, blockade of AMPA/kainate receptors for glutamate, and blockade of voltage-gated sodium channels. Although positive results were seen in one trial involving DPN,61 a combined report of three studies in DPN62 and a study with lumbar radiculopathy63 were negative. Topiramate doses up to 400 mg/day have been used in NeuP trials. The dose is typically initiated at 25 mg/day and titrated to analgesic response by increments of 25 mg per dose at weekly intervals. A variety of skin adverse effects are reported with topiramate, including rash, flushing, and alopecia. Hyperammonemia and/or a drop in serum bicarbonate level are frequently reported with topiramate treatment (9%–67% prevalence, but usually mild) and may be dose-related. Topiramate may cause loss of appetite and weigh loss in 10%–24% of patients. Dizziness, somnolence, and a variety of neurologic side effects may occur.

Lacosamide

The exact mechanism of action of lacosamide is unknown. It is a functionalized amino acid and appears to selectively enhance voltage-gated sodium channel slow inactivation, thus reducing neuronal hyperexcitability. As in the case of topiramate, several larger negative trials followed one positive trial, all in DPN. The initial dose of lacosamide is 100 mg twice a day, which can be increased weekly by 50 mg twice a day up to a total daily dose of 400 mg. Cardiovascular side effects have been reported with lacosamide, including atrioventricular blocks of various degrees, bradycardia, and atrial fibrillation/flutter. Nausea and dizziness are among the most common side effects; ophthalmic side effects such as diplopia and blurred vision may occur in 5%–10% of subjects.

Valproic Acid

Valproic acid (as valproate or divalproex sodium) has shown positive results in three trials (two DPN, one PHN) of relatively poor quality, especially for PHN. Three studies (SCI, DPN, and mixed peripheral neuropathy) have been negative. Valproic acid has multiple mechanisms of action, and those responsible for analgesic effect are unclear. This drug is also a subject of multiple drug interactions by inhibiting the hepatic metabolism of some drugs, being affected by other CYP450 inducers and inhibitors, or additional mechanisms affecting its glucuronidation pathways. 64,65 Valproic acid may cause fatal hepatotoxicity in 1 of 800 children under the age of 2; the incidence in adults is not clear, but appears to be around 1 in 10,000–40,000 patients. Thrombocytopenia has been reported in 1%–30% patients treated with valproic acid. Due to the above safety issues, the treatment for NeuP is usually not recommended. This is particularly true for women of childbearing age because of a twofold to fivefold increase in the rate of birth defects with perinatal exposure to valproic acid.

Leviteracetam

Levetiracetam has an excellent safety profile compared with other anticonvulsants and therefore has been an attractive candidate for testing its effectiveness in NeuP. Unfortunately none of the six RCTs with levetiracetam that met NeuPSIG inclusion criteria showed any difference from placebo in terms of effectiveness. Therefore levetiracetam is currently not recommended for the treatment of NeuP.

Topical Agents

Capsaicin

Capsaicin, 8-methyl-N-vanillyl-6-nonenamide, is an active ingredient in chili peppers that provokes a typical hot burning sensation. Capsaicin is insoluble in water but freely soluble in ethanol, ether, benzene, and chloroform.

Mechanism of Action

Capsaicin is a highly selective agonist of the transient receptor potential vanilloid receptor (TRPV1) a ligand-gated, nonselective cation channel preferentially expressed on small-diameter sensory neurons, especially on the nociceptors. TRPV1 is a heat-activated calcium channel that normally opens at approximately 43 degrees Celsius, but with capsaicin bound, the threshold decreases below 37 degrees Celsius or even to skin temperature. This activation, in turn, causes depolarization, the initiation of an action potential, and the transmission of pain signals to the spinal cord. After several days of capsaicin application, TRPV1-containing sensory axons are desensitized, which inhibits the transmission of pain. Capsaicin-induced defunctionalisation of cutaneous nociceptors is mediated by an increase in intracellular calcium, followed by mitochondrial dysfunction and peripheral nerve terminals death. The functionality of the peripheral endings, as measured by the ability to detect painful sensations, returns a few months after treatment.

Standard capsaicin-containing creams have been found moderately effective in PHN, but they require many applications per day and cause a burning sensation for many days before the analgesic effects start. Recently, the efficacy of a one-time application of a highly concentrated (8%) capsaicin patch (for 30, 60, or 120 min) to the painful area compared to a patch with a low concentration (0.04%) has been demonstrated from weeks 2 to 12 in PHN or HIV neuropathy [20], with safety confirmed in an open-label 48-week extension study [21].

Side Effects

Adverse effects were primarily due to local capsaicin-related reactions at the application site like pain, erythema, and sometimes oedema and itching. If inhaled, capsaicin can cause cough and/or bronchoconstriction. Accidental application to oral mucosa or eyes can cause severe stinging sensation. Moreover, careful blood pressure monitoring is necessary because of a potential risk of high blood pressure during application.

The drug does not impair sensory function, as tested with a standard sensory evaluation, in PHN and HIV neuropathy after repeated applications for up to 1 year. In human volunteers, only a transient impairment of density of epidermal fibers (lasting 1 week) has been evidenced on skin punch biopsies after a single application, but there was a 93% recovery rate after 6 months.

Dosing

Capsaicin 8% patches are applied on non-irritated and unbroken skin. Up to four patches can be applied at the same time. Topical lidocaine or tramadol premedication can be used because the application is often unpleasant or painful. The patch is applied for 30 or 60 min. The treatment may be repeated every 3 months. Capsaicin cream is applied to the painful skin area and exerts its effect locally, as the systemic uptake is limited. The cream is applied up to 4 to 5 times daily, and it requires a treatment period of approximately 4 weeks until maximum effectiveness is observed.

Capsaicin is poorly metabolized by human skin and has no significant drug interactions.

Capsaicin patches have the advantage of high compliance since the effect may last for 3 months after a single application. There is a low risk for systemic side effects and drug-drug interactions, but the effect size is modest, and the treatment is associated with high costs.

Lidocaine

Lidocaine Patch 5%

Mechanism of Action

Excited nociceptors are indeed considered a crucial part of the pathophysiology of neuropathic syndromes. Lidocaine acts through blockade of abnormally functioning (sensitized) Nav 1.7 and Nav 1.8 Na^+ channels in dermal nociceptors, thereby reducing ectopic discharges. Lidocaine has also been shown to regulate T-cell activity and inhibit nitric oxide production, thereby reducing inflammatory processes within the deep tissue, such as injured muscle, joints or constricted nerves. C ertain preclinical and clinical findings point towards the existence of additional biological effects, such as blockage of Aβ-afferents conveying allodynia and traveling adjacent to degenerating nociceptors within the affected nerve. The occurrence of a possible central negative feedback signal can be drawn from the fact that application of lidocaine patches also has been shown to demonstrate an analgesic effect in central NeP syndromes [22].

Dosing

Lidocaine-medicated patches are adhesive patches containing lidocaine 5%; they are applied on intact, dry, non-irritated skin. These patches are approved for PHN. Lidocaine may also be applied topically on the skin in a gel or spray form. Lidocaine patches cause a steady release of lidocaine, which penetrates the skin in small amounts and acts near the site of administration. Up to three to four patches can be applied to intact skin. The patches are applied for 12 h per day with a 12-h patch-free interval before new patches are applied. The patches may be cut to fit the area of pain.

Pharmacokinetics

The amount of lidocaine systemically absorbed from the adhesive patch is directly related to both the duration of application and the surface area over which it is applied. When the patch is used according to the recommended dosing instructions, only 2–3% of the dose applied is expected to be absorbed. The lidocaine concentration does not increase with daily use Lidocaine patch should be used with caution in patients receiving Class I antiarrhythmic drugs since the toxic effects are additive and potentially synergistic. Lidocaine patch when used concomitantly with other products containing local anaesthetic agents, the amount absorbed from all formulations must be considered.

Intravenous Lidocaine

One of the proposed pathophysiological mechanisms that contribute to neuropathic pain is an upregulation of sodium channels in nociceptors. The change in channel density on nociceptor membranes creates an electrochemical environment that causes neurons to reach their depolarization threshold more rapidly, which leads to increased nociceptive signalling.

Lidocaine, a sodium channel blocker, may modulate neuropathic pain by decreasing the function of these sodium channels, reversing the effects of sodium channel upregulation.

Parenteral intravenous (i.v.) lidocaine administration for the off-label treatment of resistant neuropathic pain has been occurring in clinical practice since the 1950s. Specifically, recent studies have found i.v. lidocaine therapy to be effective in treating neuropathic pain associated with spinal cord injury [23], diabetic neuropathy [24], central pain syndrome, chronic regional pain syndrome, and post herpetic neuralgia [25]. Additionally, i.v. lidocaine infusions have an opioid sparing effect during the postoperative period when administered during abdominal surgery.

Dosing

Although several studies have investigated i.v. lidocaine in neuropathic pain therapy, there is no consensus for dosing and administration of i.v. lidocaine. Various dosing regimens have been implemented, most of them in the range of 3- to 5-mg/kg infused over 30–60 min.

Although several studies have investigated i.v. lidocaine in neuropathic pain therapy, there is no consensus for dosing and administration of i.v. lidocaine. Some studies have found that the effect of lidocaine on neuropathic pain may be dose related. There is currently no best practice or recommended guideline for the use of lidocaine infusions in this patient population.

Side Effects

The safety characteristics of i.v. lidocaine have been well established. The most common adverse effects seen with i.v. lidocaine include light-headedness, dizziness and confusion, lethargy, nausea and vomiting, vision changes, and perioral numbness. Because of its antiarrhythmic effects, patients receiving lidocaine infusions are typically screened for conduction defects via electrocardiogram (ECG) prior to lidocaine administration.

Patients at a heightened risk for arrhythmia should not receive lidocaine infusions. No studies have reported arrhythmias due to i.v. lidocaine for neuropathic pain. An increase in mean blood pressure can occur but clinical relevance is not known.

Cannabinoids

Combined with growing scientific knowledge and a groundswell of public opinion regarding therapeutic benefits, the medical use of cannabinoids has been pushed onto the political agenda. Cannabis sativa has been a valuable source of hemp fibre for many thousands of years and is one of mankind's oldest recorded crops. In addition, therapeutic benefits have been described for thousands of years in China, India and the Middle East. Cannabis was introduced much later to the West following the observations of an army physician in India in 1842. The advent of superior alternative medications and concerns about abuse potential led to cannabis being withdrawn from the US and British pharmacopoeias in 1942 and 1976, respectively.

Mechanism of Action

Delta-9-tetrahydrocannabinol (Δ 9 THC) is the major active constituent of the C. sativa. Two cannabinoid (CB) receptors (CB1 and CB 2) were cloned and characterised. The CB 1 receptor is one of the most abundantly expressed neuronal receptors (hippocampus, basal ganglia, cerebellum, periaqueductal grey, rostral ventromedial medulla, superficial dorsal horn of spinal cord, primary afferent neurones) and its heterogeneous distribution accounts for several prominent pharmacological actions, including analgesia. The CB 2 receptor is primarily restricted to immune cell lines such as macrophages, lymphocytes, natural killer cells and mast cells. The location on macrophages and mast cells seems to be particularly important in curtailing inflammatory pain. The prototypical second messenger event for both CB 1 and CB2 receptor signalling is a fall in cAMP, which is mediated via negatively coupled G proteins. CB1 receptor activation also directly inhibits voltage sensitive $Ca2+$ channels, and augments inwardly rectifying $K +$ channels. The net effect of cannabinoid receptor activation is to increase membrane hyperpolarisation and inhibit neurotransmitter release.

Dronabinol and nabilone are synthetic analogs of THC available in oral tablet form; Nabiximols (sativex) is the name for a cannabis extract containing THC and CBD, available in some countries as an oromucosal spray. Various administration and delivery forms have been tested for therapeutic use. Cannabis products are commonly either inhaled by smoking/vaporization or taken orally. The oro-mucosal, topical-transdermal and rectal routes are minor, but interesting, administration routes.

Pharmacokinetics

Cannabinoids undergo metabolism in the liver and are excreted through the kidneys. Cytochrome P450 isoenzymes (CYP2D6 and CYP3A4) are inhibited. The absorption of the drugs is slow, and peak concentrations are relatively low. The plasma half-life is 24–36 h, and the pharmacodynamic effect is prolonged by oral administration. Sativex (sublingual and oropharyngeal spray) achieves its peak plasma concentration in 45–120 min. Caution must be observed when co-prescribing cannabinoids with other psychoactive drugs with sedative or neurologic side effects.

The pharmacokinetics and dynamics of cannabinoids vary as a function of the route of administration with absorption showing the most variability of the principal pharmacokinetic steps.

Absorption is affected both by intrinsic product lipophilicity and by inherent organ tissue differences (i.e., alveolar, dermal vs. gastric).

A variety of factors, such as recent eating (for oral), depth of inhalation, how long breath is held for and vaporizer temperature (for inhalation) all affect cannabinoid absorption, which can vary from 20–30% for oral administration and up to 10–60% for inhalation. A reference review detailing the pharmacokinetic and pharmacodynamic aspects of cannabinoids has been written by Grotenhermen [25].

Dosing
Typical daily dosing regimens:

- Nabilone (oral, 1e4 mg)
- Dronabinol (oral, 2.5e10 mg)
- Nabiximols [oromucosal THC-CBD spray, range 1–48 sprays (mean 8.3 sprays)]
- Cannabis (smoked or vaporised medical marijuana, containing 1.875–34 mg THC).

These doses were associated with a significant reduction in mean numerical rating scale (NRS) scores, improved Quality of Life (QoL) measures, sleep, and patient satisfaction.

Side Effects
Side effects include dizziness, drowsiness, tachycardia, dry mouth, anxiety, mood changes, disorientation, impaired memory and cognition, constipation, and diarrhoea. Smoked cannabis can exhibit neurocognitive effects—such as dizziness, euphoria, concentration difficulties, fatigue, and headaches. Cannabinoids contraindicated in patients with cardiovascular disease, epilepsy, renal or hepatic impairment, in patients with history of psychotic or substance abuse disorders.

It is expected that recent developments in pharmacological, pharmaceutical, and technological sciences will result in new therapeutic strategies using both known cannabinoids for new therapeutic strategies as well as cannabinoid synthetic derivatives.

Nanotechnology is indeed a promising approach that may bring cannabinoids closer to clinical use and administration via both the oral and pulmonary routes. Furthermore, it is at an early stage the use of well-known advanced nanomaterials in cannabinoid delivery (e.g., carbon nanotubes). Nevertheless, additional evaluation is required if the cost effectiveness and long-term safety of nano-delivery systems is to be improved.

Botulinum Toxin

Botulinum toxin A, also known as Botox, is produced by Clostridium botulinum, a gram-positive anaerobic bacterium. Botulinum toxin injections are among the most practiced cosmetic procedures in the USA. Although botulinum toxin is typically associated with cosmetic procedures, it can be used to treat a variety of other conditions like focal spasticity and dystonia, overactive bladder, hyperhidrosis, and certain pain condition like migraine and neuropathic pain. For the treatment of neuropathic, intradermal or subcutaneous injections are used.

Mechanism of Action
Botulinum toxin blocks neuromuscular transmission by cleaving SNAP-25 protein, which inhibits the vesicular release of acetylcholine from nerve terminals to paralyze muscles and to decrease the pain response. It also appears to inhibit release of neurotransmitters involved in pain transmission (including glutamate, calcitonin gene-related peptide, and substance P) and may enter CNS via retrograde axonal transport.

Dosing
Powder for injection: 100 u, 50 u. Administer every 3 months using the lowest effective dose.

Botulinum toxin has a long duration of action, lasting up to 5 months after initial treatment which makes it an excellent treatment for chronic pain patients. As of today, the only FDA-approved chronic condition that botulinum toxin can be used to treat is migraines and this is related to its ability to decrease muscle tension and increase muscle relaxation. Contraindications to botulinum toxin treatments are limited to a hypersensitivity to the toxin or an infection at the site of injection, and there are no known drug interactions with botulinum toxin.

Side Effects
Most adverse effects depend on site of injection. Injection site pain and hemorrhage, infection, fever, headache, pruritis, and myalgia. When used for cervical dystonias-dysphagia, neck weakness and upper respiratory infection can occur.

Rarely patients may experience severe dysphagia requiring a feeding tube or leading to aspiration pneumonia. Use with caution in patients with motor neuropathies or neuromuscular junctional disorders. These patients may be at greater risk for systemic weakness or respirator problems.

Botulinum toxin is an advantageous and effective alternative pain treatment and a therapy to consider for those that do not respond to opioid treatment.

Opioids

Strong opioids, such as morphine, oxycodone, and hydromorphone, and weak opioids, such as tramadol, are efficacious when compared with other drugs used for neuropathic pain and are similar to antidepressants in terms of the numbers needed to treat [6]. Nevertheless, they have always been considered second-line drugs, and more recently third-line drugs due to adverse drug reactions and concerns about abuse, diversion, and addiction.

Mechanism of Action
The analgesic effect of opioids is due to their action in the brain, brainstem, spinal cord, and, under certain circumstances, on peripheral terminals of primary afferent neurons. All endogenous opioid peptides, including β-endorphin, enkephalins, and dynorphins, bind to seven transmembrane G protein-coupled receptors, which are divided into three classes: mu, delta, and kappa receptors. Opioid receptors are coupled to inhibitor G proteins, with receptor activation inhibiting the adenylate cyclase as well as the intracellular production of cAMP. However, the coupling of opioid receptors to calcium and potassium channels is thought to be a central mechanism of analgesia production by both endogenous and exogenous opioids.

In spite of their efficacy, the role of opioids in the long-term treatment of non-malignant pain is controversial for a number of reasons, including concerns over tolerability, possible development of tolerance to the analgesic effect, and the risk of addiction [26]. A systematic review of randomized controlled trials of oral opioids for chronic non-malignant pain indicated that approximately 50% of patients experienced an adverse event with opioids and more than 20% discontinued treatment because of adverse events [27]. A more recent Cochrane review of long-term opioid management of chronic non-cancer pain reported a rate of discontinuation due to adverse events of 22.9% for oral opioids and 12.1% for transdermal opioids [28].

Side Effects
The most frequent adverse drug reactions to opioid therapy are nausea and vomiting (tend to diminish with increasing tolerance), constipation (remains a constant problem), pruritus, respiratory depression (very uncommon), dry mouth, urinary retention, drowsiness, and cognitive impairment. Drowsiness and cognitive impairment should be considered, along with constipation, the most serious adverse drug reactions to opioids, because they can seriously affect the patients' quality of life.

Nevertheless, the use of appropriate tools to identify at-risk patients prior to initiating treatment with opioids, constant vigilance on the behaviour associated with opioid assumption, and frequent re-evaluation of the balance between risks and benefits of long-term opioid therapies should become a normal attitude among physicians.

Tapentadol

Tapentadol is a single molecule agent with dual actions: mu opioid receptor agonism and selective norepinephrine reuptake inhibition. Tapentadol has a better adverse effect profile including good gastrointestinal (GI) tolerability, improved treatment adherence, and lower tolerance and abuse potential compared with older opioids. Metabolism is by hepatic glucuronidation, meaning a lower risk of adverse interactions with other drugs metabolised by CYP450 enzymes. In one study with patients with severe chronic neuropathic low back pain, monotherapy with Tapentadol was as effective as combination therapy with pregabalin [11]. The incidence of dizziness and somnolence was clinically and statistically significantly lower in the group receiving Tapentadol alone. These findings suggest a role for Tapentadol as a single agent in this difficult-to-treat group of patients.

Tramadol

Tramadol is a weak agonist of mu opioid receptors; it is used for the treatment of mild to moderate musculoskeletal pain but also inhibits the reuptake of serotonin and norepinephrine, somewhat similarly to SNRIs. In doses up to 400 mg/day, it was shown to be effective in seven RCTs, with a combined NNT of 4.7. Adult doses typically start at 25–50 mg/day (or up to 100 mg/day of an extended-release formulation); they are titrated as tolerated up to 400 mg/day. In elderly patients the initial dose should be low, and titration might need to be slower to prevent excessive drowsiness, dizziness, and falls. Both the opioidergic and serotonergic-noradrenergic effects of tramadol must be accounted for in considering its potential side effects and drug-drug interactions.

NMDA Receptor Antagonists

NMDA receptors for glutatame have been implicated in the development of neuropathic pain. Since the late 1980s, NMDA receptor antagonists have been known to decrease neuronal hyperexcitability and reduce pain, and the efficacy of several NMDA receptor antagonists has been investigated in preclinical and clinical pain studies [29]. Despite the large number of studies, there is still no consensus on the efficacy of NMDA receptor antagonist on neuropathic pain therefore the present systematic review was performed.

Mechanism of Action

Ketamine is probably the most investigated NMDA receptor antagonists for the treatment of neuropathic pain [29]. Ketamine is known to equally bind the NMDA subtypes 2A to 2D and may therefore have a more favourable effect in such a heterogenic disease as neuropathic pain, compared with NMDA receptor antagonists with more discriminative NMDA subtype selectivity. In addition, ketamine is a high affinity NMDA receptor antagonist, resulting in long-term blocking of the receptor and strong inhibiting of the neuronal hyperexcitability occurring in neuropathic pain. A disadvantage of this undiscriminating and strong binding property, however, is the higher proportions of side effects due to binding of the antagonists to neuronal structures not involved in pain. The use of the S (+) enantiomer of ketamine in clinical trials, may be favourable regarding side effects. S (+) ketamine is twice as potent in analgesic effect compared with racemic ketamine; therefore, lower doses of S (+) ketamine may reduce side effects, while providing pain reduction resembling racemic ketamine.

Several oral NMDA receptor antagonist drugs, primarily dextromethorphan and memantine, have been tested for effectiveness in this setting.

Short-term studies with intravenous administration of other NMDA antagonists such as ketamine [30] and amantadine have been positive [31] but more long-term data are needed to assess the applicability of these interventions.

The combined NNH with oral NMDA antagonists is around 8.7, suggesting limited tolerability, and there are currently inconclusive recommendations regarding the place of these drugs in the therapy of NeuP.

Future Perspective

Cebranopradol

This is a promising unique, centrally acting agent. It is a single molecule but has dual agonist action at opioid and nociception/orphanin FQ peptide (NOP) receptors [32]. Compared with traditional opioids, cebranopradol is more potent against neuropathic than nociceptive pain. In preclinical testing it showed antinociceptive, antihyperalgesic, and antiallodynic actions, with significantly higher potency than morphine. The adverse effect profile of cebranopradol is favourable compared with morphine at equianalgesic doses; it also has lower incidences of opioid-induced respiratory depression and pruritus, and delayed onset of tolerance. In addition, NOP agonism reduces dopamine release from neurones involved in reward pathways. Thus, the combination of NOP and MOP (mu opioid peptide) receptor agonism may attenuate opioid reward pathways in a similar manner to buprenorphine. The results of phase III clinical trials are awaited.

Angiotensin Ii Type 2 Receptor Antagonists

In the past two decades, there has been a collaborative global research effort on the pathophysiology of NeP. This has revealed a multitude of 'pain targets' including receptors, enzymes, and ion channels. Despite promising results in animal models this failed to translate into humans. One exception is the AT2 receptor antagonists, which represent a completely new analgesic class. EMA401 is a first-in-class orally active, highly selective, peripherally restricted AT2 receptor antagonist that has been successful in a clinical proof of-concept trial in patients with postherpetic neuralgia [33].

Conclusion

Several recommendations have recently been proposed concerning pharmacotherapy, neurostimulation techniques and interventional management, but no comprehensive guideline encompassing all these treatments has yet been issued.

A systematic review of pharmacotherapy, neuro-stimulation, surgery, psychotherapies and other types of therapy for peripheral or central neuropathic pain, based on studies published in peer-reviewed journals before January 2018 [34]. The main inclusion criteria were chronic neuropathic pain for at least 3 months, a randomized controlled methodology, at least 3 weeks of follow-up, at least 10 patients per group, and a double-blind design for drug therapy.

Based on the GRADE system, weak-to-strong recommendations for use and proposal as a first-line treatment for SNRIs (duloxetine and venlafaxine), gabapentin and tricyclic antidepressants and, for topical lidocaine and transcutaneous electrical nerve stimulation specifically for peripheral neuropathic pain; a weak recommendation for use and proposal as a second-line treatment for pregabalin, tramadol, combination therapy (antidepressant combined with gabapentinoids), and for high-concentration capsaicin patches and botulinum toxin A specifically for peripheral neuropathic pain; a weak recommendation for use and proposal as a third-line treatment for high-frequency Transcranial Magnetic Stimulation (rTMS) of the motor cortex, spinal cord stimulation (failed back surgery syndrome and painful diabetic polyneuropathy) and strong opioids (in the absence of an alternative).

Psychotherapy (cognitive behavioural therapy and mindfulness) is recommended as a second-line therapy, as an add-on to other therapies. An algorithm encompassing all the recommended treatments is proposed.

Although the mainstay of neuropathic pain management is still represented by drug therapy, particularly antidepressants and antiepileptics, the place of nonpharmacological therapy including brain-neuromodulation techniques has substantially increased in recent years. Newer study designs are also increasingly implemented, based on in depth phenotypic profiling to achieve more individualized therapy, or on screening strategies to decrease placebo effect and contribute to increase assay sensitivity. These approaches are now considered the most promising to decrease therapeutic failures in neuropathic pain.

Neuropathic pain management should not be restricted to pharmacotherapy but now encompasses multiple approaches including particularly neuromodulation techniques. Multimodal assessment can also help identify predictors of the response in clinical trials to ensure appropriate management [35]. The proposed algorithm is as shown in the diagram below (Fig. 15.1).

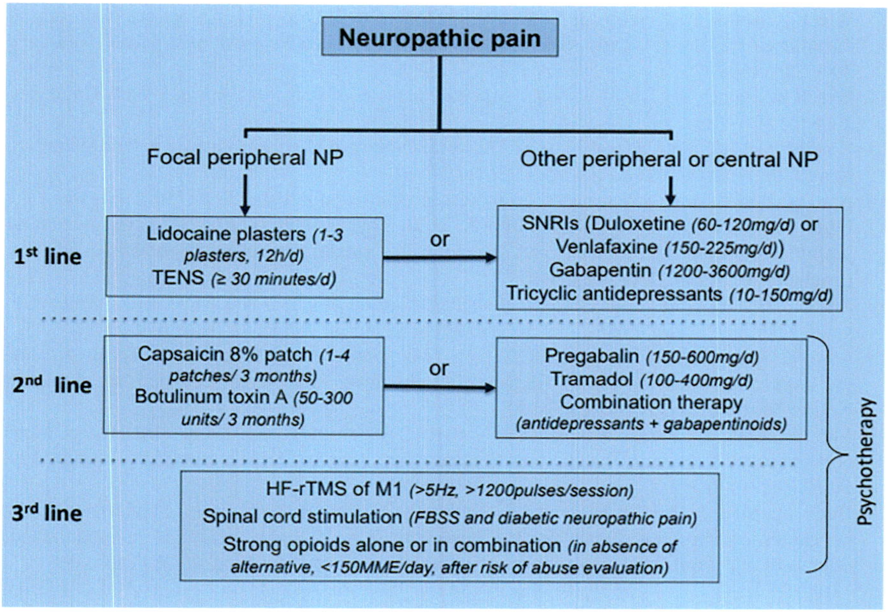

Fig. 15.1 Proposed neuropathic pain management stepwise approach. Reference: Revue Neurologique; 176:325–352,2020 [35]

References

1. Treede RD, Jensen TS, Campbell JN, et al. Neuropathic pain: redefinition and a grading system for clinical and research purposes. Neurology. 2008;70:1630–5.
2. Bouhassira D, Lanteri-Minet M, Attal N, Laurent B, Touboul C. Prevalence of chronic pain with neuropathic characteristics in the general population. Pain. 2008;136:380–7.
3. Torrance N, Smith BH, Bennett MI, Lee AJ. The epidemiology of chronic pain of predominantly neuropathic origin. Results from a general population survey. J Pain. 2006;7:281–9.
4. Alleman CJ, Westerhout KY, Hansen M, et al. Humanistic and eco–nomic burden of painful diabetic peripheral neuropathy in Europe: a review of the literature. Diabetes Res Clin Pract. 2015;109:215–25.
5. Baron R, Binder A, Wasner G. Neuropathic pain: diagnosis, pathophysiological mechanisms, and treatment. Lancet Neurol. 2010;9:807–19.
6. Finnerup NB, Attal N, Haroutounian S, et al. Pharmacotherapy for neuropathic pain in adults: a systematic review and meta-analysis. Lancet Neurol. 2015;14:162–73.
7. Woolf CJ. Central sensitization: implications for the diagnosis and treatment of pain. Pain. 2011;152:2–15.
8. Wiffen PJ, Derry S, Bell RF, et al. Gabapentin for chronic neuropathic pain in adults. Cochrane Database Syst Rev. 2017;6:CD007938.
9. Derry S, Bell RF, Straube S, et al. Pregabalin for neuropathic pain in adults. Cochrane Database Syst Rev. 2019;1:CD007076.
10. National Institute of Clinical Excellence. Neuropathic pain in adults: pharmacological management in non-specialist settings, https://www.nice.org.uk/guidance/cg173
11. Baron R, Binder A, Attal N, Casale R, Dickenson AH, Treede R-D. Neuropathic low back pain in clinical practice. Eur J Pain. 2016;20:861e3.
12. Bymaster FP, Dreshfield-Ahmad LJ, Threlkeld PG, Shaw JL, Thompson L, Nelson DL, Hemrick-Luecke SK, Wong DT. Comparative affinity of duloxetine and venlafaxine for serotonin and norepinephrine transporters *in vitro* and *in vivo*, human serotonin receptor subtypes, and other neuronal receptors. Neuropsychopharmacology. 2001;25:871–80.
13. Wiech K, Kalisch R, Weiskopf N, Pleger B, Stephan KE, Dolan RJ. Anterolateral prefrontal cortex mediates the analgesic effect of expected and perceived control over pain. J Neurosci. 2006;26:11501–9.
14. Wiech K, Ploner M, Tracey I. Neurocognitive aspects of pain perception. Trends Cogn Sci. 2008;12:306–13.
15. Knadler MP, Lobo E, Chappell J, et al. Duloxetine: clinical pharmacokinetics and drug interactions. Clin Pharmacokinet. 2011;50(5):281–94.
16. Attal N, Bouhassira D. Pharmacotherapy of neuropathic pain. Pain. 2015;156:S104–14.
17. Bauer CS, Rahman W, Tran-Van-Minh A, et al. The anti-allodynic α2δ ligand pregabalin inhibits the trafficking of the calcium channel α2δ-1 subunit to presynaptic terminals in vivo. Biochem Soc Trans. 2010;38:525–8.
18. Zhou C, Luo ZD. Electrophysiological characterization of spinal neuron sensitization by elevated calcium channel alpha-2-delta-1 subunit protein. Eur J Pain. 2014;18:649–58.
19. Suto T, Severino AL, Eisenach JC, et al. Gabapentin increases extracellular glutamatergic level in the locus coeruleus via astroglial glutamate transporter-dependent mechanisms. Neuropharmacology. 2014;81:95–100.
20. Simpson DM, Brown S, Tobias J. NGX-4010 C107 study group. Controlled trial of high-concentration capsaicin patch for treatment of painful HIV neuropathy. Neurology. 2008;70:2305–13.
21. Backonja MM, Malan TP, Vanhove GF, Tobias JK. C102/106 study group. NGX4010, a high-concentration capsaicin patch, for the treatment of postherpetic neuralgia: a randomized, double-blind, controlled study with an open-label extension. Pain Med. 2010;11:600–8.

22. Hans GH, Robert DN, Van Maldeghem KN. Treatment of an acute severe central neuropathic pain syndrome by topical application of lidocaine 5% patch: a case report. Spinal Cord. 2008;46:311–3.
23. Attal N, Gaudé V, Brasseur L, et al. Intravenous lidocaine in central pain: a double-blind, placebo-controlled, psychophysical study. Neurology. 2000;54:564–74.
24. Wallace MS, Laitin S, Licht D, Yaksh TL. Concentration-effect relations for intravenous lidocaine infusions in human volunteers: effects on acute sensory thresholds and capsaicin-evoked hyperpathia. Anesthesiology. 1997;86:1262–72.
25. Grotenhermen F. Pharmacokinetics and pharmacodynamics of cannabinoids. Clin Pharmacokinet. 2003;42:327–60. https://doi.org/10.2165/00003088-200342040-00003.
26. Labianca R, Sarzi-Puttini P, Zuccaro SM, et al. Adverse effects associated with non-opioid and opioid treatment in patients with chronic pain. Clin Drug Investig. 2012;32(Suppl 1):53–63. https://doi.org/10.2165/11630080-000000000-00000.
27. Moore RA, McQuay HJ. Prevalence of opioid adverse events in chronic non-malignant pain: systematic review of randomised trials of oral opioids. Arthritis Res Ther. 2005;7:R1046–51. https://doi.org/10.1186/ar1782.
28. Noble M, Treadwell JR, Tregear SJ, et al. Long-term opioid management for chronic noncancer pain. Cochrane Database Syst Rev. 2010;CD006605
29. Childers WE, Baudy RB. N-methyl-D-aspartate antagonists and neuropathic pain: the search for relief. J Med Chem. 2007;50:2557–62.
30. Webster LR, Walker MJ. Safety and efficacy of prolonged outpatient ketamine infusions for neuropathic pain. Am J Ther. 2006;13(4):300–5.
31. Pud D, Eisenberg E, Spitzer A, et al. The NMDA receptor antagonist amantadine reduces surgical neuropathic pain in cancer patients: a double blind, randomized, placebo controlled trial. Pain. 1998;75(2–3):349–54.
32. Raffa RB, Burdge G, Gambrah J, et al. Cebranopadol: novel dual opioid/NOP receptor agonist analgesic. J Clin Pharmacol Ther. 2017;42:8e17.
33. Smith MT, Anand P, Rice AS. Selective small molecule angiotensin II type 2 receptor antagonists for neuropathic pain: preclinical and clinical studies. Pain. 2016;157:S33e41.
34. Moisset X, Bouhassira D, Couturier JA, Alchaar H, Conradi S, Delmotte MH, Lanteri-Minet M, Lefaucheur JP, Mick G, Piano V, Pickering G, Piquet E, Regis C, Salvat E, Attal N. Pharmacological and non-pharmalogical treatments for neuropathic pain: systemic review and French recommendations. Rev Neurol. 2020;176(5):325–52. https://www.sciencedirect.com/science/article/pii/S0035378720304720
35. Moisset X, Bouhassira D, Couturier JA, Alchaar H, Conradi S, Delmotte MH, Lanteri-Minet M, Lefaucheur JP, Mick G, Piano V, Pickering G, Piquet E, Regis C, Salvat E, Attal N. Pharmacological and non-pharmacological treatments for neuropathic pain: systematic review and French recommendations. Rev Neurol. 2020;176:325–52.

Part VII
Interventional Therapy

Chapter 16
Interventional Procedures for Chronic and Neuropathic Pains

Donald Tsung-Yung Tang and Chih-Peng Lin

Chronic pain is very common and could be a very disabling problem for the sufferers. The cost of chronic pain takes preeminence among patients, their families, and society. The prevalence of chronic pain disorders is estimated to be 13–50%, while 10.4–14.3% of the chronic pain patients suffer from moderate-to-severe excruciating pain [1]. For those who do not respond to medication or other conservative treatments, interventional procedures or referral to surgery should be considered. Interventional pain management could be a transitional modality before sending a patient to surgery.

In this chapter, the image-guided technique with relevant image modalities, modalities for neuroablation and neuromodulation will be briefly reviewed. Regenerative techniques belong to another category of therapy. Conceptually, their mechanism of pain relief is opposed to neuroablation or anti-inflammation by corticosteroid injection, and will be discussed in the next chapter. Some techniques will be described for introducing different imaging or interventional modalities and the target of treatment are mainly spine-related pain. Details of all the interventional techniques are beyond the scope of this chapter.

D. T.-Y. Tang
Department of Pain Management, Taichung TZu-Chi Hospital, Taichung City, Taiwan

C.-P. Lin (✉)
Department of Anesthesiology, National Taiwan University Hospital, Taipei City, Taiwan

© The Author(s), under exclusive license to Springer Nature Switzerland AG 2022

J. de Castro, Y. El Miedany (eds.), *Advances in Chronic and Neuropathic Pain*, Contemporary Rheumatology, https://doi.org/10.1007/978-3-031-10687-3_16

Principles of Pain Management and Interventional Pain Management

Principles of successful pain management include: (1) Treating the pain generator; (2) Modifying or blockade of the nociceptive pathway; (3) Modifying the pain perception in the supraspinal level. In this chapter, we will focus on the modalities that modify or block the nociceptive signal, which is neuromodulation or neuroablation. The modalities for neuroablation include cryoneurolysis, conventional radiofrequency, cooled radiofrequency and chemical neurolysis. Chemical neurolysis could be achieved either by ethanol or phenol. Neuromodulation is usually conducted with spinal cord stimulation (SCS) or intrathecal pumps (ITP). Deep brain stimulation is another effective neuromodulating tool, however, it is beyond the scope of this chapter.

Modalities for Neuroablation

Cryoneurolysis

Cryoneurolysis is a technique that applies low temperature to destroy neural tissue in the nociceptive pathway. The cryoprobe consists of a larger hollow tube with an inner tube, in which pressurized gas travels (Fig. 16.1) [2]. The pressurized gas

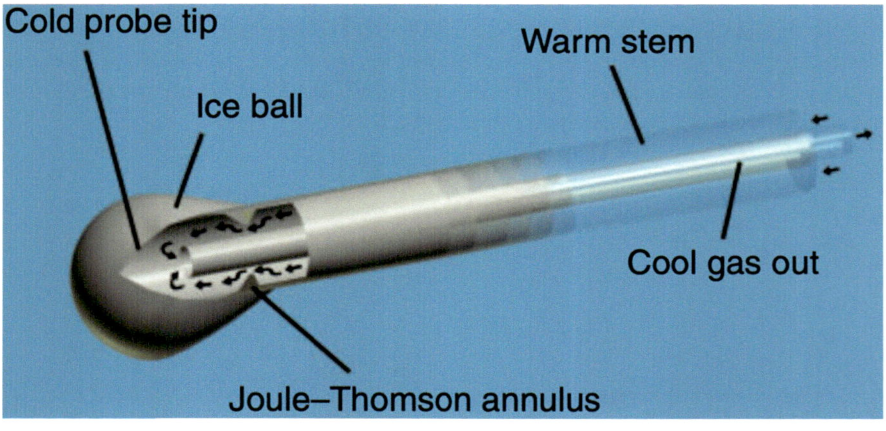

Fig. 16.1 A modern cryoneurolysis probe ('cannula') produces extremely cold temperatures at its tip because of the Joule–Thomson effect resulting from gas flowing from a high- to low-pressure chamber. *(Reprinted from British Journal of Anaesthesia 119 (4): 709–12 (2017), "Ultrasound-guided percutaneous cryoneurolysis for treatment of acute pain: could cryoanalgesia replace continuous peripheral nerve blocks?" with permission from Elsevier and Professor B. M. Ilfeld.)*

moves from the inner to the outer tube through a small aperture, expands quickly and extracts heat, and lowers the temperature to −70 °C, creating an ice ball [3].

Temperature below −20 °C could be destructive to human cells [4]. When the temperature goes down, the extracellular fluid becomes crystalized and leads to cell dehydration. As the dehydration process goes on, cell shrinkage and membrane rupture take place and induce cell death [5, 6]. The cooling effect also disrupts the blood flow around the nerves, which leads to microcirculatory stasis. These mechanisms result in Wallerian degeneration of the axon without disruption of the myelin sheath and the endoneurium [6].

Cryoneurolysis is a useful modality for peripheral nerve-related pain. It has good results in many areas like plantar nerve [7], intercostal nerve [8], genitofemoral nerve [9], pudendal nerve [10], greater occipital nerve, [11] and other peripheral nerves [12]. As a neuroablation technique, cryoneurolysis provides durable pain relief, usually in a period of 6–8 months. A distinct advantage of cryoanalgesia is that, denervation, the disrupted nerve regrows without formation of painful neuromas with full recovery of sensory and motor function is possible. Shah et al. [13] performed cryoneurolysis on common peroneal nerves of male Lewis rats where axon counts are not significantly different from control, and no post-intervention persistent motor deficit was found.

To optimize the therapeutic result, sensory stimulation and image-guidance including ultrasound and/or fluoroscopy are strongly recommended. Accurate placement of the cryoprobe optimizes the therapeutic outcomes. Additionally, it is usually recommended to do several freeze-defrost cycles, because the targeted nerve could be insulated from the probe by the ice ball.

The complications of cryoanalgesia include common procedural complications like bleeding, hematoma, infection, damage to adjacent structures like nerves or muscles. In superficial procedures, frostbite of skin is possible. During the procedure, we should always carefully inspect for any white, or waxy changes of the overlying skin. Hydro-dissection between the skin and subcutaneous layer could minimized the risk of frostbite.

Targeted Radiofrequency (RF) Techniques

RF technique is currently widely used in interventional pain management. It was used initially to treat trigeminal neuralgia in the early 1930 by a German surgeon Martin Kirschner [14]. Later, the application of RF in spinal pain was done by Shealy [15] for pain from lumbar zygapophyseal joint. This technique disrupts or modifies the nociceptive pathway from the pain generators, thus producing substantial pain relief. Although the root causes of pain are not directly treated, the lasting analgesia produced by RF is sufficient to abate the complications of chronic pain like poor sleep, hygiene, mood disorder and functional incapability. It can also significantly help the patient return to normal daily activities.

Currently, RF is conducted percutaneously by placing an insulated needle with an active tip close to the targeted neural pathway. The high-frequency alternating current generated by the metal active tip activates oscillation of molecules, produces friction in the tissue, and produces lesions in the nerve fibers. Lesioning in the nerve fibers blocks the nociceptive transmission from the pathology. RF could be performed as conventional, or continuous mode, and pulsed mode, which has been used since the mid-1970. The conventional mode RF burns all types of nerve fibers, while the pulsed mode RF delivers current in small bursts thus preventing heat accumulation, producing selective disruption of small unmyelinated fibers in a less destructive way [16–18].

During the procedure, whether conventional or pulsed mode, several technical parameter and patient response should be monitored for both avoidance of complications and precision of the techniques. The impedance should be monitored for verifying the integrity of the electric circuit. The value of impedance varies from 200 to 800 Ω and is affected by surrounding structures. The higher the tissue density, the higher the impedance. When the needle is in the scar tissue or is contacting bony structures, the high impedance would probably decrease the electric current, thus potentiate treatment failure. Injection of saline could decrease the impedance. Temperature, voltage, and current should also be monitored for the controlled lesion, especially in the pulsed mode where the temperature should be controlled and should not be higher than 42 °C. Neurostimulation, sensory or motor mode is used to check the proximity between the needle and the targeted nerve, while preventing damage to the non-targeted neural tissue. For example, when performing conventional RF lesioning of lumbar medial branches for zygapophyseal joint pain, the clinician should affirm that the lumbar spinal nerve root is not damaged. The motor stimulation is performed at 2 Hz, while the sensory one is at 50 Hz.

Conventional RF

In interventional pain management, the goal of conventional RF is to increase the temperature around the neural tissue, creating permanent damage to the nerve and blocking the nociceptive pathway. The largest lesioning area is along the long axis of the electrode, so the physician should place the needle and the nerve as parallel as possible. The lesion size produced by RF should be carefully manipulated by the physician. The lesion size is important in achieving meaningful pain relief, such that a small lesion could fall short of meaningful pain relief while an oversized lesion could lead to undesirable tissue damage other than nerve itself. The lesion size could be controlled by following factors [19, 20]:

1. Temperature: the lesion size is positively correlated with the temperature up to 90 °C. Temperature higher than 90 °C potentiates abscess formation. Additionally, the lesion size would not be larger because the charring of the tissue limits the electric current transmission and heat distribution.
2. Duration of coagulation: The lesion size increases over time, and it grows most rapidly in the first minute. When compared to the lesion size of the first minute,

the size increases 11–20% in a 2-min duration and 23–32% in 3-min duration [19]. The lesion size could keep growing less rapidly up to 10 min.
3. Tip gauge and length: To increase the size of lesioning, pick a larger gauge electrode with longer active tip. A conventional 16-gauge cannula at 80–90 °C for 2–3 min generate lesions of average width similar to that produced by the cooled RF configuration proposed for sacroiliac joint denervation [19].
4. Injection of fluids [21–23]: More energy could be distributed when the impedance gets lower. Injecting saline or local anesthetics decrease the impedance and increase the lesion size. Increasing the concentration of saline could further decrease the impedance, increase the power output and enlarge the lesion size [23].

Clinical Application of Conventional RF: Lumbar Medial Branch Radiofrequency

1. Indication: Lumbar zygapophyseal joint pain, also known as lumbar facet joint pain.
2. Positive diagnostic block before RF ablation is mandatory. Diagnostic block could be executed by either facet joint intra-articular injection or medial branch block. However, medial branch block, as a prognostic tool, is anticipated to obtain better outcomes [24, 25].
3. Relevant anatomy:

   At typical levels, L1 to L4, the course of medial branches is relatively consistent. After emerging from the neuroforamen, the nerve runs at the base of superior articular process (SAP) of the respective level (Fig. 16.2). After that, it runs dorsally and caudally and disappears under the mamillo-accessory ligament, sending its branches to the multifidi. Due to the strong constraint by the mamillo-accessory ligament, the course of medial branches is constant on the neck of SAP [26]. Radiofrequency is suggested to perform at 2 points: the deeper one is at the junction of the first and second ventral quarters of the superior articular process, while the second one is the point on the middle of the neck of the superior articular process, which could be located by withdrawing the electrode 3–5 mm from the deeper point [26]. At the L5 level, the dorsal ramus is much longer than those at the typical levels. It courses around the junction of sacral ala and the S1 SAP.

   Each facet joint is innervated by the medial branches of the nerve root above and below. For example, the L4–5 facet joint is innervated by the L3 and L4 medial branches. To denervate the joint, both medial branches should be blocked.
4. Technique:

   - RF for the lumbar medial branches is usually performed under fluoroscopic guidance. It is also possible to perform this procedure under ultrasound guidance. However, verification with fluoroscopy could optimize the precision of needle tip placement.

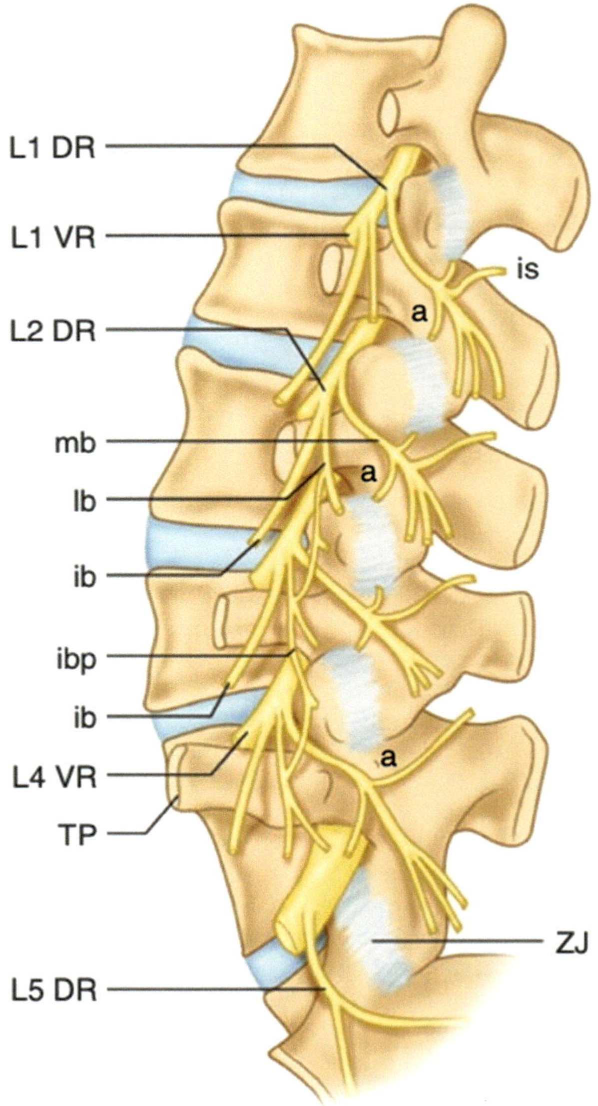

Fig. 16.2 Innervation of lumbar facet joints. Each joint is innervated by the lumbar medial branches above and below. *DR* dorsal ramus, *ib* intermediate branch, *ibp* intermediate branch plexus, *lb* lateral branch, *mb* medial branch, *TP* transverse process, *a* articular branch, *is* interspinous branch, *VR* ventral ramus, *ZJ* zygapophysial joint. *(Reprinted from "Essentials of Interventional Techniques in Managing Chronic Pain, Fig. 19.3, with permission from Springer.)*

- Neurostimulation is usually necessary in RF procedures. However, in RF of lumbar medial branch, correct anatomical placement of the electrode without neurostimulation could achieve adequate coagulation of the medial branches [27]. Nevertheless, neurostimulation could be performed to rule out the proximity between the electrode and the dorsal root ganglion.

- Brief Technical Overview:
  - The patient is placed in prone position, with firm padding under the abdomen to reduce the lumbar lordosis. Routine monitoring and aseptic technique are implemented.
  - Confirm the target level.
  - Turn the fluoroscope obliquely and ipsilaterally in the symptomatic side, 20–30° to obtain the "Scotty dog" landmark (Fig. 16.3). The oblique angle at the L5 level is smaller (10–15°), because the anatomy is different and the iliac crest may interfere the needle trajectory.
  - Others may suggest a caudal to cephalad trajectory by caudally tilting the fluoroscope. This could optimize the parallel placement of cannula and the nerve.
  - Tunnel vision technique: The target for L1 to L4 medial branches is the junction of transverse process and SAP, which is the junction of nose and ear in the Scotty dog landmark (Fig. 16.3). The target for L5 dorsal ramus is on the junction of S1 SAP and sacral ala. Infiltrate local anesthetic before introducing the RF cannula. Try to get bony contact on the target to prevent advancing the cannula too anteriorly.
  - Check the final position of the cannula tip by AP and lateral views:

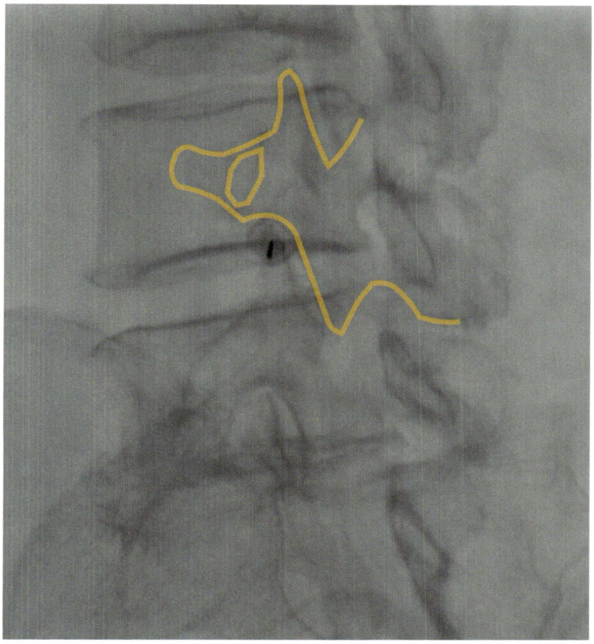

Fig. 16.3 Scotty Dog landmark for lumbar spine interventions. The nose corresponds to the transverse process, the eye corresponds to the pedicle, the ear corresponds to the superior articular process and the forefoot corresponds to the inferior articular process

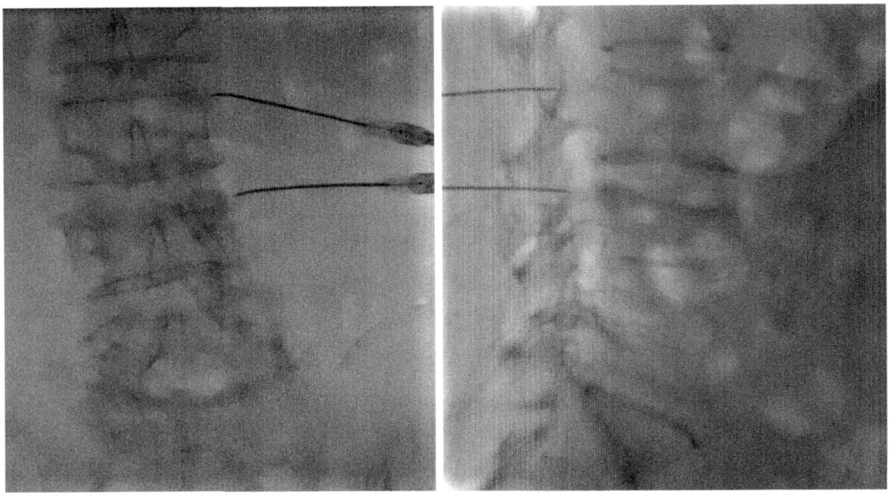

Fig. 16.4 Radiofrequency for the lumbar medial branches. Left, AP view of fluoroscopy image, the needle tip should be placed at the at the junction of transverse process and the superior articular process; right, lateral view, the needle tip is placed on the supero-posterior part of the transverse process

- In AP view, the tip of the cannula should be on the lateral margin of the SAP or slightly medial to it. In lateral view, the needle tip should be placed on the supero-posterior quadrant. The needle tip should not be too medial in the AP view or too ventral in the lateral view (Fig. 16.4).
- Perform neurostimulation: if a paresthesia is radiating to the ipsilateral lower limb, repositioning is needed.
- Inject 1 mL local anesthetic before RF protocol. The RF lesioning is generated at 80–90 °C for 60–90 seconds.

Pulsed RF

Conventional RF achieves pain relief by thermal lesioning of the nociceptive Pathway. In contrast, pulsed RF obtains pain relief by producing an intense electric field. Although pulsed RF is less destructive and its complication rate is lower than conventional RF, the mechanism of pain relief is still not fully understood.

Pulsed RF generates intense electric fields by creating quick, short currents of 20 milliseconds in duration and usually the frequency is 2 per second. Therefore, the 480-millisecond cooling periods alternate with the heating period, thus, allowing adequate heat dissipation, keeping the temperature under the neuro-destructive level, which is usually 42 °C. Theoretically, this protocol does not induce protein denaturation or neural ablation. However, damage to the neural tissue by pulsed RF was noticed in animal studies [28, 29], the temperature effect could not be completely ruled out from the therapeutic mechanism of pulsed RF.

Other possible mechanisms of pulsed RF could be structural change, modulation of genetic expression and immune-modulatory effect. Ultrastructural changes of the axons post-pulsed RF includes abnormal membranes and morphology of mitochondria, disruption and disorganization of microfilaments, and microtubules as reported by Erdine et al. [29]. These changes are more prominent in C fiber than in A-δ and A-β fibers, which could be a part of pain relief mechanism. Dorsal horn lamina I and II neurons could be activated after pulsed RF [30]. Changes in genetic or molecular level [31], including down regulation of calcitonin gene-related peptide [32], glutamate [33], IL-1β, TNF-α, spinal β-catenin [34], P2X3 receptor [35], substance P [36] and upregulation of GDNF [37] are also of clinical significance. Changes of lymphocyte in the CSF after pulsed RF on the dorsal root ganglion (DRG) are also reported [38], which means immunomodulation could be a part of the mechanism.

Clinical Application of Pulsed RF: Lumbar DRG Pulsed RF

1. Indication: Partial nerve lesion in the DRG, e.g. lumbar radicular pain, lumbar zoster associated pain.
2. Technique:
   - Procedures on the DRG are performed with fluoroscopic-guidance. Ultrasound could guide the needle into the neuroforamen [39], however, it could not affirm the adequate depth of the needle and the proximity to the DRG since the ultrasound beam is interrupted by the lamina. The final needle position is confirmed with both fluoroscopy and neurostimulation.
   - In pulsed RF technique, the needle is better placed perpendicular to the nerve instead of parallel to the nerve because the electric field is more intense at the tip of the electrode.
   - The technique for pulsed RF on lumbar DRG is similar to lumbar transforaminal epidural injection. However, in a transforaminal injection, the needle tip could be placed either in safe triangle or Kambin triangle, while for pulsed RF, the needle tip should be specifically placed in the safe triangle, where the DRG is located. In clinical practice, epidural steroid injection is usually performed simultaneously in a pulsed RF procedure.
   - Brief technical overview:
     - The patient is placed in prone position, with firm padding under the abdomen to reduce lumbar lordosis. Routine monitor and aseptic technique are implemented.
     - Confirm the target level.
     - Tilt the fluoroscopy cephalad or caudally to align the fluoroscopy beam with the superior end plate of the target level. Using the superior end plate instead of the inferior end plate facilitates an inferior-to-superior needle trajectory.

- Turn the fluoroscopy in oblique position: The fluoroscopy is rotated ipsilaterally to obtain the classic view of "Scotty dog," in which the pedicle is the dog's eye, the transverse process is the nose and the pars interarticularis is the neck. The target of the needle placement is on the junction of the transverse process and the pars interarticularis. (Fig. 16.3)
- Tunnel vision technique: the needle trajectory should be parallel to the fluoroscopy beam.
- Check the depth with lateral view. The tip of the needle should be kept in the posterior half of the neuroforamen to avoid injury to the spinal nerves. (Fig. 16.5)
- If transforaminal injection is performed in the same procedure, deliver contrast medium to affirm the spreading of the injectate then inject the solution for treatment.
- Perform sensory and motor stimulation for pulsed RF. Positive response should be obtained below 0.5 V.
- Pulse RF therapy: The treatment course

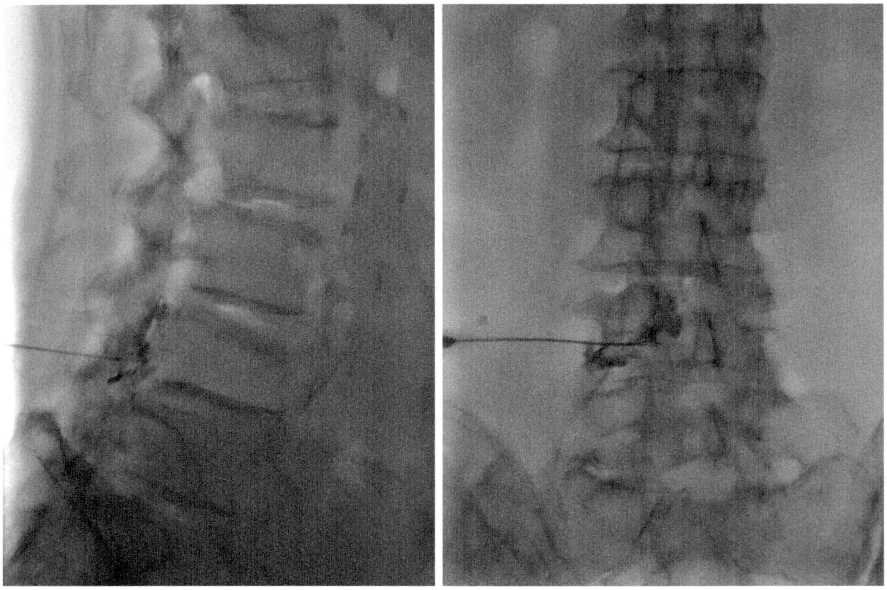

Fig. 16.5 Lumbar transforaminal epidural injection with or without pulsed radiofrequency. The needle tip is placed in the 6 o' clock direction of the pedicle in the AP view and in the posterior half of neuroforamen in the lateral view

Bipolar RF

Bipolar radiofrequency achieves tissue lesioning when the electric current passed from one electrode to another, thus, transmitting through the target tissue. The most intriguing example to illuminate the essence of bipolar radiofrequency is strap lesioning of the sacral lateral branches to treat sacroiliac joint pain (Fig. 16.6).

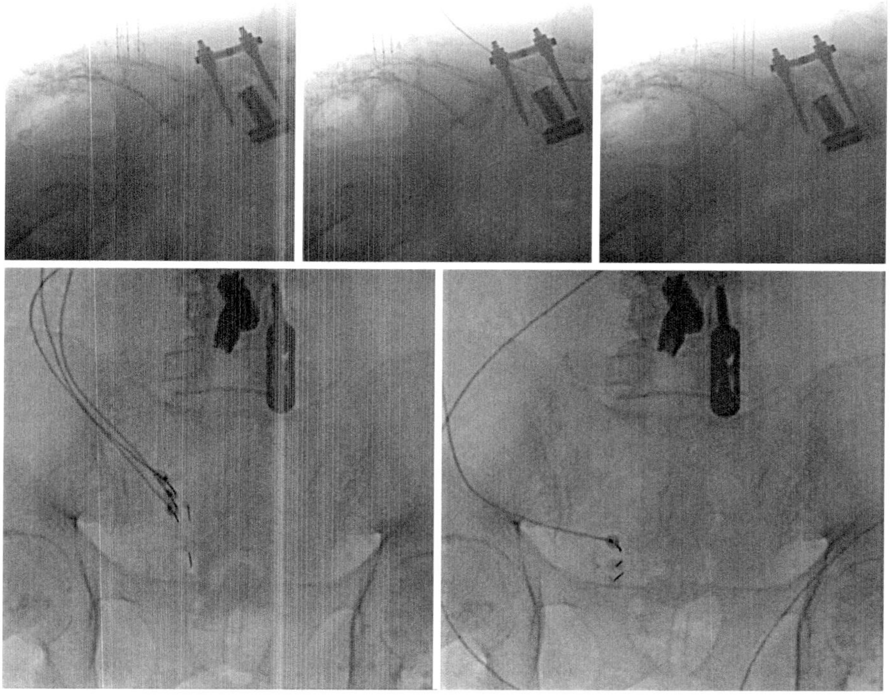

Fig. 16.6 Bipolar radiofrequency of sacral lateral branches of S1, 2, 3. In lateral view, the needles are placed parallel and perpendicular to the posterior surface of the sacrum. In AP view, the needles are placed just lateral to the posterior sacral foramina

Cooled RF

Cooled RF uses constant flow of ambient water circulated around the electrode to maintain lower tissue temperature while creating neurolysis (Fig. 16.7). The constant flow of water removes heat from tissues around the electrode, keeps the temperature to enable it to create tissue ablation and limits scar formation at the same time [40, 41]. Avoiding scar tissue formation effectively by avoiding high impedance of the tissue that blocks the electric current of radiofrequency. Therefore, the lesion size obtained by cooled RF is substantially greater than one by conventional RF [42]. Another advantage of cooled RF is that the shape of the lesioning is spheric, which means the electrodes could be placed in any angle without negatively affecting the lesion size. With its spheric, larger lesion size, it is easier to attain successful neuroablation.

Clinical Application of Bipolar or Cooled RF: sacral lateral branches neurotomy for sacroiliac (SI) joint pain (Fig. 16.8), genicular nerves ablation of the knees (Fig. 16.9) and ablation of hip articular branches.

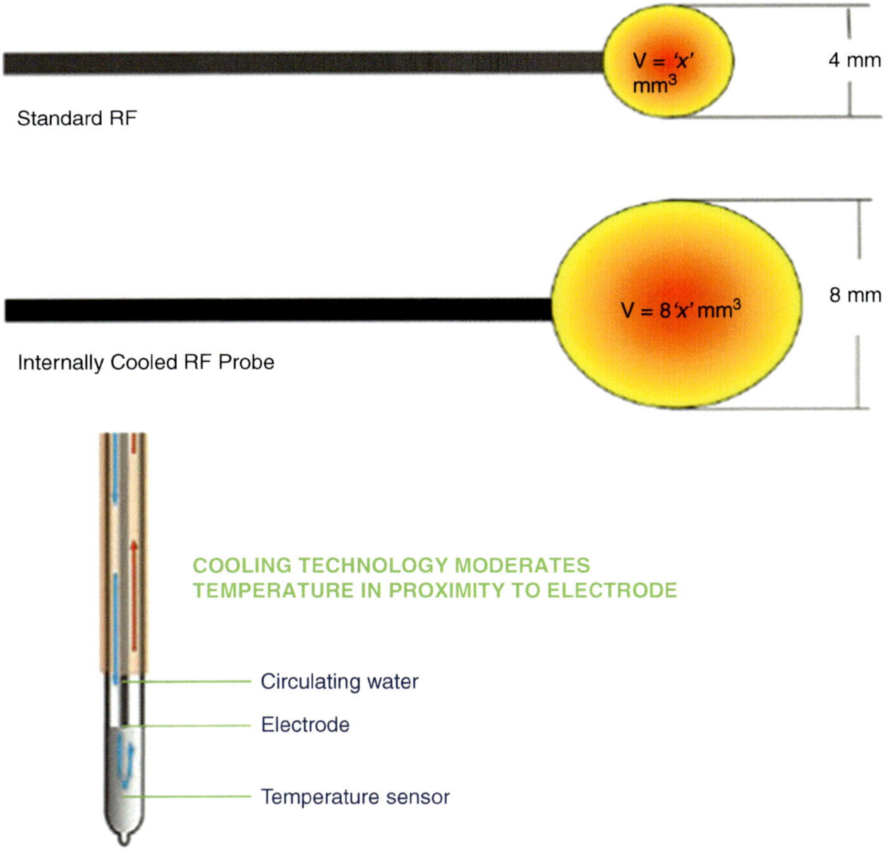

Fig. 16.7 Cooled radiofrequency probe. The inner cooled water flow decreases the temperature, preventing tissue charring thus enlarges the lesion size

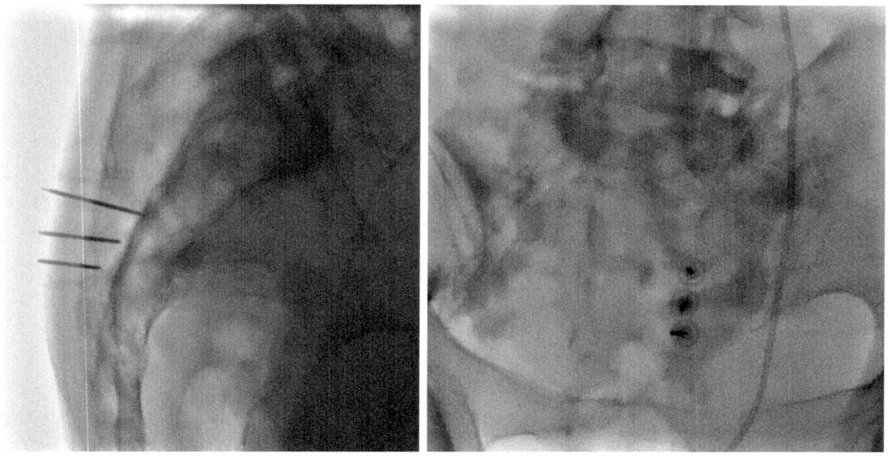

Fig. 16.8 Cooled radiofrequency of the sacroiliac joints. Similar to bipolar radiofrequency, the needles are placed parallel and perpendicular to the posterior surface of the sacrum in lateral view and just lateral to the posterior sacral foramina in the AP view

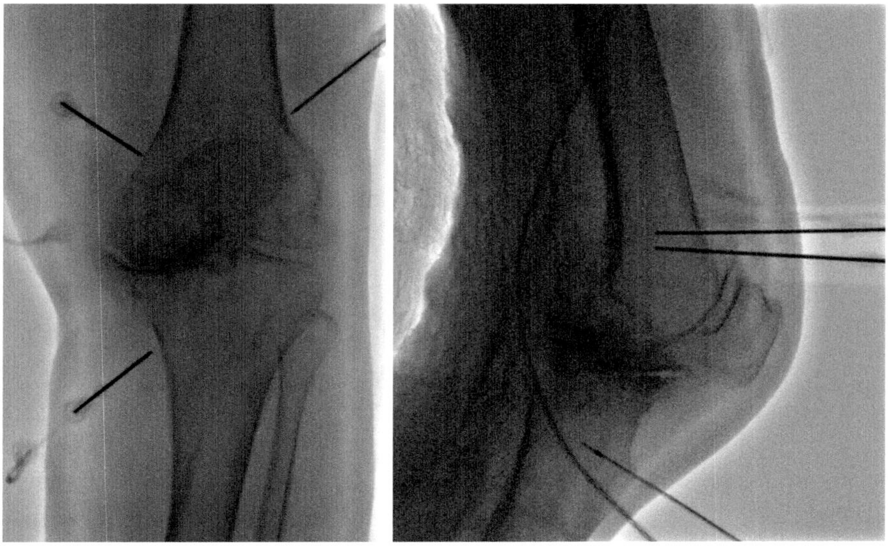

Fig. 16.9 Cooled radiofrequency of genicular nerves of the knee. Infero-lateral genicular nerve is spared to avoid damage to the common peroneal nerve

Chemical Neurolysis

Chemical neurolytic techniques are usually the last resort for intractable pain syndromes. When less destructive interventional modalities (like injection or radiofrequency) fail to obtain substantial pain relief, chemical neurolysis is considered. Due to its destructive nature, chemical neurolysis is usually utilized in cancer pain management, especially for the terminal cancer patients. The extent of tissue ablation created by chemical neurolytic agents is less predictable than RF. Inadvertent spreading to non-targeted structures may cause severe complication, including neurological deficits, tissue necrosis and vascular injury or spasm. For example, celiac plexus neurolysis, one of the most common procedure performed by chemical neurolysis, is possible to damage the artery of Adamkiewicz and subsequently induces paraplegia [43].

Alcohol

The neurolytic effect from alcohol is produced by extraction of intracellular components of neural cells. Subsequently, sclerotic changes of nerve fibers and myelin sheath leads to Wallerian degeneration. The basal lamina of the Schwann cells remains intact in chemical neurolysis, allowing nerve regrowth. Commercially available alcohol is usually anhydrous (100%), but will absorb small amount of water when exposed to room air. The effective concentration for neurolysis ranges from 45% to 100%, however, our personal experience suggests that the concentration should be more than 80% since the preceding contrast and local anesthetics on the target site will further lower the concentration.

Alcohol, as a neurolytic agent, has some disadvantages that limit its use. First, the injection of alcohol may be associated with acute injecting pain. Inject local anesthetic before alcohol would prevent this adverse event. Second, partial neurolysis or involvement of other non-targeted nerve may potentiate neuritis and induce permanent dysesthesia. Finally, tissue necrosis could occur in any chemical neurolytic technique.

Phenol

The neurolytic effect of phenol is produced by coagulation of proteins, leading to neural tissue necrosis and Wallerian degeneration. The effective concentration for neurolysis ranges from 4% to 10% [44]. The clinical application of phenol is similar to alcohol, however, the pain provoked by injection is mild and more tolerable for the patient.

Clinical application of chemical neurolysis: Denervation of refractory pain for cancer patients is the main application of chemical neurolysis. Splanchnic nerve neurolysis (Fig. 16.10) for abdominal cancer pain and superior hypogastric plexus neurolysis (Fig. 16.11) for pelvic cancer pain are two of the most common procedures.

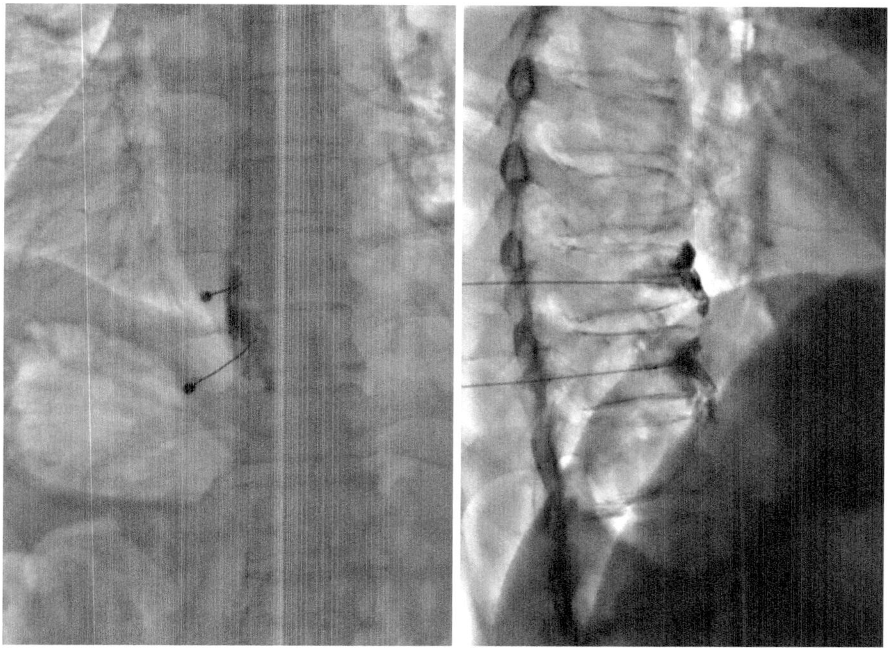

Fig. 16.10 Nerve block or chemical neurolysis of the splanchnic nerves. In this picture, the procedure is conducted at bilateral T10 and T11 levels. The needle tips are placed medial to the lateral border of the vertebral body in the AP view, and in the anterior 1/3 in the lateral view

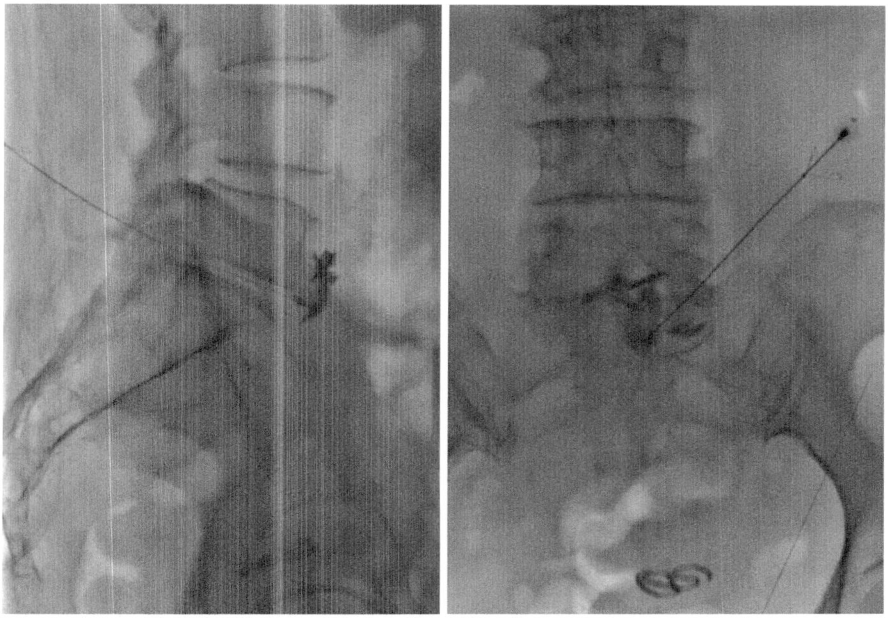

Fig. 16.11 Superior hypogastric plexus block or neurolysis, transdiscal approach. The needle tip is placed just anterior to the L5-S1 disc in lateral view and close to the midline of the L5-S1 disc in the AP view

Neuromodulation

Spinal Cord Stimulation (SCS)

When conservative therapy, injection or radiofrequency techniques fail to obtain adequate pain relief, electrical stimulation to the nerve system could be the main alternative for refractory pain. Electrical stimulation could be applied to the brain (deep brain stimulation, DBS), the spinal cord and peripheral nerves. In spinal cord stimulation, the lead-carrying electrodes are placed in the epidural space to generate electrical stimulation to the dorsal spinal cord (Fig. 16.12). The neuromodulatory effect by SCS, although is not a cure for pain syndromes, could alleviate pain symptoms in a minimally invasive way.

Anatomy

The spinal cord is a vital component of the central nervous system in the vertebral column. It extends from the foramen magnum to the first or second lumbar vertebrae. The lower nerve roots form the cauda equina. The internal structure of the spinal cord comprises H-shaped inner gray matter with cell bodies and outer white mater containing myelinated and unmyelinated fibers. The gray matter is divided into 4 parts: the dorsal horn, ventral horn, lateral horn and intermediate column. The

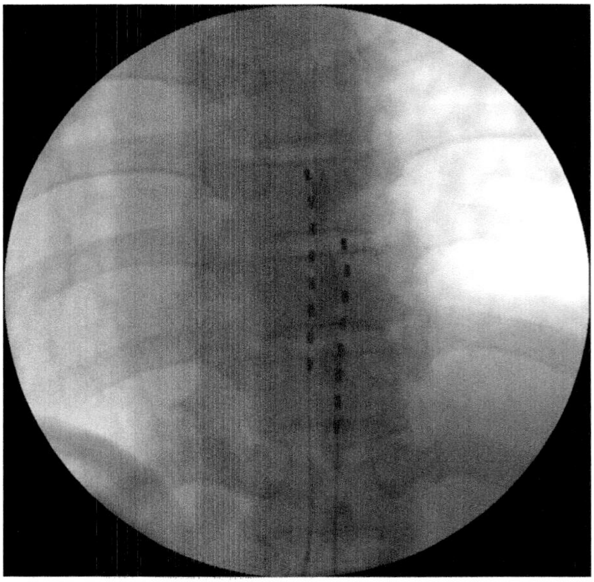

Fig. 16.12 Spinal cord stimulation. The electrode is placed in the dorsal epidural space, close to the midline

most crucial part is the dorsal horn, which transmit somatosensory signal to the supraspinal level via ascending tracts in the white matter. The white matter is divided into three area such as the dorsal column, ventral column, and lateral column. Ascending tracts in the white matter receive the signal from DRG, which is a pivotal structure for pain processing. In the dorsal column of the white matter, the gracile and cuneate fasciculi carry tactile sensation, vibration and proprioception to the brain. SCS is placed on the anatomical midline, stimulating the dorsal column to achieve substantial pain relief.

Mechanism

Melzack and Wall proposed the "gate control theory" in 1965 [45]. They suggested that pain signal could be blocked by stimulating the large A-β fibers, thus, activating the gate control system and closing the transmission of nociceptive inputs by A-δ and C fibers. The principle of gate control theory is the basis of SCS, however, the mechanism of action is still not fully elucidated. Direct suppression of sensitized C-fiber component in the dorsal horn with changes in chemical transmission is also a key component of SCS theory [46]. Additionally, modulation of the supraspinal level contributes to the pain reduction by SCS [47, 48]. Sympathetic modulation from SCS attenuates ischemic pain syndromes, like angina [49, 50] and peripheral vascular disease [51].

Indications and Evidence [52]

1. Failed back surgery syndrome in the absence of neurologic deficit requiring surgical intervention.
2. Radicular pain syndromes.
3. Cervical SCS for neuropathic pain syndromes in the upper extremities.
4. Complex regional pain syndrome, type I and type II.
5. Raynaud's syndrome and other painful ischemic vascular disorders.
6. Post-herpetic neuralgia: experimental level, high level evidence is warranted.
7. Visceral pain, e.g. angina pectoris, chronic pancreatitis or mesenteric ischemia. Experimental level, high level evidence is warranted.

Intrathecal Drug Delivery (IDD)

Intrathecal drug delivery is a technique that deliver medication for pain or spasticity directly into the cerebrospinal fluid (Fig. 16.13). Since it could deliver the medication directly to the nociceptive receptor of the spinal cord, the efficacy is enhanced and the complications of medication is attenuated [53]. Therefore, IDD is useful in refractory pain conditions, either cancerous or non-cancerous pain.

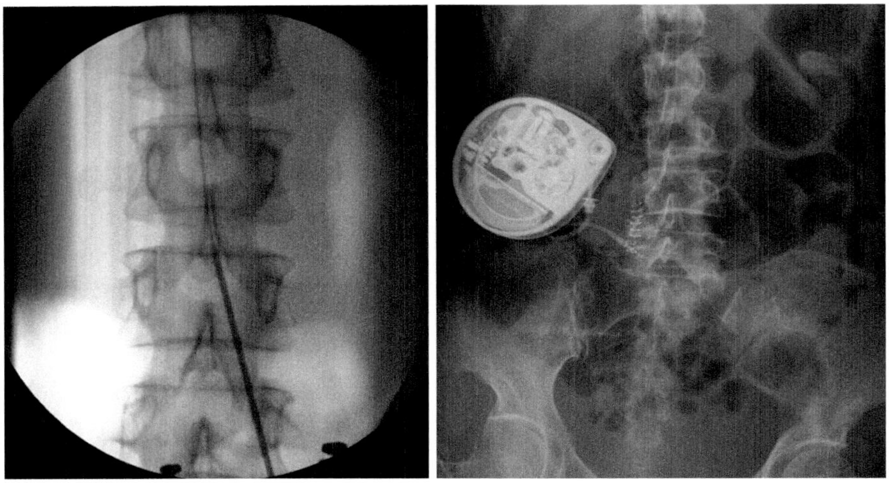

Fig. 16.13 Intrathecal drug delivery system. The catheter is directly placed in the CSF to maximize the efficacy of the medication while reducing the side effects. A pump/reservoir is implanted between the subcutaneous fat and the abdominal muscles

Indications

Currently, the indication for IDD include chronic intractable pain syndromes, either cancerous or non-cancerous pain [54]. IDD should be also be considered when the systemic pain therapy is maximized or the dose titration is limited by intolerable side effects.

The clinicians should always try to identify patients whose pain is likely to respond to IDD. Failed back surgery syndrome, complex regional pain syndrome, spinal stenosis, osteoporosis with compression fracture, pancreatitis, phantom limb pain and peripheral neuropathies are likely to be relieved by IDD, while head and neck pain and fibromyalgias are less likely to respond to this therapy [54]. The absolute exclusion criteria include systemic infection, allergy to the equipment, patient refusal, untreated drug abuse and noncompliant patient. The patient should have no contraindication before proceeding to the treatment. Noncancerous pain patient receiving IDD therapy should have a comprehensive evaluation including physical, psychological, and environmental domains followed by a trial. However, in certain population, like terminally-ill cancer patient, psychological evaluation and treatment trials are not necessary. Currently, there is no universal protocol for trialing intrathecal medication, the evidence level for single shot trialling, bolus trialling or continuous infusion are equal [55].

Medication for IDD

For pain management, there are several drugs used for intrathecal administration. Only two intrathecal agents are approved by Food and Drug Administration of the United States: preservative-free morphine and the conotoxin peptide, ziconotide.

The Polyanalgesic Consensus Conference (PACC) developed recommendations for properly application of the drugs [53].

1. Opioids are currently and commonly used in intrathecal application for intractable pain conditions. Morphine is the prototypical opioid, and is the most commonly used opioid, and the only FDA-approved opioid for intrathecal administration. It acts mostly on the μ-receptor. Due to its hydrophilic nature, it is poorly metabolized in the CSF and the duration of pain relief could be prolonged. Other commonly used opioids include hydromorphone, fentanyl and sufentanil. Hydromorphone is also a commonly used medication for intrathecal administration, and is more lipophilic than morphine thus, has less supraspinal distribution and side effects. Fentanyl and sufentanil are synthetic μ-receptor agonist. Both are highly lipophilic thus, result in segmental analgesia and rapid diffusion into the systemic.
2. Ziconotide is an FDA-approved drug for intrathecal administration. It is a selective N-type calcium channel blocker, decreasing the excitatory neurotransmitter release in the dorsal horn. It is poorly metabolized in the CSF, and the clearance of the drug is mediated by bulk flow of the CSF. The side effects of ziconotide include blurred vision, dizziness or lightheadedness, nausea and/or vomiting, nystagmus and urinary retention.
3. Other commonly used intrathecal agents are bupivacaine, clonidine for pain, and baclofen for spasticity. For the suggested doses, algorithm for intrathecal drug titration, please refer to the most updated PACC consensus guideline.

Risks and Complication

The complications of intrathecal drug administration could be divided into 2 categories: technical complications and complications associated with the therapy. Technical complications include infection, epidural hematoma, spinal cord or nerve injury, dural leak, and catheter failure. Complications associated with the therapy include drug overdose, side effects from the drug, granuloma and pain at the implant area. Granuloma is one of the most catastrophic complications. It is an inflammatory mass around the catheter tip. The mechanism of granuloma formation is still not fully elucidated, however, it is probably associated with higher concentration and higher dose of intrathecal opioids. The mass may result in the risk of spinal cord compression and neurological deficit. Clinician should consider an intrathecal granuloma when there is loss of analgesia following drug administration or new neurological deficit such as sensory or motor loss. MRI with contrast or CT myelogram could be diagnostic for the granuloma.

Image-Guided Techniques

Principles of Fluoroscopy-Guided Techniques

Fluoroscopy

Fluoroscopy is an image modality that applies X-ray to image structures. The image is obtained by the X ray sent from the X-ray tube, passing through the patient's body part and received by the image receptor. In interventional procedures, it could be utilized continuously or intermittently to demonstrate structures, verify the position of needle tip and the spread of contrast medium or implants like spinal cord stimulator.

Since the X-ray absorbed by human tissue could have certain detrimental effect, radiation safety is a concept of paramount importance. To minimize the radiation exposure to our patients, colleagues and ourselves, clinicians should try to limit the duration of exposure, maximize the distance from the X-ray, properly utilize the shield. Among the above tips for radiation safety, the most crucial one is limiting the duration of exposure. To limit the duration of exposure, use pulsed mode instead of conventional mode as much as possible. A thorough understanding of patient's anatomy by other pre-procedural image modalities, anticipating the proper C-arm localization as precise as possible, using the laser of the fluoroscope to estimate the X-ray trajectory, and obtaining multiplanar images simultaneously in multi-level procedures should be considered prior to the procedure.

Operating the Fluoroscopy

Tunnel vision technique is the key in positioning the needle in interventional pain procedures. In tunnel vision technique, the trajectory of the needle and the fluoroscopic beam are placed in parallel position. The needle is introduced toward the target with the needle demonstrating a single radiopaque dot on the fluoroscopic image (Fig. 16.14). For the orthogonal nature of tunnel vision technique, obtaining orthogonal AP and lateral views of the targeted level of the spine is a prerequisite for fluoroscopy-guided interventional procedures. Additionally, adjusting the fluoroscope by adequate oblique angle to identify the anatomic landmark (e.g., Scottie Dog in the lumbar spine, Fig. 16.3) for introducing the needle is crucial for starting an interventional procedure. These skills require a thorough knowledge of spinal anatomy, familiarity with fluoroscopy, and experience. As to the details of spinal anatomy, the normal spine curvature of the human body is the most crucial part. From the cranio-cervical junction to the coccyx, the cervical and lumbar spine are lordotic and the thoracic spine is kyphotic (Fig. 16.15).

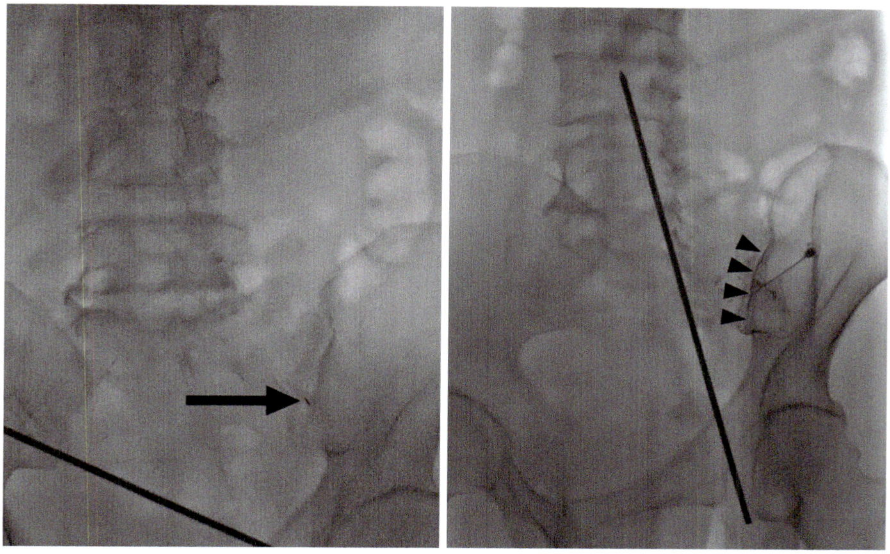

Fig. 16.14 Tunnel vision technique, sacroiliac joint injection as an example. Left, the needle tip should be a dot in the fluoroscopic image; right, contrast medium in the sacroiliac joint (arrow heads)

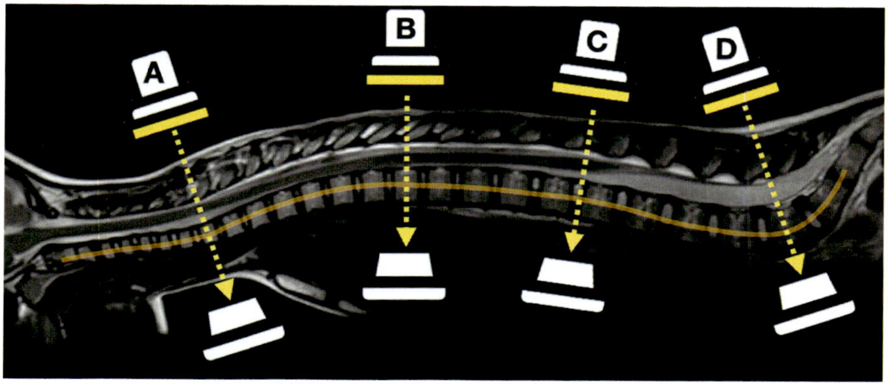

Fig. 16.15 Normal curves of the vertebral column. The thoracic spine is kyphotic while the cervical and lumbar spine are lordotic. For tunnel vision technique of fluoroscopy-guided intervention, the fluoroscopic beam should be orthogonal to the targeted spine level. For example, (**a**), the cervicothoracic junction, the fluoroscopy should be slightly cranially tilted; (**b**), middle to lower thoracic spine, minimal cranio-caudal adjustment is needed; (**c**), Thoracolumbar junction, caudal tilt is usually needed; (**d**), Lumbosacral junction, the fluoroscopy needs to be adjusted cranially (In some patient, the angle of cranial tilt could be up to 20–30°.)

Principles of Ultrasound-Guided Techniques

Ultrasound is another important imaging modality for intentional pain procedures. As a guiding image tool when compared to fluoroscopy, ultrasound has the advantage of portability, no radiation, conspicuous images of soft tissue including muscle, tendon neurovascular bundles, and real-time needle demonstration. However, the ability to detect vascular spread, demonstrate deeper tissues or tissues behind bone or air is limited, and the probability of miscalculating levels is higher than in fluoroscopy. Additionally, it is more operator-dependent than fluoroscopy, which means the image proof of the needle tip position is less objective than fluoroscopy. For interventional pain practice in the spine, ultrasound is usually used for the purpose of avoiding inadvertent damage to vital structures, and in reducing radiation exposure.

Examples of Dual-Image Guided Technique: Thoracic Transforaminal Epidural Injection

Thoracic radicular pain is a rare diagnosis, however, zoster-associated pain (ZAP) occurs most frequently in the thoracic spine level. Managing acute pain and prevention of post-herpetic neuralgia are the primary goals in ZAP management. Transforaminal epidural steroid injection with or without pulsed RF could be utilized in managing acute ZAP [56].

One of the most threatening complications in thoracic spine procedures is pneumothorax. Ultrasound could guide the needle trajectory, preventing inadvertent needle puncture to the pleura. In thoracic transforaminal epidural injection, the ultrasound transducer is placed in the transverse plane, demonstrating the thoracic paravertebral space of the targeted level (Fig. 16.16). The pleura is in the lateral border of the paravertebral space. The needle is introduced in a lateral to medial manner, and puncture of the pleura could be avoided with ultrasound guidance. As

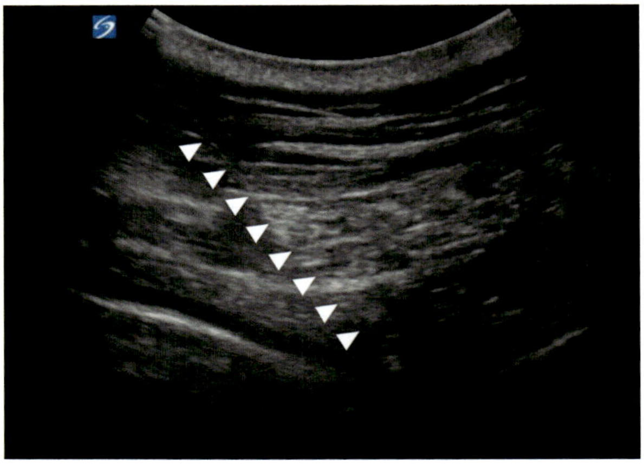

Fig. 16.16 Ultrasound guided thoracic paravertebral needle trajectory. The needle is introduced with ultrasound guidance toward the neuroforamen while avoiding puncture to the pleura

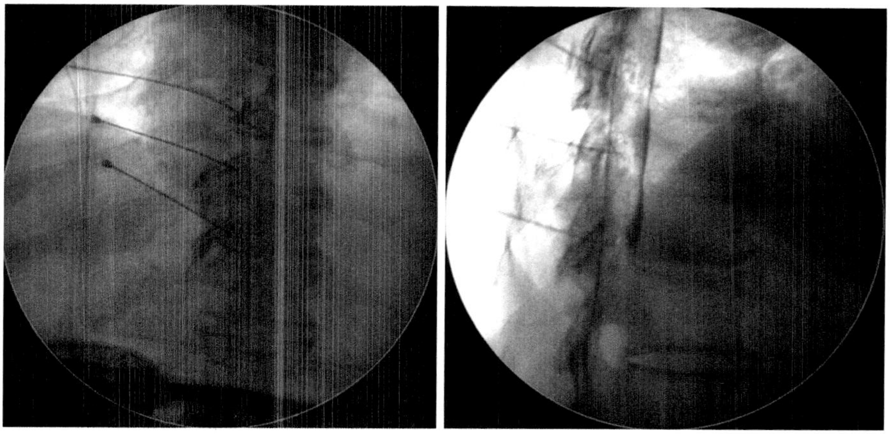

Fig. 16.17 Thoracic transforaminal epidural injection

the needle pass the dome of the pleura (Fig. 16.16), the risk of pneumothorax is significantly reduced and the clinician could proceed with fluoroscopy-guidance to check the real "transforaminal" position of the needle tip (Fig. 16.17).

Conclusion

The key of successful interventional procedures consists of: (1) Understanding of modalities or injectable drugs for neuroablation, neuromodulation or regenerative injection, (2) Good imaging facilities for guidance and the operating skills of the interventional pain physician, (3) Thorough knowledge of human anatomy for targeted interventional therapy. The interplay of these 3 factors serves as the essence of interventional pain management.

References

1. Mills SEE, Nicolson KP, Smith BH. Chronic pain: a review of its epidemiology and associated factors in population-based studies. Br J Anaesth. 2019;123(2):e273–e83.
2. Ilfeld BM, Gabriel RA, Trescot AM. Ultrasound-guided percutaneous cryoneurolysis for treatment of acute pain: could cryoanalgesia replace continuous peripheral nerve blocks? Br J Anaesth. 2017;119(4):703–6.
3. Trescot AM. Cryoanalgesia in interventional pain management. Pain Physician. 2003;6(3):345–60.
4. Rubinsky B. Cryosurgery. Annu Rev Biomed Eng. 2000;2:157–87.
5. Mazur P. Kinetics of water loss from cells at subzero temperatures and the likelihood of intracellular freezing. J Gen Physiol. 1963;47:347–69.

6. Mazur P. Freezing of living cells: mechanisms and implications. Am J Phys. 1984;247(3 Pt 1):C125–42.
7. Burke CJ, Sanchez J, Walter WR, Beltran L, Adler R. Ultrasound-guided therapeutic injection and Cryoablation of the medial plantar proper digital nerve (Joplin's nerve): sonographic findings, technique, and clinical outcomes. Acad Radiol. 2020;27(4):518–27.
8. Yasin J, Thimmappa N, Kaifi JT, Avella DM, Davis R, Tewari SO, et al. CT-guided cryoablation for post-thoracotomy pain syndrome: a retrospective analysis. Diagn Interv Radiol. 2020;26(1):53–7.
9. Campos NA, Chiles JH, Plunkett AR. Ultrasound-guided cryoablation of genitofemoral nerve for chronic inguinal pain. Pain Physician. 2009;12(6):997–1000.
10. Prologo JD, Lin RC, Williams R, Corn D. Percutaneous CT-guided cryoablation for the treatment of refractory pudendal neuralgia. Skelet Radiol. 2015;44(5):709–14.
11. Stogicza A, Trescot A, Rabago D. New technique for Cryoneuroablation of the proximal greater occipital nerve. Pain Pract. 2019;19(6):594–601.
12. Yoon JH, Grechushkin V, Chaudhry A, Bhattacharji P, Durkin B, Moore W. Cryoneurolysis in patients with refractory chronic peripheral neuropathic pain. J Vasc Interv Radiol. 2016;27(2):239–43.
13. Shah SB, Bremner S, Esparza M, Dorn S, Orozco E, Haghshenas C, et al. Does cryoneurolysis result in persistent motor deficits? A controlled study using a rat peroneal nerve injury model. Reg Anesth Pain Med. 2020;45(4):287.
14. M K. Zur Elektrochirurgie. Arch Klin Chir. 1931;167:761–8.
15. Shealy CN. Percutaneous radiofrequency denervation of spinal facets. Treatment for chronic back pain and sciatica. J Neurosurg. 1975;43(4):448–51.
16. Vatansever D, Tekin I, Tuglu I, Erbuyun K, Ok G. A comparison of the neuroablative effects of conventional and pulsed radiofrequency techniques. Clin J Pain. 2008;24(8):717–24.
17. Tun K, Cemil B, Gurcay AG, Kaptanoglu E, Sargon MF, Tekdemir I, et al. Ultrastructural evaluation of pulsed radiofrequency and conventional radiofrequency lesions in rat sciatic nerve. Surg Neurol. 2009;72(5):496–500. discussion 1
18. Erdine S, Yucel A, Cimen A, Aydin S, Sav A, Bilir A. Effects of pulsed versus conventional radiofrequency current on rabbit dorsal root ganglion morphology. Eur J Pain. 2005;9(3):251–6.
19. Cosman ER Jr, Dolensky JR, Hoffman RA. Factors that affect radiofrequency heat lesion size. Pain Med. 2014;15(12):2020–36.
20. Vinas FC, Zamorano L, Dujovny M, Zhao JZ, Hodgkinson D, Ho KL, et al. In vivo and in vitro study of the lesions produced with a computerized radiofrequency system. Stereotact Funct Neurosurg. 1992;58(1–4):121–33.
21. Provenzano DA, Lassila HC, Somers D. The effect of fluid injection on lesion size during radiofrequency treatment. Reg Anesth Pain Med. 2010;35(4):338–42.
22. Provenzano DA, Lutton EM, Somers DL. The effects of fluid injection on lesion size during bipolar radiofrequency treatment. Reg Anesth Pain Med. 2012;37(3):267–76.
23. Provenzano DA, Liebert MA, Somers DL. Increasing the NaCl concentration of the pre-injected solution enhances monopolar radiofrequency lesion size. Reg Anesth Pain Med. 2013;38(2):112–23.
24. Cohen SP, Moon JY, Brummett CM, White RL, Larkin TM. Medial branch blocks or intra-articular injections as a prognostic tool before lumbar facet radiofrequency denervation: a multicenter. Case-Control Study Reg Anesth Pain Med. 2015;40(4):376–83.
25. Cohen SP, Doshi TL, Constantinescu OC, Zhao Z, Kurihara C, Larkin TM, et al. Effectiveness of lumbar facet joint blocks and predictive value before radiofrequency denervation: the facet treatment study (FACTS), a randomized. Controlled Clinical Trial Anesthesiology. 2018;129(3):517–35.
26. Lau P, Mercer S, Govind J, Bogduk N. The surgical anatomy of lumbar medial branch neurotomy (facet denervation). Pain Med. 2004;5(3):289–98.

27. Dreyfuss P, Halbrook B, Pauza K, Joshi A, McLarty J, Bogduk N. Efficacy and validity of radiofrequency neurotomy for chronic lumbar zygapophysial joint pain. Spine (Phila Pa 1976). 2000;25(10):1270–7.
28. Arakawa K, Kaku R, Kurita M, Matsuoka Y, Morimatsu H. Prolonged-duration pulsed radiofrequency is associated with increased neuronal damage without further antiallodynic effects in neuropathic pain model rats. J Pain Res. 2018;11:2645–51.
29. Erdine S, Bilir A, Cosman ER, Cosman ER Jr. Ultrastructural changes in axons following exposure to pulsed radiofrequency fields. Pain Pract. 2009;9(6):407–17.
30. Higuchi Y, Nashold BS Jr, Sluijter M, Cosman E, Pearlstein RD. Exposure of the dorsal root ganglion in rats to pulsed radiofrequency currents activates dorsal horn lamina I and II neurons. Neurosurgery. 2002;50(4):850–5. discussion 6
31. Vallejo R, Tilley DM, Williams J, Labak S, Aliaga L, Benyamin RM. Pulsed radiofrequency modulates pain regulatory gene expression along the nociceptive pathway. Pain Physician. 2013;16(5):E601–13.
32. Ren H, Jin H, Jia Z, Ji N, Luo F. Pulsed radiofrequency applied to the sciatic nerve improves neuropathic pain by Down-regulating the expression of calcitonin gene-related peptide in the dorsal root ganglion. Int J Med Sci. 2018;15(2):153–60.
33. Huang YH, Hou SY, Cheng JK, Wu CH, Lin CR. Pulsed radiofrequency attenuates diabetic neuropathic pain and suppresses formalin-evoked spinal glutamate release in rats. Int J Med Sci. 2016;13(12):984–91.
34. Jiang R, Li P, Yao YX, Li H, Liu R, Huang LE, et al. Pulsed radiofrequency to the dorsal root ganglion or the sciatic nerve reduces neuropathic pain behavior, decreases peripheral pro-inflammatory cytokines and spinal beta-catenin in chronic constriction injury rats. Reg Anesth Pain Med. 2019;
35. Fu M, Meng L, Ren H, Luo F. Pulsed radiofrequency inhibits expression of P2X3 receptors and alleviates neuropathic pain induced by chronic constriction injury in rats. Chin Med J. 2019;132(14):1706–12.
36. Wang JA, Niu SN, Luo F. Pulsed radiofrequency alleviated neuropathic pain by down-regulating the expression of substance P in chronic constriction injury rat model. Chin Med J. 2020;133(2):190–7.
37. Jia Z, Ren H, Li Q, Ji N, Luo F. Pulsed radiofrequency reduced neuropathic pain behavior in rats associated with upregulation of GDNF expression. Pain Physician. 2016;19(2):49–58.
38. Das B, Conroy M, Moore D, Lysaght J, McCrory C. Human dorsal root ganglion pulsed radiofrequency treatment modulates cerebrospinal fluid lymphocytes and neuroinflammatory markers in chronic radicular pain. Brain Behav Immun. 2018;70:157–65.
39. Gofeld M, Bristow SJ, Chiu SC, McQueen CK, Bollag L. Ultrasound-guided lumbar transforaminal injections: feasibility and validation study. Spine (Phila Pa 1976). 2012;37(9):808–12.
40. Watanabe I, Masaki R, Min N, Oshikawa N, Okubo K, Sugimura H, et al. Cooled-tip ablation results in increased radiofrequency power delivery and lesion size in the canine heart: importance of catheter-tip temperature monitoring for prevention of popping and impedance rise. J Interv Card Electrophysiol. 2002;6(1):9–16.
41. Lorentzen T. A cooled needle electrode for radiofrequency tissue ablation: thermodynamic aspects of improved performance compared with conventional needle design. Acad Radiol. 1996;3(7):556–63.
42. Goldberg SN, Gazelle GS, Solbiati L, Rittman WJ, Mueller PR. Radiofrequency tissue ablation: increased lesion diameter with a perfusion electrode. Acad Radiol. 1996;3(8):636–44.
43. Abdalla EK, Schell SR. Paraplegia following intraoperative celiac plexus injection. J Gastrointest Surg. 1999;3(6):668–71.
44. Benzon HT, Raj PP. Raj's practical management of pain. 4th ed. Philadelphia: Mosby-Elsevier; 2008. xix, 1319
45. Melzack R, Wall PD. Pain mechanisms: a new theory. Science. 1965;150(3699):971–9.

46. Wallin J, Fiska A, Tjolsen A, Linderoth B, Hole K. Spinal cord stimulation inhibits long-term potentiation of spinal wide dynamic range neurons. Brain Res. 2003;973(1):39–43.
47. Song Z, Ansah OB, Meyerson BA, Pertovaara A, Linderoth B. Exploration of supraspinal mechanisms in effects of spinal cord stimulation: role of the locus coeruleus. Neuroscience. 2013;253:426–34.
48. Song Z, Ansah OB, Meyerson BA, Pertovaara A, Linderoth B. The rostroventromedial medulla is engaged in the effects of spinal cord stimulation in a rodent model of neuropathic pain. Neuroscience. 2013;247:134–44.
49. Moore R, Groves D, Nolan J, Scutt D, Pumprla J, Chester MR. Altered short term heart rate variability with spinal cord stimulation in chronic refractory angina: evidence for the presence of procedure related cardiac sympathetic blockade. Heart. 2004;90(2):211–2.
50. Latif OA, Nedeljkovic SS, Stevenson LW. Spinal cord stimulation for chronic intractable angina pectoris: a unified theory on its mechanism. Clin Cardiol. 2001;24(8):533–41.
51. Naoum JJ, Arbid EJ. Spinal cord stimulation for chronic limb ischemia. Methodist Debakey Cardiovasc J. 2013;9(2):99–102.
52. Deer TR, Mekhail N, Provenzano D, Pope J, Krames E, Leong M, et al. The appropriate use of neurostimulation of the spinal cord and peripheral nervous system for the treatment of chronic pain and ischemic diseases: the neuromodulation appropriateness consensus committee. Neuromodulation. 2014;17(6):515–50. discussion 50
53. Deer TR, Pope JE, Hayek SM, Lamer TJ, Veizi IE, Erdek M, et al. The Polyanalgesic consensus conference (PACC): recommendations for intrathecal drug delivery: guidance for improving safety and mitigating risks. Neuromodulation. 2017;20(2):155–76.
54. Prager J, Deer T, Levy R, Bruel B, Buchser E, Caraway D, et al. Best practices for intrathecal drug delivery for pain. Neuromodulation. 2014;17(4):354–72. discussion 72
55. Deer TR, Hayek SM, Pope JE, Lamer TJ, Hamza M, Grider JS, et al. The Polyanalgesic consensus conference (PACC): recommendations for trialing of intrathecal drug delivery infusion therapy. Neuromodulation. 2017;20(2):133–54.
56. Kim ED, Bak HH, Jo DH, Park HJ. Clinical efficacy of transforaminal epidural injection for management of zoster-associated pain: a retrospective analysis. Skelet Radiol. 2018;47(2):253–60.

Chapter 17
Regenerative Interventions for Chronic and Neuropathic Pains

Jeimylo de Castro

Introduction

Neuropathic pain (NP) is defined by the International Association for the Study of Pain (IASP) as pain caused by a lesion or disease of the somatosensory system. This definition found new modification with the newly released ICD-II classification and is organized into peripheral and/or central neuropathic pain based on whether the lesion or disease is found in the peripheral or central somatosensory nervous system [1, 2]. This nerve injury in the peripheral nerve may be in the form of demyelination or axonopathy. Or it may however affect any point along the neuroaxis causing neuropathic pain. Any lesion that has no somatosensory involvement does not qualify or is considered neuropathic pain. The older definition where it is considered a dysfunction is no longer acceptable due to its difficulty in verifying symptoms and soft signs as criteria for diagnosis [2]. In fact, chronic regional pain syndrome (CRPS I) whose symptoms mimic neuropathic pain does not qualify under this new definition since the lesion does not involve the somatosensory system. In a very simplistic view, this definition may seem easy to identify, but recently the IASP Neuropathic Pain Special Interest Group (NeuPSIG) noted that "the temporal relationship between the lesion or disease and the onset of neuropathic pain may vary" from an immediate onset after trauma to several years after the disease sets in. As noted by different authors, neuropathic pain can begin commonly as an acute injury although it is also characterized as a chronic neuropathic state. Thus, the diagnosis

J. de Castro (✉)
Department of Physical Medicine and Rehabilitation, The Medical City-South Luzon, Santa Rosa, Laguna, Philippines

SMARTMD Center for Non-Surgical Pain Interventions, Makati City, Philippines

© The Author(s), under exclusive license to Springer Nature Switzerland AG 2022

J. de Castro, Y. El Miedany (eds.), *Advances in Chronic and Neuropathic Pain*, Contemporary Rheumatology, https://doi.org/10.1007/978-3-031-10687-3_17

is very challenging [3]. In their study, Doshi and colleagues noted that acute neuropathic pain is temporally distinct but closely related to chronic neuropathic pain and is distinguishable from each other. Furthermore, it has distinct mechanisms and clinical features from non-neuropathic pain [3]. In addition, one observation shows very important paradoxical findings such as the combined sensory loss and pain either with or without sensory hypersensitivity in the painful areas, but whose distribution of the lesion does not necessarily correspond to the somatosensory system dermatomes. These symptoms include a sensory deficit (paresthesia), an exaggerated response to what is usually painless (allodynia) sensation, and/or a heightened painful response (hyperalgesia). The neuroanatomical distribution can still be recognizable although not entirely found within the territory of the peripheral nerve root affected and sometimes appear beyond its borders [1]. In central nervous system lesions, where there is an involvement of the somatosensory pathways affecting the thalamus, brainstem in the pons and medulla except for the midbrain such as occurs in stroke or any disease affecting these pathways from the cortex of the brain to the spinal cord presenting with central pain, may also lead to neuropathic pain [2, 4].

Neuropathic pain (NP) has an incidence of about 8% (6.9% to 10%) with consequent protracted pain severity and in fact, is refractory to the existing pain treatment and intervention [5–7]. It also makes up 20–25% of chronic pain patients and may vary among the different populations worldwide based on the definition of what they consider a neuropathic pain state [8]. Moreover, even with the healing of the injury or lesion, it does not necessarily reverse neuropathic pain [9]. Eventually, patients must contend with other psychological and emotional issues such as anxiety and depression that can secondarily interfere with sleeping patterns, work and social and recreational activities [6].

Historically, there are different theories proposed for the mechanism of neuropathic pain spanning more than 150 years of intensive works from great scientists and scholars, beginning from the father of Neurology in the United States, Silas Weir Mitchell [10], the works of Spanish neuroanatomist Santiago Ramon y Cajal [11], Rivers and Head [12] of London who did initial works of the consequences of nerve injury and Woolf [13] who observed that there are central mechanisms that causes hypersensitivity during a peripheral nerve injury, just to name a few. Furthermore, Woolf cited the possibility of more than one mechanism in a single patient with neuropathic pain that could possibly change over time [14, 15]. With this development, there is much to explain about its pathomechanisms, and thus optimal treatment strategy remains a challenge for neuropathic patients [15].

Biomarkers of Neuropathic Pain

The biomarkers for the diagnosis of neuropathic pain remain non-specific and can overlap with certain disease conditions as seen in post-herpetic neuralgia, painful diabetic neuropathy, and central post-stroke pain and thus can affect the treatment regimen of these patients [2, 15]. In fact, it is even more challenging to distinguish between neuropathic and non-neuropathic conditions such that there are certain mixed conditions with no studies distinguishing one from the other, especially with the multiplicity of symptoms as compared to objective signs present that one can gather [2]. With this background, it is difficult to identify objective findings to help diagnose a neuropathic condition. In the absence of reliable and discriminative clinical features, a hierarchal system [16, 17] was developed based on the abundance of evidence that is present. Thus, a neuropathic pain diagnosis is divided into three classes: possible, probable, and definite. The following parameters are used which includes the pain history of the patient, pain distribution which is neuroanatomically plausible, presence and location of sensory signs that is neuroanatomically attributable, and the use of confirmatory test confirming the sensory changes and confirming the underlying lesion or disease of the somatosensory system that explains the symptoms of the patients [17, 18]. These tests include CT or MRI scans, skin biopsy, electrophysiological tests, heat and laser evoked potentials, nerve excitability tests, R1 blink reflex, microneurography, genetic tests, intraoperative nerve lesions seen by a surgeon during an operative procedure [17], and the use of high-frequency musculoskeletal ultrasound [19–21]. With a definite or confirmed neuropathic pain, other types of pain such as tissue inflammation are not completely excluded but the symptoms can be traced from a neurological lesion that can explain the pain. Otherwise for the purpose of this discussion any pain with a non-neural origin is referred to as nociceptive pain [17, 18].

Pro-Inflammatory Mediators in Neuropathic Pain

Neuropathic pain is characterized by the presence of pro-inflammatory mediators which include TNF-α, IL-1β, IL-6, and NF-κB [22]. These immune cell-derived factors are usually found in the vicinity or within pathologic peripheral nerves infiltrating the areas in neuropathic pain states [2]. These factors are found to be released from activated microglia and astrocytes and are found to be involved in microglia-astrocyte crosstalk and in inflammation-associated pain, bone cancer pain, and neuropathic pain [8]. While microglia are responsible for the initiation process, which begins within 24 hours of neuropathic pain, astrocytes are responsible for its persistence accumulating immediately and lasting for about 12 weeks [23]. With the release of these inflammatory cytokines, the excitatory amino acid glutamate and its receptor in the spinal dorsal horn is upregulated resulting in pain hypersensitivity. This event is simultaneously activated by the release of excitatory N-methyl-d-aspartate (NMDA) and its receptor (NMDAR) [8]. Interestingly, glial cell activation which includes astrocytes, microglia, and oligodendrocytes, upregulates MAPK (mitogen-activated protein kinase) signaling which thus promotes long-term potentiation and central pain sensitization [8, 24]. Thus, in a typical nerve injury, a cascading sequence of events occurs which leads to an inflammatory response. The glial cells respond sequentially initiated by microglia surrounding a peripheral nerve injury and within minutes releases inflammatory chemokines and cytokines. Thereafter, the neutrophils come into play as the primary inflammatory cells that surround the injured nerve. Within hours to days, the monocyte (M1) comes along followed by the T cells. The T cells will not only infiltrate the injured peripheral nerve but will also go to the distal part of the nerve, the dorsal root ganglion, and finally at the dorsal horn of the spinal cord [8]. The T cells reached a peak at 21 days post-injury and can be detected even up to day 40. Among the macrophages, the M1 is associated with promoting pain sensitization while M2 inhibits pain sensitization, thus promoting healing [2]. The M1 macrophage plays a major role in Wallerian (axon) degeneration by releasing pro-inflammatory cytokines at the site of peripheral nerve injury and in the dorsal root ganglia with T cell infiltration, which are key to hyperalgesia at the site of injury [8].

Since the first contact of any nerve injury be it chemical, physical, or mechanical takes place at the peripheral nerve, activation of pain pathways occurs at this level. Once the threshold is reached, a change in the membrane potential gives way for a series of events triggering an action potential. Ion channels such as the TRP channel (transient receptor potential channels) family, sodium channels (e.g. $NA_V1.7$, $NA_V1.8$, $NA_V1.9$), ASIC-channels (acid-sensing ion channels) or ATP-gated purinergic channels (PR2), and mechanosensitive PIEZO ion channels mediate and transduce the different noxious stimuli in a lock and key fashion. These various channels respond with depolarization through sodium channels and hyperpolarization through potassium channels [2, 8]. Moreover, two types of pain-mediating neurotransmitters exist. These are the inflammatory (prostaglandins, prostacyclins, leukotrienes, adenosine triphosphate, adenosine, substance P, proton H+, nerve growth factors, 5-hydroxytryptamine, histamine, glutamate, neurokinin, nor-epinephrine, and nitric oxide) and non-inflammatory neurotransmitters (calcitonin-gene-related peptide, γ-aminobutyric acid, opioid peptides, glycine, and cannabinoids) [25].

The sodium channels such as the $NA_V1.7$ and $NA_V1.8$ are considered altered in a peripheral nerve injury. Voltage-gated sodium channels (VGSC) regulate neuronal activity in both normal and pathological conditions. $NA_V1.7$ and $NA_V1.8$ which are expressed in the dorsal root ganglion and in the nociceptors are upregulated following peripheral nerve injury together with $NA_V1.9$ and $NA_V1.3$. Of the following sodium channels, $NA_V1.7$ has a genetic link to pathological pain while $NA_V1.8$ due to its sensory neuron specificity is important in the pathophysiology of pain [26, 27]. Thus, their roles in neuronal firing and their deployment in sensory nerve endings where nociception is activated emphasized the importance of their roles in both normal pain signaling and during neuronal hyperexcitability in the development of chronic neuropathic pains where their activities are altered [26].

There are at least 8 different members of the TRP family (TRPV1, TRPV2, TRPV3, TRPV4, TRPM2, TRPM3, TRPM8, TRPA1) identified and expressed in the peripheral sensory neurons and are associated with different nociceptive transduction and thermal encoding. Of these TRPs, only TRPV1 (transient receptor vanilloid receptor 1) and TRPA1 (TRP ankyrin 1) have shown reduced pain hypersensitivity once these receptors are blocked pharmacologically with no evidence supporting the presence of mutations in the TRP channels among neuropathic pain conditions [28]. An increase in TRPV1 activity has been observed in response to an increase in TNF-α activity by sensitizing the peripheral nerve. Similarly, IL-1β upregulated $NA_V1.8$ activity. In both cases, these two events are enhanced by the p38 MAPK activity in the dorsal root ganglion. Thus, promoting pro-inflammatory responses in both the peripheral and central pain pathways in neuropathic pain [8].

Objective Measurements of Neuropathic Pain

Presently, there are several instruments that are useful in the diagnosis of neuropathic pain. These techniques provide us the opportunity to objectively assess the presence of neuropathic pains. This includes microneurography, neuroimaging like MRI, PET, and MEG (magnetoencephalography), EEG, EMG-NCV studies, genetic tests, skin biopsy, and ultrasound [15, 17].

Microneurography assesses the pathophysiology of sensory and axonal abnormalities in pain processing and is a useful tool for evaluating the presence of neuropathic pain. Although no published normative data for healthy subjects were reported as yet, the identification of spontaneous activity in the C fibers may indicate the potential peripheral mechanism of neuropathic pain [15].

While MRI provides good spatial resolution and has an indirect ability to assess neuronal activity, PET allows for the imaging of neurotransmitters and glial cells and thus is a functional imaging modality. It is a promising modality for glial activation and neuroinflammation and therefore can image neuropathic pain lesions [15, 29].

Electroencephalography (EEG) is used to study the electrical currents generated from the brain. It can record the activity of the neurons producing a synchronized electrical activity. For instance, a neuropathic pain lesion shows an increase in theta (4–8 Hz) power and a decrease in alpha (8–12 Hz) power and with increased rhythmicity in theta oscillations referred to as thalamocortical dysrhythmia [15, 30].

Electromyography (EMG) is a physiological test used to evaluate peripheral nerve lesions in cases such as spinal radiculopathies or metabolic neuropathies seen in diabetes mellitus [31, 32]. It is important to understand that abnormal findings do not appear during the early part of the disease. On average, a period of at least 3 to 5 weeks may be required to see the development of abnormal findings when using this modality.

Conventional Treatment of Neuropathic Pain

Most patients diagnosed with neuropathic pain report severe, chronic, and recurrent are often refractory to present and conventional treatment with major impact to the quality of life of the patient with subsequent untold suffering and disability. Although the symptoms may vary from patient to patient, given the same level of nerve lesions, the treatment management is challenging both in preventing neuropathic pains and more so in modifying its progress [33]. Smith and colleagues observed that not all patients with nerve lesions develop neuropathic pains. Interestingly, non-neuropathic pain conditions may also respond if given anti-neuropathic medications [34]. In a study by Perrot and colleagues, the average time it takes for the onset of pain to the diagnosis of neuropathic pain is about 23 ± 55.9 months, and an additional 20.1 ± 39.4 months is the mean interval for such patients to be referred to a pain center. Moreover, about 17.7 ± 38.5 months is noted from the diagnosis to referral to a pain center in the subgroup of patients who come for the first time [35]. This delay in the diagnosis and subsequent treatment impacts the quality of life, psychological and emotional comorbidity of the patients. Thus, there is a need to formulate an appropriate therapeutic intervention to reduce this delay [35].

The approach to effective treatment for neuropathic pain is usually multidisciplinary. Different specialties, however, approach this problem at their own pace with primary care physicians in the forefront of these patients and as such, they act as referring physicians to either neurologists or rheumatologists. For instance, as observed in the study by Perrot and colleagues, neurologists and rheumatologists are more likely to prescribe drugs that are effective for neuropathic pain such as anti-depressants and anti-epileptics with 40% of patients being given at least one anti-depressant, while 55% were given with one anti-epileptic drug before they are referred to a pain center as they feel more confident in managing neuropathic pain conditions. Fortunately, those with sick leave have three times more chances to be referred to a pain clinic within 2 years than those fully employed [35]. Oncologists who have close contact with patients undergoing chemotherapy tend to diagnose it early on as neuropathic pains, and thus reduce the time it takes to refer patients to the pain center. The delay then comes because of primary care physicians referring patients initially to the specialists who gave them non-neuropathic pain medications. In France, to avoid worrying terms while discussing the issues with patients is using other diagnoses, especially for non-neurological conditions. However, this method may cause unnecessary delay in referring patients to a pain center for appropriate treatment, and thus, prescribing anti-neuropathic drugs further cause a delay [35].

A consensus among different societies and groups using the best medications for treating neuropathic pain in diabetic neuropathies based on scientific evidence recommends the use of serotonin-norepinephrine reuptake inhibitors (SNRIs), tricyclic antidepressants (TCAs), and gabapentinoids [36]. When gabapentin failed, many practitioners use pregabalin as an alternative drug for neuropathic pain. Although opioids have proven to be effective for short-term therapies and in fact, the third line of treatment for neuropathic pain with limited efficacy [37], there is inherent risk involved which is associated with overdose, dependency, addiction, and death. In fact, the American Academy of Neurology (AAN) and the Center for Disease Control and Prevention (CDC) advised against its use for chronic non-cancer neuropathic pain [38, 39]. Despite the limited efficacy of opioids for neuropathic pain control, it is found to be more effective in nociceptive pain [40] (without somatosensory lesion), followed by peripheral neuropathic pain, spinal central pain, and is least useful in supraspinal central neuropathic pain [41].

For years, the management of neuropathic pain has been symptom-based instead of the primary pathologies such as in diabetic neuropathy since even if diabetes is controlled, the neuropathic pain persists. Thus, the approach for systemic pain control does not rely on the etiology. This applies to all types of neuropathic pain, central or peripheral, except for trigeminal neuralgia where specific pharmacologic guidelines exist. The first-line drugs include tricyclic antidepressants where Amitryptyline, 25–150 mg/day is given. Other drugs included here are SNRIs (Duloxetine, 20–120 mg/day; Venlafaxine, 150–225 mg/day), and anti-epileptics (Pregabalin, 150–600 mg/day; Gabapentin, 900–3600 mg/day) [42]. The level of evidence is high for SNRIs and Pregabalin [43]. The opioids such as Tramadol are the second-line drugs and oxycodone and morphine are the third-line drugs for neuropathic pain [42]. The details of pharmacologic treatments on neuropathic pain are beyond the scope of this chapter but will be discussed in other chapters of this book.

Regenerative Treatments for Neuropathic Pain

Cell-based therapies have recently shown potential in the treatment of the nervous system. It can originate from the bone marrow, adipose tissue, or umbilical cord [8]. This could be the key to addressing refractory pain especially as available medications and therapies do not show any lasting relief. Current therapies show insufficient evidence of pain relief with less than 50% of currently available drugs showing 50% efficacies for neuropathic pain based on the studies of Finnerup and colleagues [44]. Thus, the potential of regenerative treatments can provide the necessary solution for patients suffering from this condition. As it is right now, the combined cost of this condition with other pain conditions could reach up to $1 trillion per year [45].

In preclinical studies, stem cell therapy using bone marrow mesenchymal cells have the best potential for pain intervention because of its totipotent cellular source where the injured nerve cells are replaced with new cells and that it provides trophic factors to the affected nerve [8, 46]. It has a high expansion potential, genetic stability, and stable phenotype. It also can migrate to tissue injury sites where pain modulation can occur and has strong immunosuppressive properties for both autologous and heterologous transplantation [46]. Among the stem cell source, neural stem cells (NSC) are considered the best option for regeneration due to their capacity to differentiate into neurons, oligodendrocytes, and astrocytes and have been considered in the treatment of neuropathic pain by decreasing the mRNA and proteins levels of pro-inflammatory IL-1, thereby attenuating hyperalgesia [8, 47, 48]. However, such treatment remains under scrutiny by the FDA as it is derived from human fetal cells [48].

In a neuropathic condition, following a nerve injury, a series of inflammatory cascades follows with the subsequent release of pro-inflammatory cytokines, chemokines, and lipid mediators which then sensitizes the nociceptors. Once adipose-derived stem cells are injected, the immunomodulatory and angiogenic properties of stem cells are observed. There is downregulation of the IL-1β and IL-6 expression and an associated upregulation of the anti-inflammatory factor IL-10 with a reported increase in M2 macrophages which is inhibitory for pain and a decrease of M1 macrophage which initiates pain response [2, 8]. These reactions are due to the interaction of the stem cells and macrophages, where it promotes an anti-inflammatory effect [8]. Transplantation of human mesenchymal stem cells (hMSCs) in a spared nerve injury (SNI) in a mouse model was reported to significantly reduced mechanical allodynia and thermal hyperalgesia. This is believed to be due to the downregulation of pro-inflammatory IL-1β and IL-17 and upregulation of IL-10 as previously reported [49]. However, in the transplantation of bone marrow mesenchymal stem cells (BMMSCs) in neuropathic pain, Hosseini and colleagues reported a significantly improved allodynia but not hyperalgesia, especially during the first 4 days after the lesion in peripheral-mediated pain but not in central pain. Other variables affecting the success of transplantation include the time of injury to intervention, and the number of transplanted cells [50]. In the damaged axons, there is an activation of extracellular signal-related mitogen-activated protein kinase (MAPK) in the Schwann cells which leads to one of four basic pathways. Among the four pathways, only ERK1/2 and p38 have a significant role in pain modulation. As MSCs are injected, the expression of ERK1/2 in the dorsal root ganglion is inhibited. Moreover, VEGF, GDNF, and NGF from the stem cell serve an important role in promoting the growth of injured nerve fibers [8].

Central sensitization of pain initiated at the peripheral nerve injury is due to a series of the neuronal cascade. There is usually spontaneous activity arising from the uninjured nerve adjacent to the central nervous system that produces sensitization and is responsible for pain generation. Interestingly, the products released because of Wallerian degeneration may trigger changes in the channel and receptor expression that eventually adds to neuropathic pain [49]. In the spinal cord, the activated microglia in the dorsal root ganglion (DRG) releases pro-inflammatory cytokines such as TNF-α, IL-1β, and IL-6 immediately after a distal peripheral nerve injury and this is mediated via p38 MAPK system. Locally, at the chronic constriction sites (CCI) of a peripheral nerve, the same pro-inflammatory cytokines are released. Interleukins are likewise released from the leucocytes during this inflammatory process followed by reactions at the cellular level where the excitatory Na^+ currents are facilitated and inhibitory K^+ currents are attenuated. This triggers neuronal hyperexcitability which then causes neuropathic pain [51].

In the dorsal horn of the spinal cord, the excitatory neurotransmitter glutamate plays a significant role in central sensitization following its attachment to the glutamate receptor. Subsequently, other receptors like the N-methyl-D-aspartate (NMDA) receptor (NMDAR) , and α-amino-3-hydroxy-5-methyl-4-isoxazolepropionic acid receptor (AMPAR) are activated. These receptors finally send signals to the sensory regions of the brain [52, 53]. A study has shown that bone marrow stem cells (BMSCs) could inhibit the expression of NMDAR and therefore has a protective effect among rats from glutamate excitability and effectively reduce pain, especially for those suffering from spinal cord injury with chronic pains [54]. Further, BMSCs upregulated TGF-β1 (transforming growth factor-β1) levels in the cerebrospinal fluid. This factor is neuroprotective and neurotrophic in the neurons and therefore suppresses the neuronal excitability in a nerve injury. Stem cells release TGF-β1 that can resist central sensitization with the resulting analgesic effect with studies showing that TGF-β1 has a role in attenuating glutamate-induced excitotoxic neuronal damage in a concentration-dependent manner in the neocortical neurons [8, 55]. There are however a host of other neurotrophic factors that are released because of stem cell therapy injection which includes VEGF (vascular endothelial growth factor), BDNF (brain-derived nerve factor), and GDNF (glial cell line-derived neurotrophic factor) to name just a few. The secretion of these neurotrophic factors not only enhances neuroprotection and neuroregeneration in affected nerve cells but also prevents neurodegeneration and degradation of uninjured cells [49].

Glial cells in the spinal cord are activated following a peripheral nerve injury. As mentioned earlier microglia are present immediately after a nerve injury, while astrocytes could remain for as long as 12 weeks post-injury. They are the source of inflammatory cytokines which triggers a series of reaction and subsequently upregulates the receptor of glutamate resulting in hyperalgesia. With the transplantation of BMSCs, the activity of microglial cells is significantly reduced such as the case in disc herniation [8, 56]. In a similar study, glial cells activate MAPK signaling, which is then responsible for long-term potentiation and central pain sensitization [57]. With BMSCs transplantation, MAPK signaling, microglial and astrocytes activation are also inhibited, although the exact pain mechanisms require additional studies and investigation. There is, however, a reported improvement of motor function as seen in spinal cord injury in rats [8, 58]. Ichim and colleagues reported a significant improvement in pain scale from 10/10 among incomplete spinal cord injury (T12/L1 level with a crushed fracture of the L1 vertebral body) patients to 4/10 after administering several cycles of MSCs and CD34+ cells. In addition, there are improvements in muscle strength, improved sensation in the dermatome level, and recovery of urological and sexual function [59]. Similarly, studies have shown motor nerve conduction improvements among diabetic neuropathic patients. These improvements in the motor nerve conduction velocity and an increase in NGF (nerve growth factor) and NT-3 (neurotrophin-3) levels were reported to last only for 4 weeks with some studies showing contradictory results [60, 61]. With great and significant potential for neuropathic pain treatment, the optimal dosing remains unknown and further clinical trials are needed to demonstrate the process [8].

Platelet-Rich Plasma Therapy for Neuropathic Pains

Among the regenerative injection treatments, platelet-rich plasma (PRP) therapy is the most studied intervention for musculoskeletal conditions. A significant increase in the number of studies can be found as to its effectivity in tendons, ligaments, joints, and recently in peripheral nerves compared to existing medical treatments as shown in the study of carpal tunnel syndrome [62]. Previous studies by Farrag and colleagues have found out that PRP can enhance myelin thickness and increase axon counts with early axonal regeneration when both ends of an injured nerve are sutured [63] and similar studies also show functional improvements of the involved hands [64]. In the recent studies of Hassanien and colleagues, ultrasound-guided perineural injection of PRP among 60 DM Type II patients showed improvement at 1, 3, and 6 months compared to those treated medically. There is significant alleviation of pain, numbness, and functionality associated with marked improvement in nerve conduction velocity post-PRP treatment [65]. In a related study, Kuffler reported that PRP injection for neuropathic pain begins to take effect on the third week after injection, and its effect is sustained up to 6 years [66].

How does PRP work to reduce neuropathic pain? In a recently published article by Kuffler, he explained that the platelet-released cytokines and other mediators work through several mechanisms [67]. The immediate release of pro-inflammatory cytokines by Schwann cells, which are considered the first responders leads to enhance inflammation where the site is transformed from pro-inflammatory to an anti-inflammatory state by the aid of TGF-β. This important growth factor reactivates Schwann cell support for axonal regeneration [68]. The PRP then blocked the Schwann cells, macrophages, neutrophils, and mast cells from releasing pro-inflammatory cytokines and block gene receptors for pro-inflammatory cytokines. Third, they could eliminate cells that contribute to an inflammatory state. Lastly, the growth factors from the α-granules of platelets aid in the healing and regeneration of the affected tissue such as VEGF, PDGF, EGF, NGF, and FGF [67]. These growth factors are believed to exert a pain-relieving effect in peripheral nerve injury [69]. Interleukin-10, a potent anti-inflammatory cytokine, although not derived from platelets induced the release of IL-10 from mature dendritic cells and thereby inducing the T lymphocytes to proliferate and consequently reduce the production of interferon gamma (IFN-γ) [70]. Other cytokines such as IL-1 Ra (Interleukin-1 receptor antagonist) and IL-18 binding protein were also found to suppress the inflammatory reactions. It also has a role in NF-κB signaling pathways to reduce inflammation [67, 71].

PRP is administered perineurally under ultrasound guidance to enhance nerve repair or overcome post-traumatic or neuropathic inhibitory microenvironment that contributes to chronic and recurrent pains to deliver the growth factors and to reduce the effects of pro-inflammatory cytokines to make way for nerve regeneration to take place. It can also be used to fill up the gaps in cases where the loose ends of the nerves have retracted and serve as a bridge in a nerve gap to facilitate regeneration [72]. However, these effects of PRP are dose dependent. Zheng and colleagues have reported that a dose of 2.5–20% of PRP from baseline concentration significantly stimulated Schwann cell proliferation and migration compared to untreated controls and this was reported to be accompanied by an increase in NGF and GDNF. A high concentration of PRP of 40% from baseline caused suppression of Schwann cell proliferation [73]. Another important consideration in the treatment of PRP in neuropathic pain is the development of hyperalgesia during repeated PRP treatments in both activated and non-activated forms due to the reported increase in NGF and NGF receptors as well as the presence of increased inflammatory mediators [69]. This hyperalgesia-induced reaction due to NGF is dose-dependent at the site of injection. However, there is a decrease in neuroma formation and ectopic charges when NGF is sequestrated [74]. Nerve growth factor (NGF) has a role in peripherally mediating the sensitization of nociceptors in the musculoskeletal system [75].

Role of Interleukin-1 Receptor Antagonist (IL-1Ra) against Neuropathic Pain

Pro-inflammatory cytokines like IL-1β are expressed and activated in the glial cells of the spinal cord at the dorsal root ganglion following a peripheral nerve injury. It directly acts on the spinal neurons by potentiating nociceptive signaling through IL-1 receptor-dependent signaling and NMDAR (N-methly-D-aspartate- receptor) phosphorylation [76]. In a typical neuropathic pain condition, as shown in mice, IL-1β levels are upregulated causing an increase in these levels centrally [77]. In fact, when IL-1β is injected centrally and peripherally, there is central hyperexcitability with a proportionate increase in synaptic activity in the spinal cord [76]. The release of IL-1β is mediated by purinoceptors expressed by satellite glial cells at the dorsal root ganglia. It is the activation of P2X7 purinoceptors by ATP that helps in the maturation and release of IL-1β. Thus, inflammatory mediators at the peripheral level lead to the release of ATP at the dorsal root ganglia which results in inflammatory hyperalgesia. This further upregulates cyclooxygenase activity which then induces prostaglandin production leading to neuronal sensitization [78]. It is for this reason that blocking the release of IL-1β will significantly help patients who are suffering from any symptom of neuropathic pain such as hyperalgesia and allodynia.

Interleukin-1 receptor antagonist is a naturally occurring anti-inflammatory protein that showed significant effects against rheumatoid arthritis [79]. Recently, IL-1Ra treatment was reported to significantly reduced systemic LPS-induced (lipopolysaccharide) spinal cord inflammation, oxidative stress, thermal hyperalgesia, and mechanical allodynia in neonatal rats. Furthermore, it reduces the number of activated microglia, astrocytes, and oligodendrocytes and levels of IL-1β COX-2, PGE2, and lipid peroxidation in the neonatal rat spinal cord. It has a protective effect against pain hypersensitivity, spinal cord inflammation, and oxidative stress in neonatal rats [80].

Webster and colleagues have exploited the administration of IL-1Ra (Interleukin-1 receptor antagonist) mice by making use of an engineered blood-brain barrier (BBB) solution for use during neuropathic pain states facilitated by anti-mouse transferrin receptor (TfR) to enhance better central penetration. This study has shown that the administration of IL-1Ra is sensitive to central but not peripheral effects against the IL-1 receptor. Moreover, there is also the dose-dependent effect of IL-1Ra fusion and the affinity of the anti-TfR antibody to the TfR thus partly affecting analgesia by reducing ectopic neuronal discharge. Although there are indications that the administered IL-1Ra have reached the dorsal root ganglion through the cerebrospinal fluid to effect similar changes in the symptoms, there is no evidence that points to that hypothesis according to this study. Additionally, since the effect is dose-dependent, the greater IL-1Ra penetration in the CNS will usually result in a longer duration of analgesia [76]. It is also worth mentioning at this point that the increase in the number of microglia or DRG macrophages in the dorsal root ganglia are critical contributors in the initiation and maintenance of neuropathic pain but not those at the nerve injury site, and that the DRG macrophages are the main source of IL-1βThe release of IL-1β in both the DRG and spinal cord participate in the central sensitization process. Thus, neutralizing IL-1β by injecting IL-1Ra significantly reduces neuropathic pain [81].

Sciatic nerve injury was found to induce an early, but transient increase in IL-1β expression in the superficial dorsal horn (SDH) in lamina I-II of the ipsilateral lumbar spinal cord. It acts on the IL-1 receptor Type 1 (IL-1R1) which is found in the glial fibrillary acidic protein (GFAP- positive) astrocytes, a cytoskeletal protein in the SDH of the lumbar spinal cord. GFAP is the major component of glial cells. Interestingly, Choi and colleagues reported that the intrathecal administration of IL-1Ra causes a blockade of IL-1R1 during the early phase of peripheral neuropathy and a subsequent increase of astrocyte P_{450C17} and GFAP in the SDH of the spinal cord causing mechanical allodynia. This then causes an early increase of spinal IL-1β which has a transient analgesic role in neuropathic pain by inhibiting the expression of astrocyte P_{450C17} and GFAP-positive astrocytes in the SDH in a peripheral nerve injury. This new finding will help us understand the transient role of IL-1β in processing pain in the SDH of the spinal cord and the role of IL-1 receptor agonists in preventing the development of neuropathic pain [82].

Stem Cell Therapy for Neuropathic Pain

Neuropathic pain remains a challenging problem considering the limited efficacy of the available drugs, medications, and procedures. There are promising results reported with all the available and ongoing research on stem cell therapy as it relates to neuropathic pain. We will review the general effects and mechanisms of stem cell therapy in the treatment of neuropathic pain. With the complexity and variable etiologies of neuropathic pain, the use of drugs acting on a single mechanism is very challenging despite reported results in optimizing its effects. Stem cell therapies offer an approach addressing multiple mechanisms in the peripheral, central, or even at the spinal cord level where neuropathic pain is developed. There are different sources of stem cells, although bone marrow stem cells (BMSC), adipose tissue stem cells (ADSC), and human amniotic fluid-derived mesenchymal stem cells (hAFMSCs) remain one of the most common sources [83]. An appropriate harvesting technique for bone marrow stem cells (BMSCs) is important to acquire the resident cells from the periapical inflammatory sac wall referred to as the human

Periapical Cyst-Mesenchymal Stem Cells (hPCy-MSCs). This is characterized by its extensive proliferative ability and its potential to differentiate into different cell types [84]. Stem cells can interact within a damaged microenvironment and have the potential to block the degeneration process, inhibit apoptosis, strengthen the recovery of the injured nerve, and inhibit mechanisms promoting neuropathic pain both peripherally and centrally [83].

In a peripheral nerve injury, where peripheral sensitization occurs, adipose stem cell therapy reduced the level of pro-inflammatory factors such as IL-1β and IL-6 which are shown to accumulate in neuropathic pains and similarly increased the levels of anti-inflammatory IL-10 [85]. The interaction between stem cells and monocytes/macrophages is likewise stimulated where the expression of M2 macrophages increased after stem cell treatments favoring analgesia and at the same time decreasing the gene expression of M1 macrophages leading to anti-inflammatory effects [2, 8, 86]. In the dorsal root ganglion, intrathecal stem cell therapy acts on the mitogen-activated protein kinase (MAPK) pathway by causing an anti-inflammatory reaction during a peripheral nerve injury by inhibiting the expression of ERK1/2 in the dorsal root ganglion. Moreover, bone marrow-derived stem cells (BMSCs) counter the expression of p-p38-MAPK protein induced by PTX as well as the expression of inflammatory factors such as NF-κB, p65, TNF-α and IL-6 [83, 87, 88]. In another study, intravenous administration of adipose mesenchymal stem cells (AD-MSC) causes a reduction in CCI-induced TNF-α and GFAP expression [89]. Furthermore, stem cells also induced various growth factors that are essential in the regeneration of peripheral nerve and maintenance of its functions. These are the glial-derived neurotrophic factor (GDNF), nerve growth factor (NGF), and vascular endothelial growth factor (VEGF). These growth factors have very important roles in neuroprotection, normalizing neuropathic pain, axonal growth, neuronal maintenance and survival, and restoration of nerve functions [83].

Central sensitization, as a leading cause of chronic neuropathic pain, is subserved by excitatory response emanating from the activation of glutamate receptors in the dorsal horn. At the nociceptive afferent terminal, the excitatory amino acid glutamate is released which in turn activates the N-methyl-D-aspartate receptor (NMDAR) in the dorsal horn following a nerve injury which then sends signals to the sensory brain causing subsequent central sensitization. The prolonged upregulation of NMDAR gave rise to chronic neuropathic pain [83]. Injection of bone marrow-derived stem cells (BMSCs) inhibits the expression of NMDAR and is neuroprotective against glutamate excitotoxicity, thus relieving neuropathic pains following spinal cord injury as shown in a rat model [54]. Moreover, BMSCs increased the expression of TGF-β1 which decrease glutamate-induced neuronal hyperexcitability and reduces central sensitization following a nerve injury in a concentration-dependent manner [8, 55]. Further, glial cells which form 70% of central nervous system cells play a part in inducing neuropathic pain where proinflammatory cytokines are released from astrocytes and microglia following a nerve injury by upregulating glucocorticoids and glutamate receptors. Microglia in turn activates the MAPK pathway to enhance pain sensitivity. Intrathecal administration of BMSCs significantly reduced proinflammatory cytokines emerging from activated spinal microglia, thus directly inhibiting microglial activation and MAPK pathway activation [8, 56, 83]. The expression of CCL7 by the astrocytes which then activates the microglia is further inhibited by bone marrow-derived stem cells (BMSCs) [90]. In a related study, Teng et al. reported inhibition of the core pain signal pathway of P2X4R in microglia by reducing its expression thus, alleviating neuropathic pain [91]. This sequence of events leads to a reduction of central sensitization of neuropathic pain.

It could be seen from these studies that both peripheral and central sensitization could be inhibited by stem cells and thus promote the recovery of peripheral nerve showing significant clinical symptoms of neuropathic pain. Stem cells hold promise in the treatment of neuropathic pain assuming multiple roles such as peripheral, central, and spinal cord disinhibition with reduction of clinical symptoms characterized by hyperalgesia, allodynia, and spontaneous pain [83].

Recent reviews confirmed that stem cell therapy certainly alleviates neuropathic pain [92]. It is also known to secrete neurotrophic factors and anti-neuroinflammatory cytokines which provide neuroprotection and regenerative effect to an injured peripheral nerve [93]. Xie and colleagues have reported, however, that stem cell therapy is more responsive to peripheral neuropathic pain than SCI-induced neuropathic pain with aggravating pain above the lesion more challenging to treat [94]. Intrathecal administration of autologous bone marrow stromal cells however showed progressive benefit in pain score (VAS) for the treatment of neuropathic pain among 10 spinal cord injured patients as shown in this study after it was given during 1, 4, and 7 months and then followed up at 10 months [95].

A study by de Castro and colleagues of patient post-dorsal rhizotomy with dorsal root repair by means of platelet-rich plasma therapy combined with bioengineered human embryonic stem cell therapy showed good axonal regeneration as reported and seen by histological and functional observations. This study provides information that early root reconnection combined with engrafting of bioengineered stem cell therapy is effective and has led the way into new possibilities in translational medicine [96].

Alpha-2-macroglobulin for Neuropathic Pain

Chronic neuropathic pains pose a challenge among pain physicians and most if not, all have experienced failures in addressing pain in the patients. Admittedly, we have scoured the use of mesenchymal stem cells as a potential agent for treating neuropathic conditions. Although it is still in its infancy stage, the potential for such treatment can usher in more research with the goal of understanding its mechanisms and how stem cell therapy can be used to counteract its effects. One of the derivatives of plasma is found in the platelet poor component and is identified as alpha-2-macroglobulin.

Alpha-2-macroglobulin (A2M) is a broad-spectrum proteinase inhibitor found in the serum and synovial fluid of the joints which blocks different kinds of proteinases by forming an A2M-proteinase complex and is eventually removed from the serum by the endocytosis of the macrophage. It acts against both endogenous and exogenous inflammatory injuries [97]. The presence of A2M in the synovial joints is limited such that its inhibitory effect against the inflammatory mediators is inadequate. To wit, one or two molecules of proteinase will cost one molecule of A2M [98]. Although most research focuses on the effect of A2M on degenerative joints and intraarticular inflammation by delaying the degeneration of articular cartilage, the inflammatory mediators found in an inflamed joint, namely, IL-1β, IL-6, IL-8, and TNF-α are the same inflammatory mediators found in an injured peripheral nerve as in the case of chronic neuropathic pains [97–99]. In fact, the proinflammatory mediator TNF-α serves as a biomarker for Wallerian degeneration in the distal part of peripheral nerve injury. It is also identified during the progression of Wallerian degeneration and in the development of painful neuropathies [98, 99]. Furthermore, A2M was reported to be deficient in the serum of murine neuropathic pain model, suggesting that it could be used up in a nerve chronic constriction injury [100]. Although the exact mechanism of A2M remains to be identified, Zhu and colleagues reported that the major mechanism of its inhibitive effect on the inflammatory mediators is the transformation of its molecular structure. Moreover, it remains to be determined where the exact location of its active site is so that the action of its activity can be predicted [97].

In a peripheral nerve injury, the distal stump of the nerve rapidly produces proinflammatory cytokines IL-1β and TNF-α in a biologically active form [101]. These cytokines as previously described participate in the wider spectrum of inflammatory reactions that eventually produces pain characteristics of neuropathic pain. In fact, the inflammation that follows increases nerve damage leading to neuropathic pain. Other proinflammatory cytokines that are activated in a peripheral nerve injury include IL-6, interferon-gamma (IFN-γ), and IL-18 [98]. These cytokines once released, can activate a series of reactions, not only at the site of peripheral nerve injury but also at the spinal cord level. For instance, TNF-α activates p38 mitogen-activated protein kinase (MAPK) in the Schwann cells of the spinal cord and subsequently leads to increase IL-1β expression, which is produced in the spinal cord and dorsal root ganglion [102, 103]. Microglial activation and proliferation in the dorsal root ganglion in a peripheral nerve injury resulting in the release of these inflammatory cytokines with mediators such as prostaglandin E_2 acting to facilitate the response leading to neuropathic pain [8]. How these reactions are inhibited by alpha-2-macroglobulin in a peripheral nerve injury is interesting to note.

A big number of proinflammatory cytokines and growth factors bind to A2M in the protein-interaction site or by its receptor, the low-density lipoprotein receptor-related protein (LRP-1), or to its cell surface-associated Grp78 [98]. It is known to bind with several cytokines such as IL-1β, IL-6, and TNF-α and growth factors such as platelet-derived growth factor (PDGF), fibroblast growth factor (FGF), and nerve growth factor (NGF) [104]. By these different mechanisms, A2M can regulate neuroinflammation and regulate cell physiology [105]. Alpha-2-macroglobulin exists in the plasma in the native conformation due to the rapid clearance of LRP-1 when it is fully transformed. This conformational change also happens when it interacts to inhibit the proteases. In the case of peripheral nerve injuries, A2M binds to proinflammatory cytokines such as TNF-α and IL-1β to counteract its inflammatory effects [98, 99]. In the study of Arandjelovic and colleagues, A2M and its derivatives showed positive results in terms of outcome and were reported as a potential agent in regulating the progression of nerve injury [98]. In a recent study by Jordan and colleagues in the neurogenic thoracic outlet syndrome and other forms of the cervical brachial syndrome, A2M which is found at the platelet-poor component of the plasma showed good outcome when injected among patients with thoracic outlet syndrome as compared to those with complex regional pain syndrome (CRPS) and fibromyalgia achieving about 61% clinical endpoints of success compared to 35% success rate, respectively [106]. Similar results were reported by Brooks and colleagues when A2M was used as an adjunctive treatment option using the hydrodissection injection technique in the Alcock's canal [107].

Alpha-2-macroglobulin is a powerful protease and proinflammatory cytokines inhibitor. It is synthesized principally in the liver and for some patients suffering from chronic stroke and cardiovascular disease, increase serum level can serve as a biomarker for endothelial dysfunction [104]. Different techniques of preparation are presently available right now, with the A2M concentration technique from autologous plasma was originally developed to treat cartilage degenerative problems [97, 108]. Two variants of A2M namely CYT-98 and CYT-108 showed the best inhibitory effects, with CYT-108 showing the finest inhibition of TNF-α and IL-1β, in this case for cartilage catabolism inhibition. The activation of the A2M molecule is determined by its conformational or molecular change [97]. Since peripheral nerve injury shows the same pro-inflammatory cytokines that cause neuropathic pain, the use of A2M for nerve injuries is very relevant as shown in preclinical studies [99]. Like platelet-rich plasma, the use of corticosteroids and anesthetics shall be avoided during its administration [97].

Other uses of A2M include patients with discogenic pain who are FAC+ (fibronectin-aggrecan complex) diagnosed with degenerative disc disease. Clinical improvement was demonstrated as shown in a study by Montesano and colleagues following intradiscal autologous A2M injection emphasizing the need for patient selection when using this intervention [109]. In a related study, Huang and colleagues evaluated the cartilaginous endplates (CEP) of the spine and its role in intervertebral disc degenerative disease. Alpha-2 macroglobulin inhibited the expression and activity of MMP-13 or MMP-3 which are elevated in the degenerative discs of the spine in a dose-dependent manner, but its presence promoted the expression of SOX-9, aggrecan, and type II collagen in CEP. Administering a supplemental A2M provides the necessary protection in the spine against intervertebral disc (IVD) degeneration by counteracting the effects of proinflammatory cytokines. Additionally, in this study, TNF-α and IL-1β upregulated the gene expression of MMP-13, MMP-3, and ADAMTS-5 which leads to the degenerative changes in the CEP and downregulates the gene expression of SOX-9, Col II of ECM, and ACAN confirming the findings in degeneration in CEP. Autologous administration of A2M is thus a protective factor in the degeneration of the CEP. Moreover, A2M can suppress the nuclear translocation of TNF-α-induced NFκB p65 in CEP cells which in turn upregulate MMP-13 which is responsible for the degenerative changes in the CEP of the spine [110].

Exosomes as a Treatment for Neuropathic Pain

Exosomes are membrane-bound extracellular vesicles secreted by many cells in the body, with an ability for intercellular communication via paracrine, juxtacrine, and endocrine signaling. The extracellular vesicles, of which the exosomes are derived are surrounded by a phospholipid bilayer in both normal and pathological cells [111]. It is generated by the inward budding of the membrane of the multivesicular endosome containing intraluminal vesicles to the plasma membrane. Thus, the shredded intraluminal vesicles are referred to as exosomes [112]. Basically, the extracellular vesicles exist in three forms: the exosomes, the microparticles, and the apoptotic bodies. Exosomes have a size ranging from 30 to 100 nm and it originates from the cell membrane during endocytic internalization. Although exosomes were originally differentiated based on their size, one other characteristic of exosomes that determines their identity from other forms is their protein composition [111]. These specific proteins include tetraspanins (CD9, CD63, CD81, and CD82) heat shock proteins (HSP60, HSP70, and HSP90) tumor susceptibility gene 101 protein (TSG 101), and ALG-2-interacting protein X (ALIX) . Other differentiating features include lipids composition, content, and cellular origin [113]. Exosomes contain RNAs, DNAs, mRNAs, microRNAs (miRNA), proteins, and lipids and their cargo molecules reflect the composition of the parent cell. These cargo molecules can be transported unaltered in nearby and distant target sites [111]. Interestingly, the mRNAs can silence gene expression and regulate posttranscriptional processes through exosome-cell interaction once it integrates into the recipient cell [114]. Moreover, the bilayer phospholipid membranes of the exosomes control and protect the internal microenvironment and can migrate to different cells without being degraded or altered [115].

There is an increasing interest in using exosomes for pain states as shown in different studies such as in chronic [116, 117] and neuropathic pain [118] conditions. In fact, studies have demonstrated their ability to improve painful symptoms with fewer side effects with potential immuno-protective and anti-inflammatory effects. Moreover, exosome is a good biomarker of different diseases and pain and a tool for therapeutic intervention [113].

The effect of exosomes on chronic neuropathic pain conditions is premised on its existence in the mesenchymal stem cells (MSCs) exerting analgesic effects with fewer side effects [119]. The exosomes in the MSCs can transfer miRNAs cargo to target nerves to facilitate axonal growth and neural survival [120, 121]. The efficacy of exosomes against peripheral nerve injury is believed to be due to the release of different neurotrophic factors inherent in the MSCs such as GDNF (glial-derived neurotrophic factor), FGF-1 (fibroblast growth factor), BDNF (brain-derived neurotrophic factor), IFG-1 (insulin-like growth factor), and NGF (nerve growth factor) although the exact mechanism is still unclear up to the present [120].

Exosomes play a crucial role in neuropathic pain because of their ability in interneuronal communication. It can cross the blood-brain barrier and as such can serve both as a biomarker for specific diseases and/or can mediate pain threshold and allodynia in neuropathic pain states [113]. A chemokine, CCL3 which mediates both peripheral and central sensitization in neuropathic pain is transported via exosomes from Schwann cell to the peripheral blood [122]. As to its effect on specific pain conditions, a macrophage-derived exosomes injection can alleviate thermal hyperalgesia in chronic regional pain syndrome [113]. A recent study reported that exosomes regulate mechanisms in the sensory process which includes nociception [123]. As exosomes are ubiquitous in most cells in the body, the mesenchymal stem cells from bone marrow, adipose tissue, and umbilical cord remain to be the best source during a treatment session with very distinct effects. Bone marrow-derived exosomes showed superior tissue regeneration ability, adipose tissue-derived exosomes played a significant role in immune regulation while umbilical cord-derived exosomes were more effective in tissue damage repair [124]. In another related study, adipose tissue-derived exosomes reportedly improve and enhance nerve regeneration after peripheral nerve injury [125]. Other effects of exosomes include that of spinal cord injury (SCI) where exosomes relieved SCI by regulating the GFAP expression and suppressing glial scar formation. It showed neuroprotective effects by reducing SCI-induced astrocytosis and by inhibiting inflammation [126]. Moreover, studies have shown that early treatment of SCI by bone marrow-derived exosomes attenuates neuronal cell apoptosis [127].

Another interesting secondary effect of exosomes is the miRNA contained in the cargo of exosomes. These single-stranded, small non-coding RNAs regulate genes such as those involved in nociceptive signaling. It can exert its effects both intracellularly or extracellularly, the latter of which can be released either as an unbound molecule or attached to an exosome [128]. It can either act as an activator or inhibitor of spinal microglia in neuropathic conditions. For instance, the miR-124, reverses neuropathic pain by keeping microglia quiescent, while miR-155 promotes neuropathic pain following microglial activation. The study by Tang and colleagues implies the role of exosomes with their microglial-derived exosomal miRNA providing new potential for neuropathic pain treatment. This effect was demonstrated in post-brain trauma of microglial exosomal miR-124-3p where it reduces neurodegeneration and subsequently improves cognitive function [129].

Conclusion

Diagnosing neuropathic pain conditions is crucial in ensuring that correct interventions are given. The use of objective clinical biomarkers and tools are necessary guides to obtain a definitive diagnosis, such as the one suggested by Treede and colleagues [16]. A wrong diagnosis is damaging to the patients because the specific treatment takes place over a period, not to mention the deleterious side effects that go with it, which subsequently disturb the daily activities of everyday life. Moreover, the use of nociceptive drugs may prove ineffective if one is dealing with neuropathic pain [130].

Although originally used in diagnosing polyneuropathy, DN4 (Douleur Neuropathique en 4 questions) [131] remained to be the first step in the grading system of neuropathic pain and where Treede also derived his grading system [16].

In fact, it is the best diagnostic tool for neuropathic pain among nonspecialist physicians. It has a sensitivity of 83% and a specificity of 90% in various forms of neuropathic pain [130]. Recently, the use of c-miRNA (circulation microRNA) types was used as biomarkers to distinguish between neuropathic and nociceptive pain as they are potent players in the control of protein expression [130].

The treatment of chronic and neuropathic pains remains a challenge for most pain practitioners. Although first-line drugs like tricyclic anti-depressants (desipramine and amitriptyline) SNRIs (selective noradrenaline reuptake inhibitors) such as duloxetine and venlafaxine, anti-convulsant acting at calcium channels (gabapentin and pregabalin) and second- and third-line drugs like opioids such as morphine, oxycodone and tramadol and topical lidocaine were used as drugs for neuropathic pains from different causes, concerns about adverse reactions, abuse, diversion and addiction were observed in its use especially among opioid users [132]. And since most of these drugs act centrally, they usually produced central side effects such as dizziness and sedation [83]. Thus, an effective but with reduced side effects could be the key in addressing neuropathic pain conditions.

The advent of regenerative interventions as a treatment for neuropathic pain has the advantage of multiple roles, such as peripheral, central, and spinal cord disinhibition, and can decrease the occurrence of clinical symptoms such as spontaneous pain, allodynia, and hyperalgesia. Stem cells in neuropathic pain interact with resident cells to block degeneration, inhibit apoptosis, and enhance the survival and recovery of both injured and uninjured nerves [83]. Having possessed strong immunosuppressive and anti-inflammatory effects in different microenvironments, stem cells have the potential to provide the necessary ingredients for the recovery of damaged tissues in neuropathic pain as shown in preclinical studies. With good results arising from different sources like bone marrow, adipose tissue, and peripheral blood and its derivatives, it carries with it the potential of becoming the needed treatment in the twenty-first century for chronic and neuropathic pains.

Acknowledgement I would like to thank God for His constant guidance and wisdom while I was preparing this manuscript, my supportive wife Kyna de Castro and my two children, Rafael Bennett de Castro, and Zarah Francine de Castro.

References

1. Scholz J, Finnerup NB, Attal NA, Baron R, Bennett MI, et al. Classification committee of the neuropathic pain special interest group (NeuSIG). The IASP classification of chronic pain for ICD-II: chronic neuropathic pain. Pain. 2019;160:53–9.
2. Finnerup N, Kuner R, Jensen T. Neuropathic pain: from mechanisms to treatment. Physiol Rev. 2021;101(1):259–301.
3. Doshi T, Dworkin R, Polomano R, Carr D, Edwards R, Finnerup N, Freeman R, Paice J, Weisman S, Raja S. AAAPT diagnostic criteria for acute neuropathic pain. Pain Med. 2021;22(3):616–36.
4. Riddoch G. The clinical features of central pain. Lancet. 1938;231:1093–8.
5. Nadine A. Neuropathic pain: mechanisms, therapeutic approach, and interpretation of clinical trials. Continuum (Minneap Minn). 2012;32(2):512–32.

6. Wang H, Huo X, Han C, Ning J, Chen H, Li B, Liu J, Ma W, Li Q, Yu Y, Shi K. Ferroptosis is involved in the development of neuropathic pain and allodynia. Molecular and Cellular Biochemistry. Online First. 2021:1–13.
7. Van Hecke O, Austin SK, Khan RA, Smith BH, Torrance N. Neuropathic pain in the general population: a systematic review of epidemiological studies. Pain. 2014;155(4):654–62.
8. Joshi H, Jo H, Kim Y, An S, Park C, Han I. Stem Cell Therapy for Modulating Neuroinflammation in Neuropathic Pain. Int J Mol Sci. 2021;22(9)
9. Baad-Hansen L, Benoliel R. Neuropathic orofacial pain: facts and fiction. Cephalalgia. 2017;37(7):670–9.
10. Mitchell SW. Injuries of nerves and its consequences. Philadelphia, PA: Lippincott; 1872.
11. Ramon y Cajal S, DeFelipe J, Jones EG, May RM. Cajal's degeneration and regeneration of the nervous system. Oxford, UK: Oxford Scholarship; 1991.
12. Rivers WHR, Head H. A human experiment on nerve division. Brain. 1908;31:323–450.
13. Woolf CJ. Evidence for a central component of post-injury pain hypersensitivity. Nature. 1983;306:686–8.
14. Woolf CJ, Mannion RJ. Neuropathic pain: etiology, symptoms, mechanisms, management. Lancet. 1999;353(9168):1959–64.
15. Fisher A, Lanigan M, Upton N, Lione L. Preclinical neuropathic pain assessment; the importance of translatability and bidirectional research. Front Pharmacol. 2021;11
16. Treede RD, Jensen TS, Campbell JN, Cruccu G, Dostrovsky JO, Griffin JW, Hansson P, Hughes R, Nurmikko T, Serra J. Neuropathic pain: redefinition and a grading system for clinical and research purposes. Neurology. 2008;70:1630–5.
17. Finnerup NB, Haroutounian S, Kamerman P, Baron R, Bennett DL, Bouhassira D, Cruccu G, Freeman R, Hansson P, Nurmikko T, Raja SN, Rice AS, Serra J, Smith BH, Treede RD, Jensen TS. Neuropathic pain: an updated grading system for research and clinical practice. Pain. 2016;157:1599–606.
18. Rosenberger DC, Blechschmidt V, Timmerman H, Wolff A, Treede RD. Challenges of neuropathic pain: focus on diabetic neuropathy. J Neural Transm. 2020;127:589–624.
19. Rbia N, Nijhuis THJ, Roukema GR, Selles RW, van der Vlies CH, Hovius SER. Ultrasound assessment of the sural nerve in patients with neuropathic pain after ankle surgery. Muscle Nerve. 2018;57(3):407–13.
20. Huang H, Wu S. Application of high-resolution ultrasound on diagnosing diabetic peripheral neuropathy. Diabetes Metab Syndr Obes. 2021;14:139–52.
21. Chang K, Wu WT, Ozcakar L. Ultrasound imaging and guidance in peripheral nerve entrapment: hydrodissection highlighted. Pain Management. 2020;10(2)
22. Rao P, Mainkar O, Bansal N, Rakesh N, Haffey P, Urits I, Orhurhu V, Kaye A, Urman R, Gulati A, Jones M. Flavonoids in the Treatment of Neuropathic Pain. Current Pain and Headache Reports. 2021;25(7)
23. Davies AJ, Kim HW, Gonzalez-Cano R, Choi J, Back SK, Roh SE, Johnson E, Gabriac M, Kim MS, Lee J, et al. Natural killer cells degenerate intact sensory afferents following nerve injury. Cell. 2019;176:716–28.
24. Ji RR, Gereau RW IV, Malcangio M, Strichartz G. MAPK and pain. Brain Res Rev. 2009;60:135–48.
25. Yam MF, Loh YC, Tan CS, Adam SK, Manan NA, Basir R. General pathways of pain sensation and the major neurotransmitters involved in pain regulation. Int J Mol Sci. 2018;19:2164.
26. Hameed S. Nav1.7 and Nav1.8: role in the pathophysiology of pain. Mol Pain. 2019;15
27. Dib-Hajj SD, Binshtok AM, Cummins TR, Jarvis MF, Sammad T, Zimmermann K. Voltage-gated sodium channels in pain states role in pathophysiology and target for treatment. Brain Res Rev. 2009;60:65–83.
28. Basso L, Altier C. Transient receptor potential channels in neuropathic pain. Curr Opin Pharmacol. 2017;32:9–15.
29. Albrecht DS, Granziera Z, Hooker JM, Loggia ML. In vivo imaging of human neuroinflammation. ACS Chem Neurosci. 2016;7(4):470–83.

30. Llinas RR, Ribary U, Jeanmonod D, Kronberg E, Mitra PP. Thalamocortical dysrhythmia: a neurological and neuropsychiatric syndrome characterized by magnetoencephalography. Proc Natl Acad Sci U S A. 1999;96(26):15222–7.
31. Rabbi MF, Ghazali KH, Altwijri O, Alqahtani M, Rahman SM, Ali A, Sundaraj K, Taha Z, Ahamed NU. Significance of electromyography in the assessment of diabetic neuropathy. J Mech Med Biol. 2019;19(3)
32. Andrasinova T, Kalikova E, Kopacik R, Srotova I, Vickova E, Dusek L, Bednarik J, Adamova B. Evaluation of neuropathic component of chronic low back pain. Clinical J Pain. 2019;35(1):7–17.
33. Aminoff MJ. Aminoff's electrodiagnosis in clinical neurology. p. 233–59.
34. König S, Prusak M, Pramhas S, Windpassinger M. Correlation between the neuropathic pain DETECT screening questionnaire and pain intensity in chronic pain patients. Medicina. 2021;57(4)
35. Perrot S, Pickering G, Lantéri-Minet M, Attal N. Real-life management pathways for chronic peripheral neuropathic pain at tertiary pain clinics in France. Pain Med. 2021;22(4):875–82.
36. Callaghan B, Reynolds E, Banerjee M, Kerber K, Skolarus L, Burke J. Longitudinal pattern of pain medication utilization in peripheral neuropathy patients. PAIN. 2019;160(3)
37. Vickers E, Karsten E, Flood J, Lilischkis R. A preliminary report on stem cell therapy for neuropathic pain in humans. J Pain Res. 2014;7:255–63.
38. Franklin GM. American academy of neurology. Opioids for chronic non-cancer pain: a position paper of the American Academy of Neurology. Neurology. 2014;83:1277–84.
39. Dowell D, Haegerich TM, Chou R. CDC guideline for prescribing opioids for chronic pain–United States, 2016. JAMA. 2016;315:1624–45.
40. Mercadante S, Gebbia V, David F, Aielli F, Verna L, Casuccio A, et al. Tools for identifying cancer pain or predominantly neuropathic origin and opioid responsiveness in cancer patients. J Pain. 2009;10(6):594–600.
41. Smith H, Meek P. Pain responsiveness to opioids: central versus peripheral neuropathic pain. J Opioid Manag. 2011;7(5):391.
42. Schembri E. Are opioids effective in relieving neuropathic pain? SN Comprehensive Clin Med. 2018;1(1):30–46.
43. Balshem H, Helfand M, Schunemann H, Oxman A, Kunz R, Brozek J, et al. GRADE guidelines: 3. Rating the quality of evidence. J Clin Epidemiol. 2011;64(4):401–6.
44. Finnerup NB, Sindrup SH, Jensen TS. The evidence for pharmacological treatment of neuropathic pain. Pain. 2010;150(3):573–81.
45. Stewart WF, Ricci JA, Chee E, Morganstein D, Lipton R. Lost productive time and cost due to common pain conditions in the US work force. JAMA. 2003;290(18):2443–54.
46. Siniscalco D, Rossi F, Maione S. Stem cell therapy for neuropathic pain treatment. J Stem Cells & Regen Med. 2007;3(1):2–11.
47. Bassio C, Mastrangelo R, Morini R, Tonna N, Coco S, Verderio C, Matteoli M, Bianco F. A simple method to generate adipose stem cell-derived neurons for screening purposes. J Mol Neurosci. 2013;51:274–81.
48. Franchi S, Castelli M, Amodeo G, Niada S, Ferrari D, Vescovi AL, Brini AT, Panerai AE, Sacerdoti P. Adult stem cell as new advanced therapy for experimental neuropathic pain treatment. Biomed Res Int. 2014:1–10.
49. Fortino V, Pelaez D, Cheung H. Concise review: stem cell therapies for neuropathic pain. Stem Cells Transl Med. 2013;2(5):394–9.
50. Hosseini M, Yousefifard M, Aziznejad H, Nasirinezhad F. The effect of bone marrow-derived mesenchymal stem cell transplantation on allodynia and hyperalgesia in neuropathic animals: a systematic review with meta-analysis. Biol Blood Marrow Transplantation. 2015;21(9):1537–44.
51. Guha D, Shamji MF. The dorsal root ganglion in the pathogenesis of chronic neuropathic pain. Neurosurgery. 2016;63(CN_suppl_1)

52. Kamp J, Van Velzen M, Olofsen E, Boon M, Dahan A, Niesters M. Pharmacokinetic and pharmacodynamic considerations for NMDA-receptor antagonist ketamine in the treatment of chronic neuropathic pain: an update of the most recent literature. Expert Opin Drug Metab Toxicol. 2019;15:1033–41.
53. Chen J, Li L, Chen SR, Chen H, Xie JD, Sirrieh RE, Maclean DM, Zhang Y, Zhou MH, Jayaraman V, et al. The α2 δ-1-NMDA-receptor complex is critically involved in neuropathic pain development and gabapentin therapeutic actions. Cell. 2018;22:2307–21.
54. Guo W, Chu YX, Imai S, Yang JL, Zou S, Mohammad Z, Wei F, Dubner R, Ren K. Further observations for the behavioral and neural effects of bone marrow stromal cells in rodent pain models. Mol Pain. 2016;12:1744.
55. Chen NF, Huang SY, Chen WF, Chen CH, Lu CH, Yang SN, Wang HM, Wen ZH, Chen CL. TGF-β1 attenuates spinal neuroinflammation and the excitatory amino acid system in rats with neuropathic pain. J Pain. 2013;14:1671–85.
56. Huang X, Wang W, Liu X, Xi Y, Yu J, Yang X, Ye X. Bone mesenchymal stem cell attenuate radicular pain by inhibiting microglial activation in a rat non-compressive disk herniation model. Cell Tissue Res. 2018;374:99–110.
57. Ji RR, Gereau RW IV, Malcangio M, Strichartz G. MAPKinase and pain. Brain Res Rev. 2009;60:135–48.
58. Watanabe S, Uchida K, Nakajima H, Matsuo H, Sugita D, Yoshida A, Honjoh K, Johnson WE, Baba H. Early transplantation of mesenchymal stem cells after spinal cord injury relieves pain hypersensitivity through suppression of pain-related signaling cascades and reduced inflammatory cell recruitment. Stem Cells. 2015;33:1902–14.
59. Ichim T, Solano F, Lara F, et al. Feasibility of combination of allogeneic stem cell therapy for spinal cord injury: a case report. Int Arch Med. 2010;3:30.
60. Shibata T, Naruse K, Kamiya H, et al. Transplantation of bone marrow-derived mesenchymal stem cells improves diabetic polyneuropathy in rats. Diabetes. 2008;57:3099–107.
61. Kim B, Jin H, Bae J. Bone marrow-derived mesenchymal stem cells improved the functioning of neurotrophic factors in a mouse model of diabetic neuropathy. Lab Anim Res. 2011;27:171–6.
62. Wu YT, Ho TY, Chou YC, et al. Six-month efficacy of platelet-rich plasma for carpal tunnel syndrome: a prospective randomized, single-blind controlled trial. Sci Rep. 2017;7(1):94.
63. Farrag TY, Lehar M, Verhaegen P, Carson KA, Byrne PJ. Effect of platelet-rich plasma and fibrin sealant in facial nerve regeneration in a rat model. Laryngoscope. 2007;117(1):157–65.
64. Sariguney Y, Yavuzer R, Elmas C, Yenicesu I, Bolay H, Atabay K. Effect of platelet-rich plasma on peripheral nerve regeneration. J Reconstr Microsurg. 2008;24(3):159–67.
65. Hassanien M, Elawamy A, Kamel EZ, Khalifa WA, Abolfadl GM, Roushdy AI, El Zohne RA, Makarem YS. Perineural platelet-rich plasma for diabetic neuropathic pain, could it make a difference? Pain Med. 2020;0(0):1–9.
66. Kuffler D. Platelet-rich plasma and the elimination of neuropathic pain. Mol Neurobiol. 2013;48(2):315–32.
67. Kuffler D. Mechanisms for reducing neuropathic pain. Mol Neurobiol. 2020;57(1):67–87.
68. Sulaiman OA, Gordon T. Transforming growth factor-beta and forskolin attenuate the adverse effects of long-term Schwann cell denervation on peripheral nerve regeneration in vivo. Glia. 2002;37:206–18.
69. Ince B, Yıldırım MC, Kilinc I, Oltulu P, Dadaci M. Investigation of the development of hypersensitivity and hyperalgesia after repeated application of platelet-rich plasma in rats: an experimental study. Aesthetic Surgery Journal. 2019;39(10)
70. Hagihara M, Higuchi A, Tamura N, Ueda Y, Hirabayashi K, Ikeda Y, Kato S, Sakamoto S, et al. Platelets, after exposure to high shear stress, induced IL-10 producing mature dendritic cells in vitro. J Immunol. 2004;172:5297–303.
71. Park JS, Lee EJ, Lee JC, Kim WK, Kim HS. Anti-inflammatory effects of short chain fatty acids in IFN-gamma stimulated RAW 264.7 murine macrophage cells: involvement of NF-κB and ERK signaling pathways. Int Immunopharmacol. 2007;7:70–7.

72. Sanchez M, Garate A, Delgado D, Padilla S. Platelet-rich plasma, an adjuvant biological therapy to assist peripheral nerve repair. Neural Regen Res. 2017;12(1):47–52.
73. Zheng C, Zhu Q, Liu X, Huang X, He C, Jiang L, Quan D, Zhao X, Zhu Z. Effect of platelet-rich plasma concentration on proliferation, neurotrophic function, and migration of Schwann cells in vitro. Tissue Eng Regen Med. 2016;10(5):428–36.
74. Chang DS, Hsu E, Hottinger DG, Cohen SP. Anti-nerve growth factor in pain management: current evidence. J Pain Res. 2016;9:373–83.
75. Mizumura K, Murase S. Role of nerve growth factor in pain. In: Schaible HG, editor. Pain control, Handbook of experimental pharmacology, vol. 227; 2015. p. 57–77.
76. Webster C, Hatcher J, Burrell M, Thom G, Thornton P, Gurrell I, Chessell I. Enhanced delivery of IL-1 receptor antagonist to the central nervous system as a novel anti–transferrin receptor-IL-1RA fusion reverses neuropathic mechanical hypersensitivity. Pain. 2017;158(4):660–8.
77. del Ray A, Yau H, Randolf A, Centeno MV, Wildman J, Martina M, Besedovsky HO, Apkarian AV. Chronic neuropathic pain-like behavior correlates with IL-1β expression and disrupts cytokine interaction in the hippocampus. Pain. 2011;152:2827–35.
78. Neves AF, Farias FH, de Magalhaes SF, Araldi D, Pagliusi M, Tambeli CH, Sartori CR, da Cruz Latufo CM, Parada CA. Peripheral inflammatory hyperalgesia depends on P2X7 receptors in satellite glial cells. Front Physiol. 2020; https://doi.org/10.3389/fphys.2020.00473.
79. Arend WP, Malyak M, Guthridge CJ, Gabay C. Interleukin-1 receptor antagonist: role in biology. Annu Rev Immunol. 1998;16:27–55.
80. Hsieh CT, Lee YJ, Lee JW, Lu S, Tucci MA, Dai X, Ojeda NB, Lee HJ, Fan LW, Tien LT. Interleukin-1 receptor antagonist ameliorates the pain hypersensitivity, spinal inflammation and oxidative stressinduced by systemic lipopolysaccharide in neonatal rats. Neurochem Int. 2020;135 https://doi.org/10.1016/j.neuint.2020.104686.
81. Yu X, Liu H, Hamel KA, Morvan MG, Yu S, Leff J, Guan Z, Braz JM, Basbaum JI. Dorsal root ganglion macrophages contribute to both the initiation and persistence of neuropathic pain. Nature Communications. 2020, 11(264)
82. Choi SR, Han HJ, Beitz AJ, Lee JH. Spinal interleukin-1β inhibits astrocyte cytochrome P450c17 expression which controls the development of mechanical allodynia in a mouse model of neuropathic pain. Front Mol Neurosci. 2019; https://doi.org/10.3389/fnmol.2019.00153.
83. Liu M, Li K, Wang Y, Zhao G, Jiang J. Stem cells in the treatment of neuropathic pain: research progress of mechanism. Stem Cells Int. 2020:1–13.
84. Marelli M, Paduano F, Tatullo M. Cells isolated from human periapical cysts express mesenchymal stem cell-like properties. Int J Biol Sci. 2013;9(10):1070–8.
85. Mert T, Kurt AH, Altun I, Celik A, Baran F, Gunay I. Pulsed magnetic field enhances therapeutic efficiency of mesenchymal stem cells in chronic neuropathic pain model. Bioelectromagnetics. 2017;38(4):255–64.
86. Guo W, Imai S, Yang JL, et al. In vivo immune interactions of multipotent stromal cells underlie their long-lasting pain-relieving effect. Sci Rep. 2017;7(1):10107.
87. Xie J, Ren J, Liu N, et al. Pretreatment with AM1241 enhances the analgesic effect of intrathecally administered mesenchymal stem cells. Stem Cells Int. 2019;7025473:1–17.
88. Al-Massri KF, Ahmed LA, El-Abhar HS. Mesenchymal stem cells therapy enhances the efficacy of pregabalin and prevents its motor impairment in paclitaxel-induced neuropathy in rats: role of notch 1 receptor and JAK-STAT signaling pathway. Behav Brain Res. 2019;360:303–11.
89. Forouzanfar F, Amin B, Ghorbani A, Ghazavi H, Ghasemi F, Sadri K, Mehri S, Sadeghnia H, Hosseinzadeh H. New approach for the treatment of neuropathic pain: fibroblast growth factor 1 gene-transfected adipose-derived mesenchymal stem cells. Eur J Pain. 2018;22(2):295–310.
90. Li J, Deng G, Wang H, et al. Interleukin-1β pre-treated bone marrow stromal cells alleviate neuropathic pain through CCL-7-mediated inhibition of microglial activation in the spinal cord. Scientific Reports. 2017;7(1)
91. Teng Y, Zhang Y, Yue S, et al. Intrathecal injection of bone marrow stromal cells attenuates neuropathic pain via inhibition of P2X4R in spinal cord microglia. J Neuroinflammation. 2019;16(1):271.

92. Asgharzade S, Talaei A, Farkhondeh T, Forouzanfar F. A review of stem cell therapy for neuropathic pain. Curr Stem Cell Res Ther. 2020;15(4):349–61.
93. Han YH, Kim KH, Abdi S, Kim TK. Stem cell therapy in pain medicine. Korean J Pain. 2019;32(4):245–55.
94. Xie F, Yue Y, Guan Y, Wang Y. Stem cells for the treatment of neuropathic pain. J Anesth Perioperative Med. 2017;10(10):1–9.
95. Vaquero J, Zurita M, Rico MA, Aguayo C, Fernandez C, Gutierrez R, Rodriguez-Boto G, Saab A, Hassan R, Ortega C. Intrathecal administration of autologous bone marrow stromal cells improves neuropathic pain in patients with spinal cord injury. Neurosci Lett. 2018;670:14–8.
96. de Castro M, da Silva M, Chiarotto G, Santana M, Luzo ACM, Kyrylenko S, de Oliveira A. Spinal reflex recovery after dorsal Rhizotomy and repair with platelet-rich plasma (PRP) gel combined with bioengineered human embryonic stem cells (hESCs). Stem Cells International, 2020.
97. Zhu M, Zhao B, Wei L, Wang S. Alpha-2-macroglobulin, a native and powerful proteinase inhibitor, prevents cartilage degeneration disease by inhibiting majority of catabolic enzymes and cytokines. Curr Mol Biol Rep. 2021;7:1–7.
98. Arandjelovic S, Drajovlovic N, Li X, Myers RR, Campana WM, Gonias SL. A derivative of the plasma protease inhibitor alpha-2-macroglobulin regulates the response to peripheral nerve injury. J Neurochem. 2007;103(2):694–705. https://doi.org/10.1111/j.1471-4159.2007.04800.x.
99. de Castro J. Alpha-2-macroglobulin: the new weapon of neuropathic pains. J Clinical Research and Anesthesia. 2018; https://doi.org/10.31579/JCRA/002.
100. Vincenzetti S, Pucciarelli S, Huang Y, Ricciutelli M, Lambertucci C, Volpini R, Scuppa G, Soverchia L, Ubaldi M, Polzonetti V. Biomarkers mapping of neuropathic pain in a nerve chronic constriction injury mice model. Biochimie. 2019;158:172–9.
101. Nadeau S, Filali M, Zhang J, Kerr BJ, Rivest S, Soulet D, Iwakura Y, Vaccari JPR, Keane RW, Lacroix S. Functional recovery after peripheral nerve injury is dependent on the pro-inflammatory cytokines IL-1β and TNF: implications for neuropathic pain. J Neurosci. 2011;31(35):12533–42.
102. Lee JC, Laydon JT, McDonnell PC, et al. A protein kinase involved in the regulation in the regulation of inflammatory cytokine biosynthesis. Nature. 1994;372:739–46.
103. Myers RR, Sekiguchi Y, Kikuchi S, Scott B, Medicherla S, Protter A, Campana WM. Inhibition of p38 MAP kinase activity enhances axonal regeneration. Exp Neurol. 2003;184:606–14.
104. Shimomura R, Nezu T, Hosomi N, Aoki S, Sugimoto T, Kinoshita N, Araki M, Takahashi T, Maruyama H, Matsumoto M. Alpha-2-macroglobulin as a promising biological marker of endothelial function. J Atheroscler Thromb. 2018;25(4):350–8.
105. Armstrong PB, Quigley JP. Alpha-2-macroglobulin: an evolutionarily conserved arm of the innate immune system. Dev Comp Immunol. 1999;23:375–90.
106. Jordan S, Iovine J, Kuhn T, Gelabert H. Neurogenic thoracic outlet syndrome and other forms of cervical brachial syndrome treated with plasma concentrate enriched for alpha 2 macroglobulin. Pain Physician. 2020;23(2):229–33.
107. Brooks B, Leishear K, Aronson R, Howell M, Khakshooy A, Pico M, Shrikhande A. The use of alpha-2-macroglobulin as a novel treatment for patients with chronic pelvic pain syndrome. Int J Obstetric Gynecol. 2020; https://doi.org/10.1002/ijgo.13423.
108. Cuellar JM, Cuellar VG, Scuderi GJ. Alpha-2 macroglobulin: autologous protease inhibition technology. Phys Med Rehabil Clin N Am. 2016;27(4):909–18.
109. Montesano PX, Cuellar JM, Scuderi GJ. Intrasdiscal injection of an autologous alpha-2 macroglobulin concentrate alleviates back pain in FAC-positive patients. Orthoped Rheumatol Open Access J. 2017;4(2)
110. Huang B, Chen J, Zhang X, Wang J, Zheng Z, Shan Z, Liu J, Zhu Z, Zhao F. Alpha-2 macroglobulin as dual regulator for both anabolism and catabolism in the cartilaginous endplate of intervertebral disc. Spine. 2019;44(6):E338–47.
111. Wu X, Wang Y, Xiao Y, Crawford R, Mao X, Prasadam I. Extracellular vesicles: potential role in osteoarthritis regenerative medicine. J Orthop Translation. 2020;21:73–80.

112. Stoorvogel W, Kleijmeer MJ, Geuze HJ, Raposo G. The biogenesis and functions of exosomes. Traffic. 2002;3:321–30.
113. D'Agnelli S, Gerra MC, Bignami E, Arendt-Nielsen L. Exosomes as a new pain biomarker opportunity. Mol Pain. 2020; https://doi.org/10.1177/1744806920957800.
114. Valadi H, Ekstrom K, Bossios A, Sjostrand M, Lee JJ, Lotvall JO. Exosome-mediated transfer of mRNAs and microRNAs is a novel mechanism of genetic exchange between cells. Nat Cell Biol. 2007;9(6):654–9.
115. Eldh M, Ekstrom K, Valadi H, Sjostrand M, Olsson B, Jernas M, et al. Exosomes communicate protective messages during oxidative stress; possible role of exosomal shuttle RNA. PLoS One. 2010;5(12):e15353.
116. Ju C, Liu R, Zhang Y, Zhang F, Sun J, Lv XB, Zhang Z. Exosomes may be the potential new direction of research in osteoarthritis management. Biomed Res Int. 2019;2019:7695768.
117. Tavasolian F, Moghaddam AS, Rohani F, Abdollahi E, Janzamin E, Momtazi-Borojeni AA, Moallerm SA, Jamialahmadi T, Sahebkar A. Exosomes: effectual players in rheumatoid arthritis. Autoimmun Rev. 2020;19:102511.
118. Gupta A, Pulliam L. Exosomes as mediators of neuroinflammation. J Neuroinflammation. 2014;11:68.
119. Ren J, Liu N, Sun N, Zhang K, Yu L. Mesenchymal stem cells and their exosomes: promising therapeutics for chronic pain. Curr Stem Cell Res Ther. 2019;14(8):644–53.
120. Dong R, Liu Y, Yang Y, Wang H, Xu Y, Zhang Z. MSC-derived exosomes-based therapy for peripheral nerve injury: a novel therapeutic strategy. Biomed Res Int. 2019;2019:6458237.
121. Kosik KS. The neuronal microRNA system. Nat Rev Neurosci. 2006;7:911–20.
122. Chen CC, Liu L, Ma F, Wong CW, Guo XE, Chacko JV, Farhoodi HP, Zhang SX, Zimak J, Ségaliny A, Riazifar M, Pham V, Digman MA, Pone EJ, Zhao W. Elucidation of exosome migration across the blood-brain barrier model in vitro. Cell Mol Bioeng. 2016;9:509–29.
123. Cata JP, Uhelski ML, Gorur A, Dougherty PM. Nociception and pain: new roles for exosomes. Neuroscientist. 2021; https://doi.org/10.1177/10738584211027105.
124. Wang Z, He Z, Liang S, Yang Q, Cheng P, Chen A. Comprehensive proteomic analysis of exosomes derived from human bone marrow, adipose tissue, and umbilical cord mesenchymal stem cells. Stem Cell Res Ther. 2020;511 https://doi.org/10.1186/s13287-020-02032-8.
125. Rau CS, Kuo PJ, Wu SC, Huang LH, Lu TH, Wu YC, Wu CJ, Lin CW, Tsai CW, Hsieh CH. Enhanced nerve regeneration by exosomes secreted by adipose-derived stem cells with or without FK506 stimulation. Int J Mol Sci. 2021;22(16):8545.
126. Gabr H, Elkheir WA, Fares AE, Farghali HAM, Mahmoud BE, Madbouly MA, Gamal N, Hamaad AM, Elkheir AA, Hassan RM. Free mesenchymal stem cell-associated exosomes induced better neuroregeneration than mesenchymal stem cells and neural differentiated mesenchymal stem cells in canine model of spinal cord injury. J Stem Cells Res & Ther. 2020;10(463):1–8.
127. Feng J, Zhang Y, Zhu Z, Gu C, Waqas A, Chen L. Emerging exosomes and exosomal miRNAs in spinal cord injury. Front Cell Dev Biol. 2021; https://doi.org/10.3389/fcell.2021.703989.
128. Montague-Cardoso K, Malcangio M. The role of microRNAs in neurons and neuroimmune communication in the dorsal root ganglia in chronic pain. Neurosci Lett. 2020;735 https://doi.org/10.1016/j.neulet.2020135230.
129. Tang S, Jing H, Song F, Huang H, Li W, Xie G, Zhou J. MicroRNAs in the spinal microglia serve critical roles in neuropathic pain. Mol Neurobiol. 2020;58(1):132–42.
130. Dayer C, Luthi F, Carré J, Vuistiner P, Terrier P, Benaim C, Giacobino J, Léger B. Differences in the miRNA signatures of chronic musculoskeletal pain patients from neuropathic or nociceptive origins. PLoS ONE. 2019;14(7)
131. Bouhassira D, Attal N, Fermanian J, Alchaar H, Gautron M, Masquelier E, et al. Development and validation of the neuropathic pain symptom inventory. Pain. 2004;108(3):248–57.
132. Fornasari D. Pharmacotherapy for neuropathic pain: a review. Pain Ther. 2017;6:25–33.

Index

© The Editor(s) (if applicable) and The Author(s), under exclusive license to Springer Nature Switzerland AG 2022
J. de Castro, Y. El Miedany (eds.), *Advances in Chronic and Neuropathic Pain*, Contemporary Rheumatology, https://doi.org/10.1007/978-3-031-10687-3

O

GPSR Compliance

The European Union's (EU) General Product Safety Regulation (GPSR) is a set of rules that requires consumer products to be safe and our obligations to ensure this.

If you have any concerns about our products, you can contact us on ProductSafety@springernature.com

In case Publisher is established outside the EU, the EU authorized representative is:

Springer Nature Customer Service Center GmbH
Europaplatz 3
69115 Heidelberg, Germany

Batch number: 10756376

Printed by Printforce, the Netherlands